NEURORADIOLOGY

Neuroradiology

NICER Series on Diagnostic Imaging

Edited by

Derek C. Harwood-Nash, M.B.,Ch.B., F.R.C.P.(C.)

Professor of Radiology
The Hospital for Sick Children
Toronto, Canada

Holger Pettersson, M.D.

Professor and Chairman
Department of Radiology
University of Lund, Sweden

Merit Communications

ISBN 1 873413 30 0

Published by
Merit Communications
7 Salisbury Place
Langton Road
London SW9 6UW
England

Printed by Butler and Tanner Ltd., Frome and London

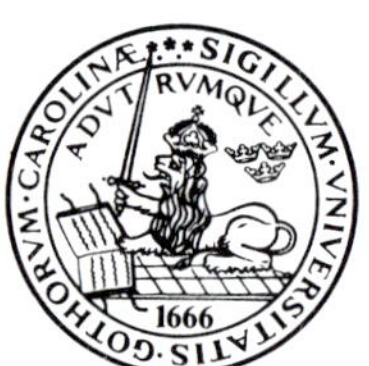

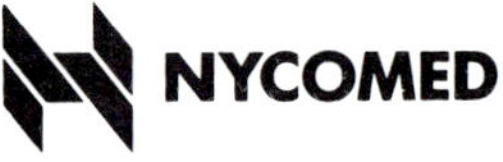

Contents

Contributors

Paul E. Berger, M.D.
Chairman, Department of
Radiology
Long Beach Memorial
Hospital
Long Beach, California
USA

Francis Brunelle, M.D.
Professor of Radiology
Hôpital des Enfants Malades
Paris
FRANCE

Olof Flodmark, M.D.
Professor of Radiology
Head, Clinical Neuroradiology
Karolinska Institutet
Stockholm
SWEDEN

**Derek C. Harwood-Nash,
M.B., M.Ch.**
Professor of Radiology
Department of Diagnostic
Imaging
University of Toronto
The Hospital for Sick Children
Toronto, Ontario
CANADA

Anton A. Hasso, M.D.
Professor of Radiology
Loma Linda University
Head Neuroradiology
Department of Radiation
Science
University of Loma Linda
Loma Linda, California
USA

Michael S. Huckman, M.D.
Professor of Radiology
Rush-Presbyterian University
Director of Neuroradiology
Rush-Presbyterian St. Luke's
Medical Center
Chicago, Illinois
USA

Ian Isherwood, M.D.
Professor of Radiology and
Chairman, Department of
Diagnostic Radiology
University of Manchester
Manchester
ENGLAND

Anne G. Osborn, M.D.
Professor of Radiology
Department of Radiology
University of Utah
College of Medicine
Salt Lake City, Utah
USA

Giuseppe Scotti, M.D.
Professor of Radiology
University of Milan
Director, Neuroradiology
Instituto Scientifico
H S Raffaele
Milan
ITALY

Preface

I keep six honest men.
(They taught me all I knew).
Their names are What and Why and When.
And How and Where and Who.

(The elephant's child. Rudyard Kipling)

In these two books, Neuroradiology and Pediatric Radiology born of the second and third segments of the NICER series on Diagnostic Imaging and the NICER course programme first presented in New Delhi, India, is contained basic and up-to-date neuroradiology and paediatric radiology. Paediatric neuroradiology is both a bridge between them and common to both. The first NICER Lecture is also included, a lecture detailing the place of imaging in Egyptology.

In both neuroradiology and imaging in infants and children are the sophistication and safety of ultrasound and magnetic resonance imaging having a major impact. In both is angiography also adding to its anatomical artistry an interventional influence. In both are "six honest men" (and women) representing the best of the best joining their colleagues worldwide to provide a unique opportunity for all to share in the art and science of radiology. To enhance and enjoy different cultures and philosophies. To add to each's medical talents.

These large numbers of remarkably erudite and current chapters deal with virtually all major organ systems, diseases and techniques in the child and in all the facets of neurological diseases at all ages. These chapters provide a more complete yet permanent aide memoire of the guest presentations at the Course. They provide to those not fortunate enough to hear the presentations an opportunity to avail themselves of the valuable contents of each. They provide the collective experience of a group of physicians, second to none in all of radiology, each a senior and renowned authority and teacher, coming from Europe and North America.

These two books, each representing a component of the combined Course are thus, in reality, two new up-to-date text books succinctly and expertly presented. The clinical and radiological contents are neither singularly simple nor excessively exotic but primarily practical.

The efforts of the authors are sincerely appreciated and acknowledged; as is the foresight and innovation by NICER; and the warm hospitality of our overseas colleagues. In this unique educational endeavour we will all be richer professionally and personally; we will make new friends and thus will we add to the strength of radiology both clinically and internationally.

Thus may we respond to Kipling and to his Devil's question - "Is it clever, is it pretty, is it an art"? To the devil we may say, for radiology - indubitably.

Derek C. Harwood-Nash
Holger Pettersson
Toronto and Lund, March 1992

Some Aspects of Tissue Characterization

Ian Isherwood

Department of Diagnostic Radiology, University of Manchester, UK

Medicine is essentially a search for the resolution of uncertainty. The diagnostic process traditionally has relied on a combination of educated observation, experience and logical induction. Quantification is relatively recent. Phrenology, the study of skull shape, was the first serious attempt to differentiate the normal from the abnormal brain by observation, induction and then quantification. Phrenology was popular from the middle of the 18th to the middle of the 19th centuries. One of its principal proponents was Franz Gall, a Viennese physician. The premise of phrenology was that the brain was not only the organ of the mind but a collection of organs topographically distinct, the size of each being a measure of its function, and its development being reflected in the local shape of the cranium. In Britain phrenology was advocated and some may still support the notion as the most rational method for selecting politicians! An Edinburgh lawyer, George Combe, described 33 organs and deployed an instrument to measure the phrenometrical angle as an index of intellectual development; a wide angle for murderers and a narrow angle for the highest moral type - in fact Combe himself. The very controversial nature of these attempts stimulated some of the most significant advances in the understanding of cerebral anatomy and clinical neurology and indeed was influential in the educational and social development of Britain in the 19th century. The outcome of craniometry led logically to skull indices and might be regarded as the antecedent of modern stereotaxis. By the end of the 19th century phrenology was discredited but in the words of Thomas Kuhn "phrenology shifted the paradigm of science and paved the way for the great developments of 19th century neurology and functional localisation."

The search for scientific unity by Faraday, Maxwell and others during the 19th century, together with the pursuit of the vacuum phenomena led inexorably to in vivo biological imaging. In 1883 Sir William Thomson later Lord Kelvin in a lecture to the Institute of Electrical Engineers declared "I often say that when you can measure what you are speaking about and express it in numbers you know something about it. When you cannot measure it in numbers your knowledge is of a meagre and unsatisfactory kind." For contemporary workers in the natural sciences Kelvin's exhortation seemed entirely appropriate. Burgeoning technology and new instrumentation were providing new means of measurement and of standardization. Nevertheless many major advances from Darwin to Virchow, and indeed Röntgen himself, were rather triumphs of verbal description than numerical expression. It is not without interest that Kelvin, that scientific giant of the 19th century, was not only extremely skeptical at Röntgen's announcement and considered it an elaborate hoax but also wrote in 1896 "I have not the smallest molecule of faith in aerial navigation other than ballooning." Even now radiological images, whatever their derivation, still rely heavily on a traditional hierarchy of clinical judgement and logical analysis of morphological features for their interpretation. Shape, size and relationship to other structures, together with density or signal variations, are all important features in the diagnosis and monitoring of disease. The ability, quantitatively, to locate disease before structural change becomes apparent, to detect any response and end points in treatment, and to identify relapse during clinical remission from radiological images would be major advances [1].

Kelvin demanded numbers. There are 3 ways of expressing numbers:

1. *Mensuration* - a dimension on an established scale, e.g. I weigh 150 lbs.
2. *Enumeration* - a number in an identifiable group, e.g. I have 3 children.
3. *Proportionality* - e.g. 60% of a radiological audience may have a higher qualification.

In Medicine and Radiology in particular the opportunities for detailed and scaled observations of diagnostic features, or statistically designed trials and latterly for computerized handling of data, have offered some solutions to the problems of enumeration and proportionality. The phenomena providing Kelvinistic metrics, however, have, up to the 1970's, been largely laboratory based and outside the patient. The shift of the radiological paradigm in 1972 with the advent of Computed Tomography (CT) and the subsequent explosion of microtechnology have provided an opportunity to express and to quantify in detail the content of an image and in particular the ability of biological tissue to interact with various forms of radiation. Access to quantitative data, sophisticated interactive display systems, and powerful image processing facilities have further facilitated approaches to both tissue characterization and cellular metabolism. In X-ray CT the liner attenuation value of small volumes of tissue can be calculated and expressed in Hounsfield numbers.

The chance finding of a solitary low attenuation lesion in the liver on CT of the abdomen for example raises several numerical issues. Enumeration is simple - there is one lesion. The literature tells us that the commonest solitary hepatic lesion in a patient without known malignant disease is a hemangioma - a benign vascular tumor. Thus proportionality has been incorporated into the analysis. The clinical problem is that only 1 in 40 hepatic lesions will be a hemangioma. Hemangiomas are described as generally of low attenuation and surrounding liver with peripheral enhancement on dynamic contrast enhanced scanning, finally becoming isodense with surrounding liver on delayed post contrast scanning. If all these criteria are met then the positive predictive value and the specificity approach 100%, though in fact only 55% of all hemangiomas fulfil all the criteria. In a patient with known malignant disease, a lesion with all these characteristics will still have a 14% chance of being a metastasis. The features said to characterise an hepatic hemangioma are therefore all descriptive, despite the CT image being entirely representational numbers. The attenuation of hemangiomas, however, does have a strong correlation with that of blood in the inferior vena cava, thus a good choice of comparator within the image is of importance.

The lack of clear correlation between tissue type and CT attenuation values has led to a search for signatures which can be derived from these values. Four such signatures have been considered - quantitative, spatial, chemical and temporal. The quantitative signature relates to the distribution and probability of occurrence of attenuation values. The spatial signature describes the distribution of attenuation values in space and can be measured for example by autocorrelation function analysis. The chemical signature is a means of expressing the atomic composition of biological tissue and can be measured by the subtraction of information obtained from two different X-ray energies. Such dual energy techniques make use of the fact that the photoelectric interaction of X-rays with tissue is highly dependent on atomic number. The method has proved of particular value in improving the accuracy of bone mineral measurement in trabecular bone. Computed Tomography is unique amongst the non-invasive methods in permitting a separate assessment of trabecular and cortical bone. Although the correlation between CT attenuation values and the concentration of mineral in cortical bone is of a high order (r = 0.98) this is not so for metabolically active trabecular bone (r = 0.67) due to the presence of variable amounts of fat in the marrow spaces. The estimation of high atomic number calcium by dual energy quantitative CT enables a high degree of correlation (r = 0.97) with trabecular bone mineral content to be achieved, thereby providing a sensitive and accurate method for measuring bone mass [2,3]. Single energy quantitative CT has greater precision (1-3%) and offers a reliable and reproducible method for longitudinal studies of bone mass in health and disease [4]. Osteoporosis is a major health problem throughout the world, particularly affecting those over 65 years, an age group destined in the UK to double in number by the year 2000. The temporal signature is one which in theory can be derived from rapid sequence studies of iodine transit time in tissue. Many factors influence the distribution of detectable iodine but the two principal obstacles to the effective use of this signature are firstly the rapid diffusion of intravenously administered contrast medium into the extravascular space (over 50% in less than 1 minute), and secondly the inadequate sampling frequency available despite segmentation of the quantitative data.

Temporal and energy subtraction are currently used in digital vascular imaging to exploit the difference in attenuation properties between iodine and surrounding tissue. Both methods have their limitations, the one by movement and the other by available X-ray flux and the polychromatic nature of the X-ray beam. Traditional X-ray sources have not changed significantly since the Coolidge tube in 1913. Synchrotron radiation, i.e. radiation from an electron accelerator, provides a new source of nearly monoenergetic X-rays, the energy which can be finely tuned to the K edge of iodine. Digital subtraction of two energies to isolate iodine in an image is then feasible. At present the technique requires an accelerator and storage rings 50 metres in diameter! The challenge is to reduce high energy storage rings to hospital proportions. Experiments to develop Computed Tomography to micrometre spatial resolution with synchrotron generated X-rays have been attempted. In theory a high atomic number probe bound to nerve membrane or attached with a metabolic precursor could be explored with a monochromatic source to detect K edge shifts with neural activity. The problem is one of sensitivity, not to mention finance.

Estimation of blood flow in cerebral tissue is possible with single photon (SPECT) and positron emission tomography (PET) but limited by spatial resolution. The use of stable Xenon gas and X-ray CT can provide parameter images for local cerebral blood flow with relatively high spatial resolution and excellent anatomical correlation. Xenon has a high atomic number (54) and is highly lipid soluble, enabling it to cross the normal blood brain barrier following inhalation. Radiological enhancement can be monitored as a function of time by sequential CT. Partition coefficient images together with flow images thus combine tissue and flow information. Xenon CT has been applied in a variety of conditions from cerebrovascular disease to dementia. There are systematic and random errors in such a system related to technique and to patient handling where useful clinical information can be obtained, for example in enabling differentiation to be made between Alzheimer's and Pick's disease by the use of differential blood flow observations.

The ability to reformat numerical data in alternative planes to obtain volume information is routinely exploited in clinical practice. The technique is now being further advanced with appropriate algorithms to provide gray scale weighting for depth and the production of true 3-dimensional images. The method, which relies on the acquisition of multiple very thin (1.5 mm) sections and the selection by the operator of pixel threshold values below which structures will not appear in the final image, has particular applications in extracranial, pelvic, and spinal disorders. 3-dimensional reformatted images do not contain any information not already present in the original CT sections but they do present selected volume data in easily assimilated and familiar anatomical format with demonstration of spatial relationships readily perceived by the non-radiologist [5,6,7,8]. A significant reduction in exposure factors and consequently radiation dose can be achieved without loss of 3-dimensional bone image quality. A reduction for example from 400 to 80 mAs results in the reduction of skin dose from 16 mGy to 12 mGy. Rapid sequential acquisition of contiguous sections enables the total patient scanning time for such examinations to be reduced to less than 5 minutes. Objective studies of craniofacial anomalies, facial trauma and abnormalities of the sella and parasellar region have found 3-dimensional imaging diagnostically superior in some circumstances to conventional CT sections. Intracranial and soft tissue structures, because of their similar attenuation values, are more difficult to differentiate and display 3-dimensionally. The problem can to some extent be overcome for vascular structures by the use of intravenous contrast. The technique then provides a potential alternative to invasive angiography for the display of some aneurysms, arteriovenous malformations and tumours.

The speed of data acquisition by conventional CT is restricted by conventional tube and detector technology, though a deflectable focal spot tube in a continuously rotating gantry has recently been made available to reduce inter scan delay times. Multiple X-ray tubes and detectors arrays have been proposed but inhibited by cost. One innovative advance in temporal resolution has been achieved by the use of a circumferential target and a focussed electron beam. Such a system (Imatron) is now in commercial use and is successfully providing millisecond CT sections for cardiac and other organ studies.

The remarkable achievements in CT, and indeed in radiological imaging generally, have been made possible to a large degree by the rapid advances in micro technology and computing. A million functions per chip are confidently forecast by 1990, perhaps one billion by 2000. The next generation of memory chips or DRAMS (64 megabyte dynamic random access memories) are likely to be less than 0.5 micrometres in size and produced by X-ray lithography, the X-rays being generated by compact storage rings for synchrotron radiation. CT scanners in the next decade should be compact, faster, lower dose instruments with dual energy and real time 3-dimensional imaging capabilities.

Magnetic Resonance (MR) proton imaging with its high contrast multiplanar facilities and absence of ionising radiation is currently without doubt the most sensitive and least invasive modality for the investigation of structural change in the central nervous system. It seems likely in the developed world to become the primary investigative tool for intracranial disease and many musculo-skeletal disorders. It is already replacing myelography in the management of disorders affecting the spine and providing valuable clinical information in a variety of neurological problems. The absence of bone artifacts in the posterior fossa compared with CT is particularly valuable.

The characterization of tissue and the assessment of its functional capacity by MR Imaging can be approached in a number of ways - the source image, the quantification of image parameters or from derived properties, e.g. texture, the use of biological markers, and microscopy, i.e. the highest achievable resolution of the imaging method.

The multiplicity of measureable MR parameters, including proton density, relaxation times, blood flow, chemical shift, diffusion, perfusion and paramagnetic contrast agents provides unprecedented opportunities to explore morphology, pathology, physiology and biochemistry [9]. Proton imaging alone provides a rich source of these opportunities to explore the interface between form and function.

The measurement of relaxation times has perhaps been the most commonly used approach in MRI towards tissue characterization since Damadian's original observations on isolated tissue in 1971 [19]. Relaxation times depend not only on the biological structure and water content of the tissue concerned but also on the technical circumstances of measurement, the use of multiple data points to express exponential decay and the need to correct for the relatively short repetition times of clinical practice [11,12]. T1 is field dependent and generally monoexponential. T2 is less dependent on field strength but multiexponential. Most measurements have been obtained from regions of interest which are subject to considerable tissue averaging. Nevertheless useful clinical data can be obtained by careful calibration and optimization. Changes of the order of 5% have been observed in white matter of brain and an excellent discrimination obtained between recurrent carcinoma rectum and fibrosis post-operatively [13]. It is clear however that region of interest techniques do not use all the discriminative information available. Relaxation time maps, where individual pixels are assigned values by multiple data point analysis and a user-defined sub image, can substantially increase tissue discrimination. Spatial variation of relaxation time values provides a means for example of studying the distribution of glycosaminoglycans, the colloid gels responsible for the resilience of the intervertebral disc [14,15].

The organization of water in biological tissues can be represented by crystalline water, in restricted motion locations, e.g. macromolecular protein matrices and cellular membranes, free bulk water with unrestricted motion in intra- and extra-cellular spaces and an intervening hydration layer. Contrast in MRI is a complex function of spin density and spin relaxation. The relaxation properties of water proteins in biological tissue may involve a number of mechanisms. One such mechanism is that of Magnetization Transfer between the motion restricted protons of bound water and the highly mobile free water protons. In such a model, protons in the surface layer interact with the macromolecular matrix by both chemical exchange and by dipole-dipole interaction. The surface layer then communicates with the free water by diffusion. Such pathways can be exploited to enhance the relaxation behavior of solvent water.

Magnetization transfer or exchange can be observed in living tissues using saturation transfer techniques where the proton spins of the macromolecular bound water are selectively saturated with a relatively strong radiofrequency irradiation 5-10 kH off resonance from free water in a modified gradient echo sequence. The transfer magnetization between free and bound water pools gives rise to a decrease in magnetization of the free water and a decrease in T1 relaxation time with consequent loss of signal intensity. This type of contrast governed by the magnetization transfer process has been termed Magnetization Transfer Contrast (MTC) [16]. Application of MTC in muscle before and after exercise has been studied. Substantial signal loss can be observed in all muscles using pre-irradiation and attenuations of over 65% have been observed. After exercise the signal intensity of the active muscle groups show a significant enhancement of the anticipated increase in signal from exercised muscle [17]. Quantification of magnetization transfer is possible and the potential for differentiation of biological tissue where tightly bound nuclei prevail is considerable. The method has been used to measure magnetization exchange in the kidney and in the brain. Recent experimental studies [18] suggest that lipid bilayers may contribute to water relaxation processes in biological tissue. This may explain the differential relaxation behavior of white and gray matter of brain. White matter has a higher membrane concentration due to the presence of lipid bilayers in myelin.

Chemical information is provided by both Magnetic Resonance Imaging (MRI) and Magnetic Resonance Spectroscopy (MRS). In MRI chemical shift and relaxation times through MTC provide information about the physiochemical environment. The derivation of chemical information by MR processes represents an area of overlap between MRS, where spectral data are extracted from an array of contiguous voxels, and MRI, where components with different chemical shifts can be displayed.

The short TI-IR sequence (STIR) is perhaps the simplest of the fat suppression techniques. Spectroscopic techniques are now being exploited in imaging with selective saturation or selective excitation of either the water or fat lines using binary RF pulse patterns.

Contrast agents act as biological markers [19]. Clinical interest in contrast agents is centred on the paramagnetic Gadolinium complexes. The principal effect of a paramagnetic agent in MR imaging is to reduce T1 relaxation times at the target site and many clinical studies have demonstrated the value of such agents [20,21, 22,23,24]. The current focus is on increasing specificity, the targeting effect and the half-life whilst reducing the dose required. Paramagnetic Gadolinium-DTPA (Gd-DTPA) is widely available. Its pharmacokinetics are similar to those of iodinated contrast agents. Gd-DOTA is an example of the higher molecular weight polychelated complexes being explored. DOTA chelation and protein conjugation are extending observed vascular enhancement. A new paramagnetic tissue specific agent for hepatobiliary imaging, Gd-BOPTA, is also being investigated. In combination with fast imaging techniques this agent is providing information on the early kinetics of hepatocyte uptake and represents a powerful approach to the assessment of dynamic processes. Low osmolar non-ionic complexes of Gadolinium may permit higher doses of contrast to be used with potential clinical advantage.

Superparamagnetic agents e.g. Magnetite and Iron Oxide are those which give rise to a significant T2 effect with loss of signal notably when taken up by the reticulo endothelial system. The conventional superparamagnetic agent is particulate iron oxide which has a relatively short half-life [25]. Recent developments in superparamagnetic agents include ferrosomes, small (80 nm) liposomes loaded with superparamagnetic iron oxide crystals which appear to be stable with a relatively long half-life (11 hours). Ultrasmall superparamagnetic iron oxide particles (USPIO) have been developed that retain superparamagnetic characteristics but are small enough to migrate across the capillary wall [26], a prerequisite in the design of targetable pharmaceuticals. USPIOs have been specifically directed to asialoglycoprotein receptors on hepatocytes enabling lower dose and better homogeneity to be obtained. Further surface modifications of these particles should enable development of a variety of receptor and antibody specific agents.

Techniques involving phase mapping and angiography for recording and measuring flow information are now well established. Magnetic Resonance Angiography (MRA) is non-invasive and requires no contrast injection. Two acquisition methods are generally described - segmental time of flight (TOF) and phase contrast (PC). 2DPC has the advantage of speed 3DPC achieves better spatial resolution and allows vessels to be viewed retrospectively from any angle [27,28]. Anisotropic flow sensitivity currently limits the generalized application of sequential 2D TOF. Time resolved PC methods are good in the absence of motion. ECG gating makes PC techniques less sensitive to pulsatility and motion and therefore provides better quality images in the abdomen.

Diffusion directly reflects molecular mobility, a process which in a homogeneous fluid may be truly random and unrestrictive. The phenomenon is not an MR parameter and varies with the direction of measurement [29]. The Diffusion coefficient is a measure of mobility at molecular level and varies inversely with viscosity. In biological tissues of course diffusion is restricted by barriers and cell boundaries. Diffusion may be more restricted in one direction than another, e.g. in myelinated white matter, while cross diffusion is more restricted than longitudinal. This is referred to as anisotropic diffusion (ARD) [30]. By deliberately applying large magnetic field gradients, usually pulsed gradient spin echoes in particular directions, anisotropic diffusion can be made the dominant image contrast mechanism enabling variations including direction to be visualized. Perfusion may be studied separately from diffusion using an intra-voxel incoherent motion (IVIM) model [31,32]. IVIM is randomly orientated and probably reflects capillary flow for which there are potentially useful values not quite the same as the classic perfusion measurements of nuclear medicine nomenclature where deposition of radioactivity is the measure.

Texture, a secondary parameter of any image, is quite different from shape or contrast and is derived by specialized image analysis techniques. Texture involves the repetition of a pattern which may vary randomly from one position to the next. The repetition and frequency can be fine or coarse and the pattern intricate or anisotropic (e.g. the grain of wood). Analysis of texture requires three stages - feature detection, feature extraction and classification. A significant separation of benign and malignant tissue in the prostate has been obtained by this technique with an 80% classification. In a recent prospective study of bone mineral disease where differentiation of MR images was impossible by human vision or by Region of Interest studies, a significant separation and high order of individual classification in three groups of disease - osteoporosis, osteomalacia, and hyperparathyroidism has been obtained [33]. The increased discrimination achieved with textural analysis and pattern recognition processing is expected to apply to a large range of clinical disease states.

"Vision," it is said, "is the extraction from an image of just such information as is required." In normal vision the eye perceives areas and spacial frequencies which neurones code for brightness and edges through from the retina to the visual cortex. Indeed much of the information used by the eye can be contained in edges, a fact well known to the artist and cartoonist. Edge detection has important applications in tissue characterization and classification of disease. Edges described by gradient magnitude have been shown to correlate with T1 relaxation rates. Texture feature maps which optimize edge information are encouraging.

High resolution MR means optimizing spatial and contrast resolution in a clinical setting. Higher spatial resolution can be obtained, for example by modification of the radio frequency coils and their surface application. Endoluminal coils can provide high resolution images of the prostate via the rectum [34]. Phased arrays of surface coils increase both the field of view and the signal to noise ratio. Higher resolution imaging requires the highest attainable signal to noise ratio. Closely fitting RF probes are required with small volume gradients of sufficient strength and fast enough switching times to allow minimization of unnecessary T2 decay. In vivo images of experimental tumors with a resolution of 100 microns at 4.7 Tesla and 200 microns at 0.26 Tesla have been obtained whilst resolution of four microns in living plant tissue has been achieved using very high field systems [35].

The quest for precision and accuracy in quantitative MR imaging raises important issues of in vivo links with histopathology. These links are complicated by the opportunities which MRI offers as a non-invasive method to investigate both the sick and the healthy, raising new ambiguities about the meaning of "normal." Whether one regards Kelvin's dictum of mensuration as a curse or a blessing the observations he made in 1871 are still relevant.

"All the grandest discoveries of science have been but the rewards of accurate measurement and patient long-continued labour in the minute sifting of numerical results."

Selected References

1. Isherwood I. Tissue characterization in computed tomography. Diagnostic imaging 1984;6:5-47.
2. Adams JE, Chen SZ, Adams PH, Isherwood I. Measurement of trabecular bone loss as determined by quantitative computed tomography. Journal of Bone Mineral Research 192;4:249-257.
3. Adams JE. Quantitative computed tomography. In Imaging techniques in orthopaedics. Ed Galasko CSB, Isherwood I. Springer Verlag. 1989:259-268.
4. Cann CE. Quantitative computed tomography for bone mineral analysis: technical considerations. In: Genant HK, ed. Osteoporosis update 1987. University of California Printing Services, 1987:131-144.
5. Gillespie JE, Isherwood I. Three-dimensional anatomical images from computed tomographic scans. BJR 1986;59:289-292.
6. Gillespie JE, Quayle AA, Barker J, Isherwood I. Three-dimensional CT reformations in the assessment of congenital and traumatic cranio-facial deformities. British Journal of Oral & Maxillo-facial Surgery 1987;25:171-177.
7. Gillespie JE, Adams JE, Isherwood I. Three-dimensional computed tomographic reformations of sellar and para-sellar lesions. Neuroradiology 1987;29,30-35.

8. Gholkar A, Isherwood I. Three-dimensional computed tomographic reformations of intracranial vascular lesions. BJR 1988;61:258-261.

9. Young IR. Considerations affecting signal and contrast in MR imaging. Brit Med Bull 1984;40:139-147.

10. Damadian R. Tumour detection by nuclear magnetic resonance. Science 1971;171:1151-1153.

11. Hickey DS, Checkley DR, Aspden RN, Naughton A, Jenkins JPR, Isherwood I. A method for the clinical measurement of relaxation times in magnetic resonance imaging. BJR 1986;59:565-570.

12. Tofts PS, du Boulay EPGH. Towards quantitative measurements of relaxation times and other parameters in the brain. Neuroradiology 1990;32:407-415.

13. Johnson RJ, Jenkins JPR, Isherwood I, James RD, Schofield PF. Quantitative MR imaging in rectal carcinoma. BJR 1987;60:761-764.

14. Isherwood I, Prendergast DJ, Hickey DS, Jenkins JPR. Quantitative analysis of intervertebral disc structure. Acta Rad 1987;369:239-241.

15. Jenkins JPR, Stehling M, Sivewright G, Hickey DS, Hillier VF, Isherwood I. Quantitative magnetic resonance imaging of vertebral bodies - a T1 and T2 study. Mag Res Imaging 1989;7;17-23.

16. Wolff SD, Balaban RS. Magnetic transfer contrast (MTC) and tissue water proton relaxation in vivo. MR in Medicine 1989;10:135-144.

17. Zhu XP, Zhao S, Isherwood I. Magnetic transfer contrast (MTC) imaging of skeletal muscle at 0.26 Tesla - changes in signal intensity following exercise. BJR-In press.

18. Fralix TA, Ceckler TL, Wolff SD, Simon SA, Balaban RS. Liquid bilayer and water proton magnetization transfer: effect of cholesterol. MR in medicine 1989;18:214-223.

19. Runge VM. Enhanced MR imaging. CV Mosley Co, St Louis, Washington, Toronto, 1989.

20. Stark DD, Bradley WG. Magnetic resonance imaging, CV Mosley, St Louis, 1988.

21. De Roos A, Doornbos J, Baleriaux D, Bloem HL, Falke THM. Clinical applications of GdDTPA in MRI. In:HY Kressel, ed. Magnetic Resonance Annual, 1988:113-145.

22. Stack JP, Antoun NM, Jenkins JPR, Metcalfe R, Isherwood I. Gadolinium DTPA as a contrast agent in magnetic resonance imaging of the brain. Neuroradiology 1988;30:145-154.

23. Stack JP, Ramsden RT, Antoun NM, Isherwood I, Jenkins JPR. Magnetic resonance imaging of acoustic neuromas: the role of Gd-DTPA. BJR 1988;61:800-805.

24. Isherwood I, Hawnaur JM, Jenkins JPR. Gadolinium DTPA in magnetic resonance imaging of spinal tumours and angiomas. In:M Jadjmi, ed. XV Congress Europ Soc of Neuroradiology. Springer Verlag. 1989:77-86.

25. Weissleder R, Stark DD, Engelstad BL et al. Superparamagnetic iron oxide: pharmacokinetics and toxicity. BJR 1989;152:167-173.

26. Weissleder R, Reimer P, Lee P, Witteberg J, Bardis TJ. MR receptor imaging: ultrasmall iron oxide particles targetted to asialoglycoprotein receptors. AJR 1990;155:1161-1167.

27. Dumoulin CL, Hart HR. Magnetic resonance angiography. Radiology 1986;161:717-720.

28. Dumoulin CL, Yucel EK, Vock P et al. 2D and 3D phase contrast MR angiography of the abdomen. J CAT 1990;14:779-784.

29. Chien D, Buxton RB, Kwong KK, Brady TJ, Rosen BR. MR Diffusion imaging of the human brain. JCAT 1990;14:514-520.

30. Hajnal JV, Doran M, Hall AS et al. MR imaging of anisotropically restricted diffusion of water in the nervous system. JCAT 1991;15:1-18.

31. Le Bihan D, Lallemand D, Grenier P, Cabanis E, Laval-Jeantet M. MR imaging of intravoxel incoherent motions : application to diffusion and perfusion in neurological disorders. Radiology 1986;161:401-407.

32. Le Bihan D, Breton E, Lallemand D, Aubin M-L, Vignal J, Laval-Jeantet M. Separation of diffusion and perfusion in intravoxel coherent motion MR imaging. Radiology 1988;168:492-505.
33. Jenkins JPR, Zhu XP, Whitehouse RW, Isherwood I, Adams JE, Adams PH. Textural analysis and quantitative magnetic resonance imaging in metabolic bone disease :an approach to tissue characterization. In: Higer HP, Bielke G, eds. Tissue Characterization in MR Imaging. Springer Verlag, 1990;170-173.
34. Schatt MD, Leakinski RE, Pollack HM, Imai Y, Kressel HY. Prostate in MR imaging with an endorectal gil. Radiology 1989;172:570-574.
35. Bowtell RS, Brown GD, Glover PM, McJury M, Mansfield P. Resolution of cellular structures by NMR microscopy at 11.7T. In: P Mansfield, EL Hahn, eds. NMR imaging, the Royal Society, London, 1990:457-467.

CT and MR Findings in Common Phakomatoses

Michael S. Huckman

*Rush-Presbyterian University and St. Luke's Medical Center,
Chicago, Illinois, USA*

Introduction

The term *phakoma* comes from the Greek word *phacos* which refers to the lens of the eye [1]. This evolved to mean a *wart*, since skin moles or warts are often lens-shaped. Hence, a phakomatosis came to be a disease characterized by the presence of a skin lesion. Phakomatoses are congenital and hereditary developmental anomalies with tumor-like malformations and angiomas or pigment patches in organs of ectodermal origin, especially skin, eye, and central and peripheral nervous system [2]. Occasionally, they may involve tissues derived from embryonic mesoderm (blood vessels, bone, cartilage) and ectoderm (epithelial lining of the GI tract) [3]. There are excellent reviews of cranial CT [2] and MR [3] findings in these diseases.

Neurofibromatosis

Neurofibromatosis consists of two different diseases [4,5]. These are neurofibromatosis-1 (NF-1) or von Recklinghausen's disease and Neurofibromatosis-2 (NF-2) which is characterized by bilateral acoustic Schwannomas. NF-2 is linked with a disorder of chromosome #22 and NF-1 is linked to a disorder of chromosome #17. MR findings in these two diseases have been recently reported [3,4,6,7].

Clinical criteria for distinguishing NF-1 and NF-2 are as follows [5]:

NF-1 may be diagnosed if two or more of the following are present:

a. Six or more cafe-au-lait spots (5-15 mm).
b. Two or more neurofibromas or one plexiform neurofibroma.
c. Axillary or inguinal freckles.
d. Optic glioma.
e. Two or more iris hamartomas (Lisch nodules).
f. A distinctive osseous lesion (orbital dysplasia or thinning of a long bone cortex).
g. Parent, sibling, or child with NF-1 according to the above criteria.

NF-2 may be diagnosed when one of the following are present [5]:

a. Bilateral eight nerve masses seen on CT or MR.
b. Parent, sibling, or child with NF-2 and either unilateral eighth nerve mass or two of the following:
   1. Neurofibroma.
   2. Meningioma.
   3. Glioma.
   4. Schwannoma.
   5. Juvenile posterior subcapsular lens opacity.

Cranial lesions of NF-1 are optic gliomas, other gliomas such as pilocystic astrocytoma of the hypothalamus [3], hamartomas, plexiform neurofibromas, cranial nerve tumors, internal auditory canal ectasia and sphenoid dysplasia. Optic gliomas (Fig. 1) are usually isointense to hypointense on T1-weighted image and strongly hyperintense on T2-weighted image [4].

The *Lisch nodule* was the subject of a recent report by Lubs et al. [8]. Lisch nodules are melanocytic hamartomas that appear as dome shaped elevations on the iris. They are clear to yellow or brown. They are the most common clinical feature in neurofibromatosis-1 in adults, and are found only in patients with von Recklinghausen's disease [8]. Only 5% of children less than 3 years of age with NF-1 have these nodules, but the incidence rises to 42%

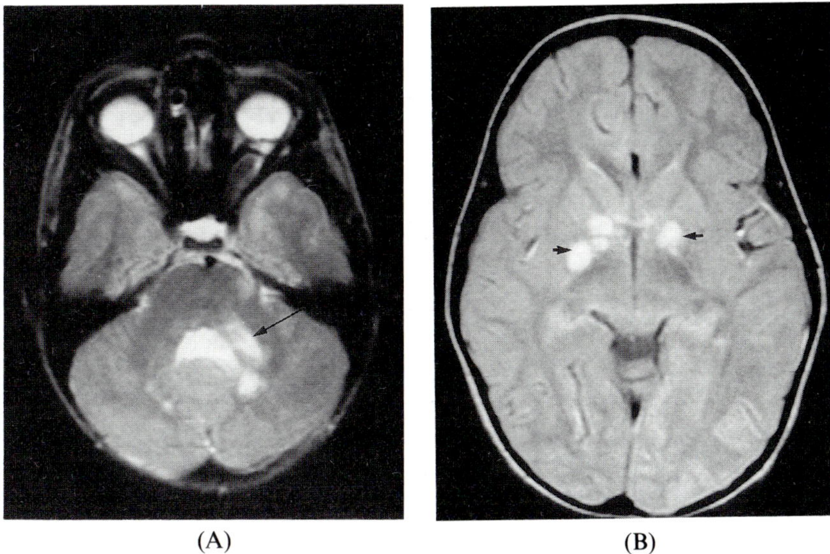

(A)   (B)

Figure 1. *NEUROFIBROMATOSIS 1. Neurofibromatosis 1 patient with bilateral optic gliomas and scattered high intensity lesions in basal ganglia and cerebellum. (A) T2 weighted axial MR image shows high intensity optic gliomas behind the globes bilaterally and also shows high intensity lesions in the cerebellum (arrow). (B) Proton density MR scan shows high intensity lesions in the basal ganglia (arrows).*

in children aged 3-4, and to 55% in 5-6 year olds. One hundred percent of adults over age 21 with NF-1 have Lisch nodules [8]. However, these are never the only sign of NF-1. They are more likely to be present in younger patients than are neurofibromas. The observation that all patients above age 20 have Lisch nodules is felt to be useful for genetic counselling, since it should enable distinction between minimally affected and unaffected patients [8].

There may be swelling of optic nerves and of the chiasm [4]. Foci of increased intensity of T2-weighted image without mass effect (Fig. 1) are seen throughout the brain, especially in the basal ganglia, brainstem and peduncles [4,5,6,7]. These lesions are most likely to occur in the globus pallidus, although the thalamus and internal capsule also may be involved [9]. These areas are not adjacent to foci or tumor and are not associated with mass effect. CT does not demonstrate these lesions, and they are not associated with neurologic abnormalities [6]. Their imaging appearance is most suggestive of widespread hamartomas or low grade gliomatosis [6].

17

These lesions may be seen in the cerebellar peduncles, cerebellar white matter, and pons [7]. Bognanno et al. suggest that these are possibly heterotopias such as meningioangiomatous malformations, atypical glial nest cells, subependymal glial nodules, ependymal ectopias or intramedullary schwannomas [7]. The high intensity lesions have an age related incidence seeming to be more common in patients over 20 years [4]. This raises the possibility that these may be the pathologic correlate, in brain parenchyma, of the Lisch nodule.

Mirowitz et al. [9] have described areas of high signal on T1-weighted image in NF-1. These have no mass or edema and do not enhance with Gd-DTPA. They believe that the high signal on T1-weighted image represents either ectopic Schwann cells or melano-cytes or both within hamartomas since either of these cells can shorten T1 relaxation. T2-weighted image shows smaller lesions at these areas [9].

The osseous orbital dysplasia of NF-1 (Fig. 2) is felt to be due to a mesodermal dysplasia. There is no associated neoplasm [3]. The temporal lobe herniates through an osseous defect into the orbit. The sella may slope toward the involved side and there is exophthalmos and displacement of the internal carotid artery toward the midline (Fig. 2) [10].

Extra-axial lesions of NF-1 are usually of intermediate intensity on T1-weighted image and markedly hyperintense on T2-weighted image [4]. These may also be associated with vascular lesions in NF-1. There may be vascular stenosis with subsequent *Moya-Moya* changes or arteriovenous fistulas [11]. Deans et al. review the theories relating neurofibromatosis-1 to arteriovenous malformation [11]. Some reports suggest that there is intimal proliferation, frag-mentation of the elastica, and thinning of the media in arteries in NF-1 leading to aneurysm formation. Such lesions, seen in half the autopsies of patients with this disease suggest that Schwann cells may grow in the arterial walls of NF-1 patients [11].

Deans et al. put forth two theories of arteriovenous malfor-mation formation in NF-1. One suggests that dysplastic smooth muscle in the arterial wall gives rise to aneurysms which leak and eventually rupture into adjacent veins. The other suggests that AVM's arise in this disease as congenital mesodermal dysplasias [11].

In NF-2, the acoustic Schwannomas show enlargement of the 7th

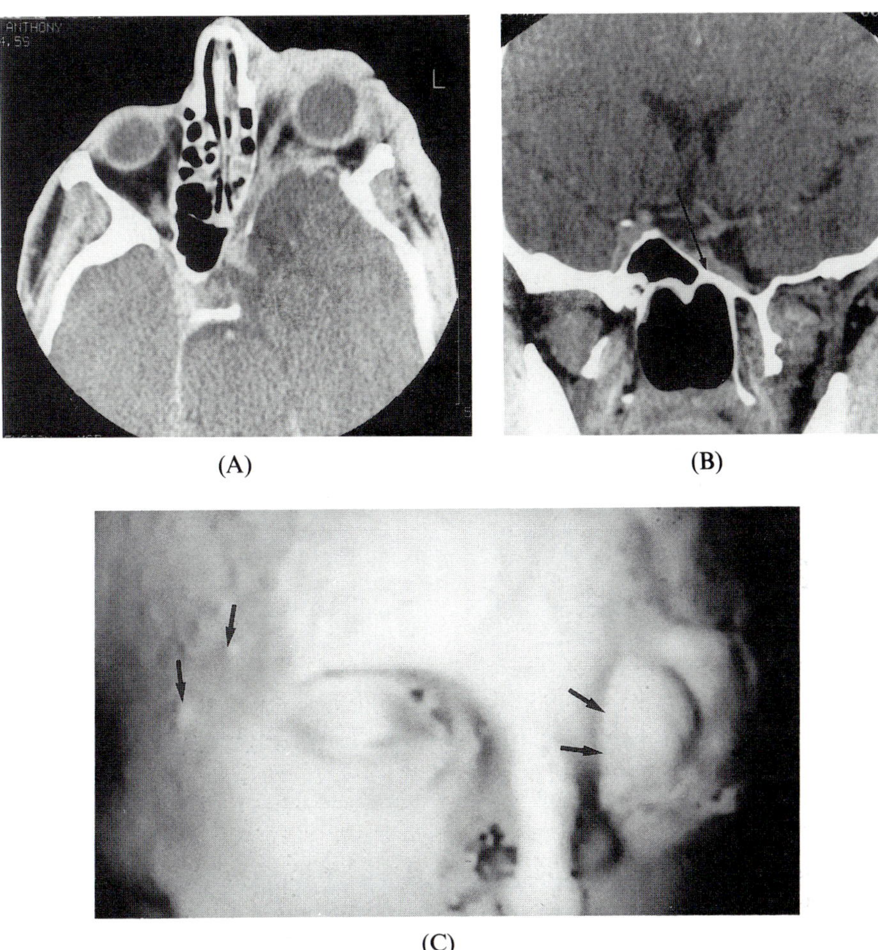

(A)

(B)

(C)

Figure 2. *ORBITAL DYSPLASIA OF NEUROFIBROMATOSIS. (A) Axial post contrast CT scan showing herniation of the left temporal lobe anteriorly causing left exophthalmos. (B) Axial post contrast CT scan showing sloping of the floor of the sella turcica downward toward the left (arrow). (C) Reformatted soft tissue image showing exophthalmos and multiple small plexiform neurofibromas over the skin of the face and the scalp (arrows).*

and 8th nerve complexes. There is intermediate intensity of the Schwannoma on T1-weighted image and increased intensity on T2-weighted image and post-enhancement study (Fig. 3). Associated cranial nerve Schwannomas are found in approximately 80% of patients with bilateral acoustic Schwannomas, especially of cranial

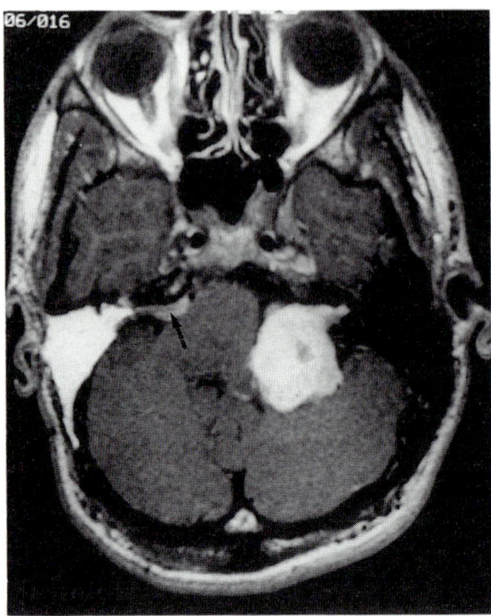

Figure 3. *NEUROFIBROMATOSIS-2. Axial post contrast T1 weighted MR scan shows a large left acoustic Schwannoma and a surgical remnant of a smaller right acoustic Schwannoma (arrow).*

nerves of V-XII (Fig. 4) [4]. Optic gliomas and hamartomas are rare in NF-2, and meningiomas are present in a little over half of patients [4]. MR of the spine in NF-2 may occasionally detect asymptomatic cord and brainstem lesions [12].

The importance of CT and MR in neurofibromatosis lies mainly in their ability to screen the families of affected patients and affected individuals looking for additional asymptomatic lesions. The frequency of CNS tumor occurrence in patients with NF-1 is 5-10%. Typical tumors include optic gliomas, acoustic and trigeminal Schwannomas, astrocytomas, ependymomas, hamartomas and glioblastomas [13]. Additional CNS tumors may be present in 45% of NF-2 patients.

According to Cammarata et al. [14], MR is the best method of screening for additional asymptomatic lesions in NF-1 and NF-2. Post Gd-DTPA imaging should be included so as to identify small intracanalicular neuromas and meningiomas.

Tuberous Sclerosis (TS)

Tuberous Sclerosis involves multiple organs [15], but a firm diagnosis is usually made by detecting the triad of epilepsy, mental

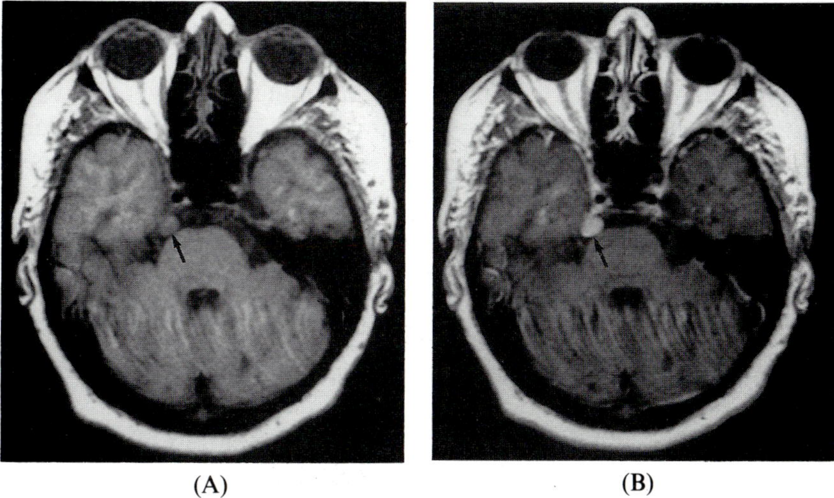

(A)   (B)

Figure 4. *SCHWANNOMA OF 5TH NERVE. Schwannoma of the cisternal portion of the right 5th nerve. (A) Pre contrast T1 weighted MR axial acquisition (arrow). (B) Post contrast T1 weighted axial acquisition (arrow).*

retardation and characteristic skin lesions. TS is much rarer than neurofibromatosis. It may be inherited as an autosomal dominant or it may result from a mutation [3]. The abnormal gene is located on the long arm of chromosome #9 [16]. Lesions occur in almost any body organ and most are hamartomas [3].

The presence of two or more of the following is pathognomonic of tuberous sclerosis [2]:

a.   Cortical tubers by neuroimaging.
b.   Subependymal glial nodules by neuroimaging.
c.   Subependymal giant cell astrocytoma at the foramen of Monro.
d.   Retinal hamartomas.
e.   Multiple facial angiofibromas (adenoma sebaceum).
f.   Peri- or sub-ungual fibromas.
g.   Forehead plaques.
h.   Multiple renal angiomyolipomas.

Presumptive signs of the disease include spasms, seizures, focal areas of increased attenuation in cerebral and cerebellar cortex on

21

CT, wedge shaped calcified cortical and subcortical lesions, hypome-lanotic macules, Shagreen patches, peripapillary retinal hamartoma, gingival fibromas, dental enamel pits, multiple renal tumors or cysts, cardiac rhabdomyoma, pulmonary lymphangiomatosis, radiographic honeycomb lung, and any immediate relative with tuberous sclerosis [3].

Three types of brain lesions are seen in tuberous sclerosis. They are: 1) *superficial cortical tubers* consisting of abnormal astrocytes and neurons, which are present in most cases. They may occasio-nally calcify. 2) *Ventricular lesions* are calcified subependymal nodules of the larger benign giant cell tumors which originate near the foramen of Monro and which may cause obstructive hydroce-phalus. 3) *White matter* may show areas of glial cell replacement. Some believe that the cortical, ventricular, and white matter lesions are the result of disordered migration and differ only in their location [17].

CT shows calcified subependymal nodules (Fig. 5) that usually do not enhance with iodinated contrast infusion, and which usually lie along the lateral aspect of the body of the lateral ventricle [15].

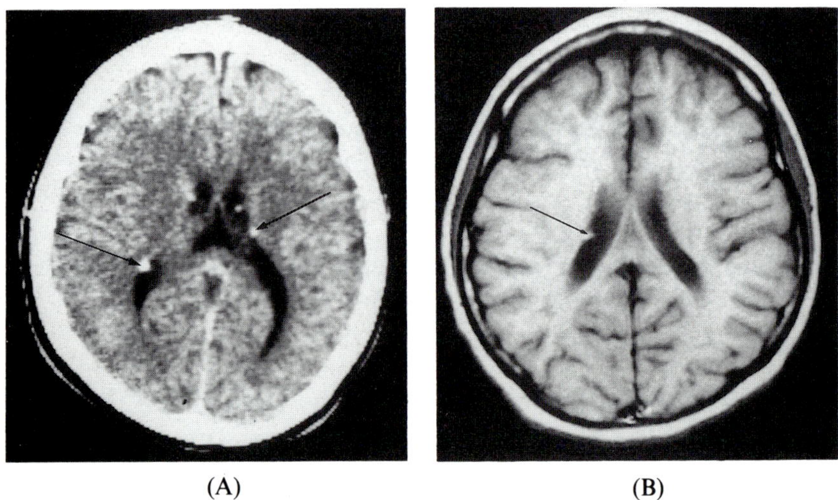

(A)   (B)

Figure 5. *TUBEROUS SCLEROSIS.* (A) *Post contrast CT scan shows mul-tiple calcified subependymal nodules (arrows).* (B) *Non contrast T1 weighted axial MR acquisition shows nodule as iso-intense filling defect in lateral ventricle (arrow).*

There may also be associated atrophy [18]. Calcification may occur in tubers, or they may be hypodense on CT. These generally do not enhance on iodinated contrast infusion whereas giant cell tumors usually do (Fig. 6) [11].

On MR, four characteristic findings are seen in tuberous sclerosis. These are 1) *Subependymal nodules* (Fig. 10), best seen on T1-weighted image as nodules isodense to brain. Calcification is difficult to detect but nodules are easily detected with T1-weighted imaging as with CT. Nodules are slightly hyperintense on T2-weighted image. When nodules are astrocytomas (Fig. 7), signal intensity increases on the T2-weighted image; 2) *cortical and subcortical foci* of increased signal intensity on T2-weighted image (Fig. 8). Anywhere from three to innumerable lesions may be seen. Most are difficult to see on CT, even in retrospect (Fig. 9). Biopsy usually shows these to be hamartomas; 3) *distortion of normal cortical architecture* which is best seen on T1-weighted image; 4) *dilated*

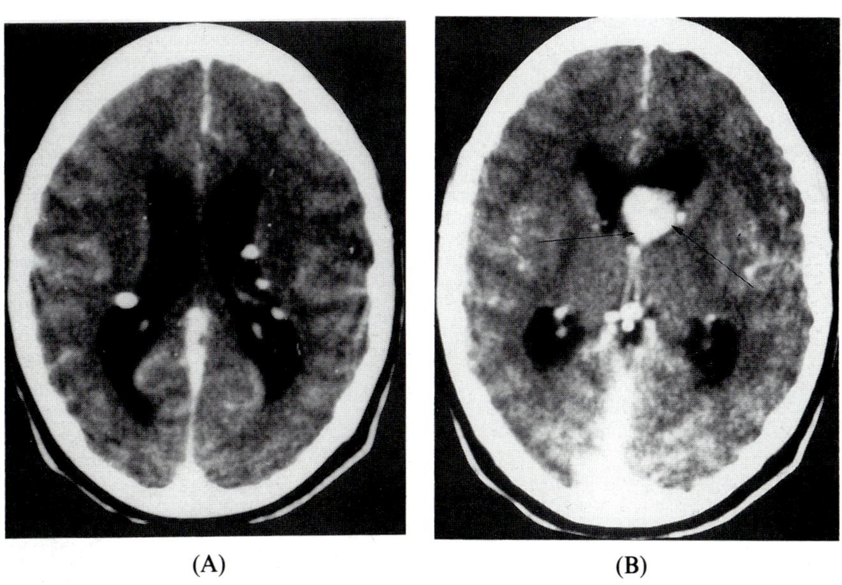

(A)   (B)

Figure 6. *TUBEROUS SCLEROSIS. Patient with tuberous sclerosis and giant cell astrocytoma·obstructing the left foramen of Monro. (A) Axial post contrast CT scan shows multiple subependymal calcified nodules and generalized ventricular enlargement. (B) Post contrast CT scan shows enhancing giant cell tumor obstructing the left foramen of Monro (arrows).*

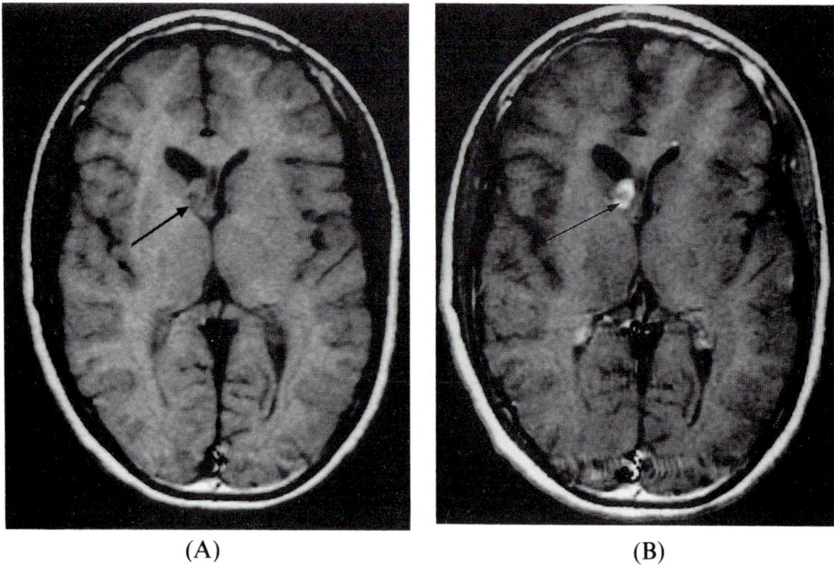

(A)   (B)

Figure 7. *SUBEPENDYMAL GIANT CELL ASTROCYTOMA.* (A) *Pre contrast axial T1 weighted MR acquisition shows an iso-intense mass (arrow).* (B) *Post contrast T1 weighted axial acquisition shows an enhancing giant cell tumor (arrow).*

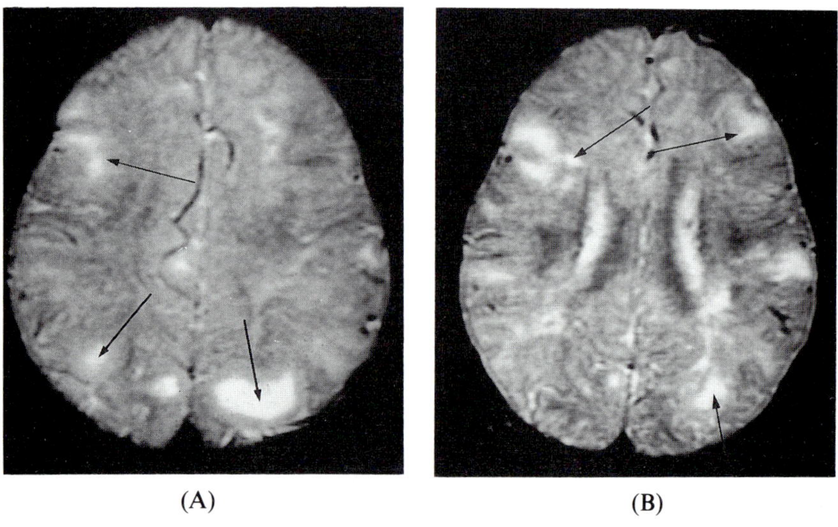

(A)   (B)

Figure 8. *TUBEROUS SCLEROSIS.* (A) *Axial T2 weighted MR acquisition shows multiple high intensity cortical tubers (arrows).* (B) *Axial T2 weighted MR acquisition shows high intensity cortical and subcortical tubers (arrows).*

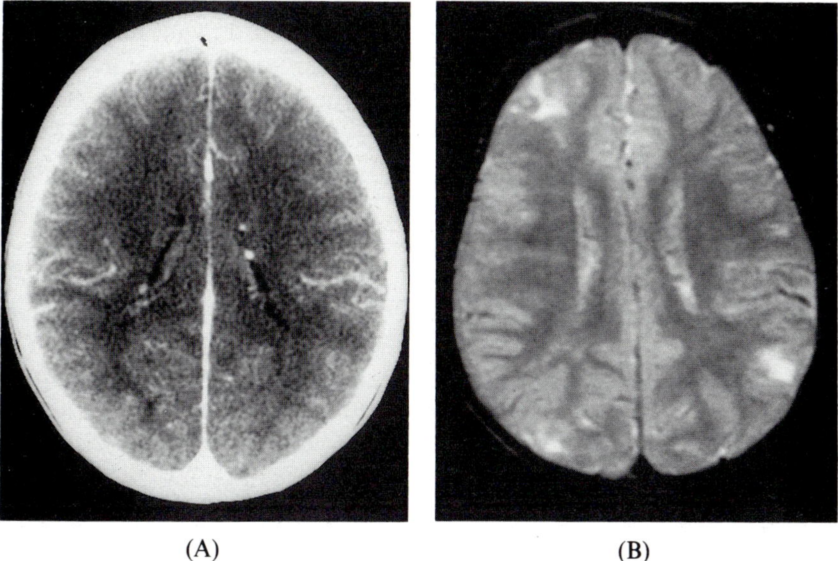

(A)   (B)

Figure 9. *TUBEROUS SCLEROSIS.* (A) *Axial post contrast CT scan shows on enhancing calcified subependymal nodules but no evidence of cortical tubers.* (B) *T2 weighted axial MR shows the presence of multiple high intensity tubers.*

ventricles with or without an obstructive lesion at the foramen of Monro [19]

The greater number of cortical tubes, the more severely affected is the patient [20]. According to Nixon et al. [21], who assessed post mortem brains of TS patients with pathologic examination and MRI, the prolonged T2 relaxation in cerebral gyri was felt to be actually due to hypomyelination of these areas. The white matter, lacking the usual number of myelinated axons, was much looser in microscopic appearance than the compact cortex with its interlacing astrocytic fibers. This looseness of tissue was felt to allow more intestinal water to accumulate in the subcortical white matter.

Since the neuronal population is decreased in tubers, the expanded appearance of involved gyri lying over some tubers is due to the increased number of astrocytes and their fibrous processes. A recent paper from Japan [22] revealed linear abnormalities in cerebral white matter connecting subependymal nodules to sub-cortical lesions. These are of increased intensity on T2-weighted image and decreased intensity in T1-weighted image. These were not seen on CT examination. The linear abnormalities suggest either a disorder of myelination or perhaps lines of a migrational disorder.

Sturge-Weber Syndrome (SWS)

Sturge-Weber Syndrome (SWS) is also called encephalotrigeminal angiomatosis. It is congenital with facial and leptomeningeal angiomatosis and atrophy of the subjacent cortex and intracerebral calcification. The facial angioma has a prediction for the territory of the superior branch of the trigeminal nerve. Ocular choroid may also be involved. Ninety percent of patients with this disease have seizures [2].

C shows cortical gyral shaped calcifications (Fig. 10). They are usually posterior. Atypical SWS may have only seizures and no cutaneous manifestations. Gyrial calcification may be the only finding in some cases [23]. Cortical calcification may be bilateral in 15% of cases [2] (Fig. 11). CT also shows ipsilateral hemiatrophy [2]. Cortical lucency may surround calcification suggesting chronic ischemia. Cranial asymmetry, secondary to hemiatrophy (Fig. 11),

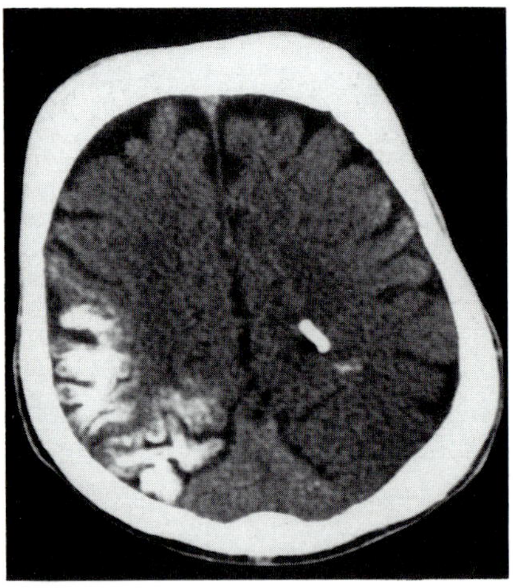

Figure 10. *STURGE-WEBER SYNDROME. Axial CT scan shows cortical gyral-shaped calcification and calcification in the choroid plexus (Case furnished by Dr. Thomas Naidich).*

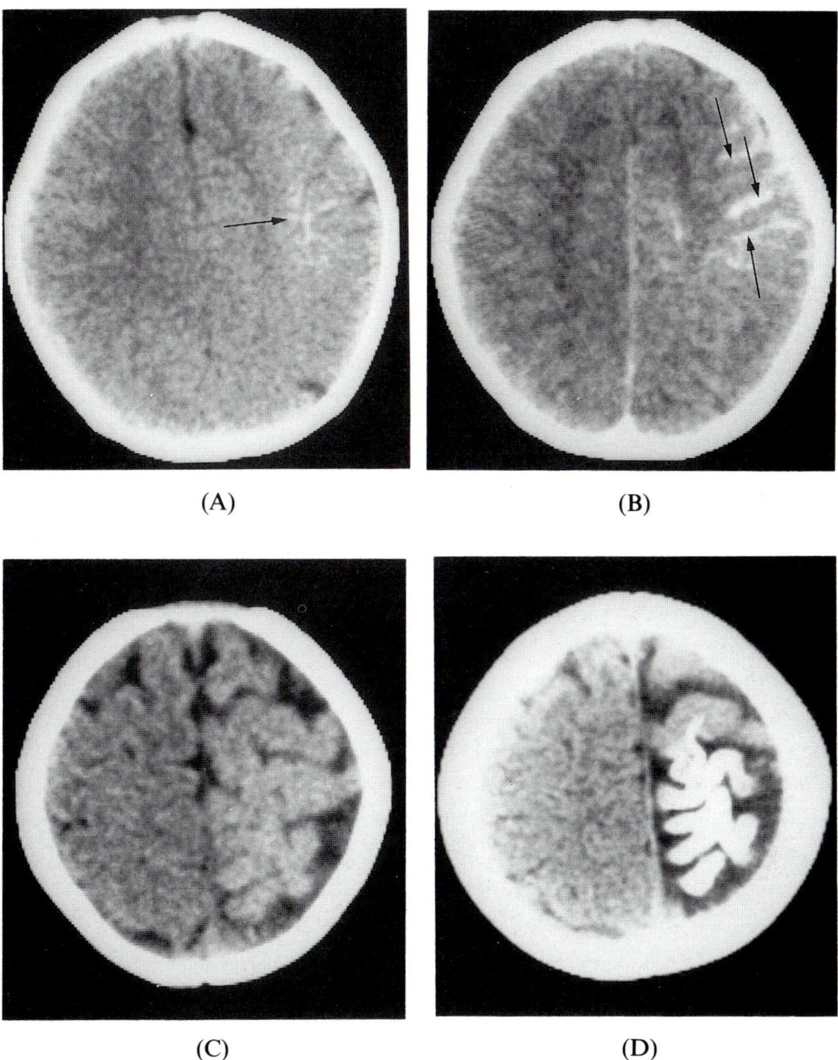

(A)

(B)

(C)

(D)

Figure 11. *STURGE-WEBER SYNDROME. (A) Non-contrast axial CT at age three months shows slight hyperdensity in the left hemisphere (arrow). (B) Post contrast axial CT age three months shows a gyral pattern of enhancement (arrows). (C) Post contrast CT at the age three months shows left hemiatrophy. (D) Non contrast CT at age two years shows heavy gyral calcification and hemiatrophy.*

may occur. The disease rarely may present with intracerebral hemorrhage [2].

Iodinated contrast CT delineates the extent of disease before calcification occurs by showing the area of gyral enhancement (Fig. 11) [24]. The cause of this is either congested cerebral veins or a defect in the blood-brain barrier. There may be abnormal enhancement of the choroid plexus within the atrium [2,23].

MR also shows cerebral atrophy and bone hypertrophy. MR shows lens shaped areas of increased signal consistent with subacute hemorrhages in cases of retinal detachment [25]. Calcification is seen on gradient recalled echo sequences [25,26]. MR also shows large (7-10 mm) choroid plexuses on the side of the atrophy [25]. Post Gd-DTPA MR scan can show enlarged deep veins, meningeal thickening, retinal angiomatosis, and gyral enhancement. Gradient recalled echo sequences and paramagnetic contrast materials make MR equal to or better than CT for the detection and delineation of the abnormalities in SWS [25,26,27].

Von Hippel Lindau Disease

Von Hippel-Lindau Disease (vHLD) is an autosomal-dominant disorder characterized by tumors of the central nervous system and abdominal viscera including cerebellar hemangioblastoma in 30-60% of cases, retinal angiomatosis, renal cell carcinoma, pheochromocytoma and medullary and spinal cord hemangioblastomas in less than 5% of cases [18]. Retinal angiomatosis occurs in over half of the affected patients and is usually the first manifestation of the disease. While the retinal lesions are difficult to image, abnormalities in the globe may be seen on CT and MR if there is resultant chronic retinal detachment [28].

Hemangioblastomas are present in 63% of patients with vHLD and they are overwhelmingly found in the cerebellum (in 47% of patients) [29]. Supratentorial hemangioblastomas present like other supratentorial intra-axial tumors except that there may be associated polycythemia [30]. They may be solid or cystic and most often occur in the parietal lobes [31]. Their imaging characteristics are similar to infratentorial hemangioblastomas [32].

Cerebellar hemangioma blastomas are rare, benign, and usually solitary. They are usually located in the cerebellar hemispheres, vermis, or medulla near the area postrema [33]. The typical cerebellar hemangioblastoma includes a small, highly vascular mural nodule associated with a much larger fluid-filled cyst situated near the surface of the cerebellum [28]. Spinal hemangioblastoma is rarer and may go unrecognized, especially when cerebellar hemangioblastoma is present [28].

Angiography, hemangioblastoma presents as a dense nodule or tangle of vessels (Fig. 12), although cysts without these nodules have been reported [34]. These may be associated with an enlarged tentorial artery [35]. The nodules or tangles may be homogenous or have a central lucency [36]. Erythropoietic fluid has been found in the cystic portions of the tumors and is felt to be responsible for the polycythemia that often accompanies this disease [37]. Spinal hemangioblastomas may have associated cord widening with serpiginous feeding vessels [34]. Seeger et al. reported that, in their experience, vertebral angiography was better able to characterize cerebellar hemangioblastomas than was CT when the CT picture was nonspecific [38].

Non-contrast CT scanning shows cysts and nodules as well defined areas of hypodensity. Solid nodules are iso to hyper dense. There is usually mass effect and obliteration of the fourth ventricle if the lesion is cerebellar. There is homogeneous enhancement of the solid nodules (Fig. 12). Cystic lesions become bordered by a dense ring [39]. Highly vascularized lesions of the spinal cord are also seen on the post-contrast CT scan [39].

MR is superior to CT in imaging of cerebellar hemangioblastoma. This is attributed to degradation of the CT image in the posterior fossa by bone hardening artifact [28]. On MR, hemangioblastomas appear early as ill-defined focal lesions with prolonged T1 and T2 relaxation times, often indistinguishable from other enhancing cerebellar lesions [28]. Subsequently they develop large cystic components with long T1 and T2 and smaller peripheral tubular structures demonstrating flow void due to dilated afferent and efferent vessels [28] (Fig. 13). Three morphologic appearances on MR have been described for cerebellar hemangioblastoma [33]. They are as follows:

A. *Cyst with small mural nodule.* Cysts measure 2.56 cm in diameter and are iso-hyperintense on T1WI and hyperintense

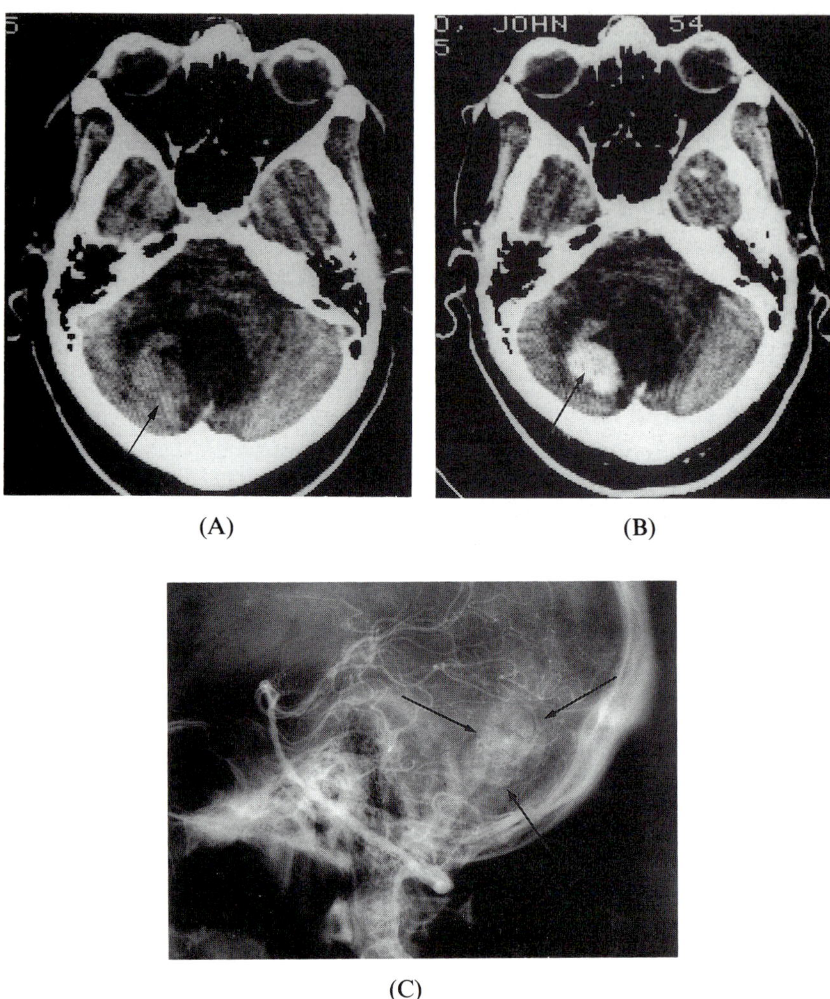

(A)   (B)

(C)

Figure 12. *RIGHT CEREBELLAR HEMANGIOBLASTOMA.* (A) *Axial CT scan shows slightly hyperdense mass in the right cerebellar hemisphere (arrow).* (B) *Post contrast CT shows enhancement of neural nodule (arrow)* (C) *Lateral vertebral arteriogram shows staining of mass (arrows).*

on T2WI compared to CSF. The mural nodule is isointense on T1WI and hyperintense on T2WI. Surrounding parenchyma is hyperintense on T2WI due to edema, and the nodule enhances brightly on post-contrast scan.

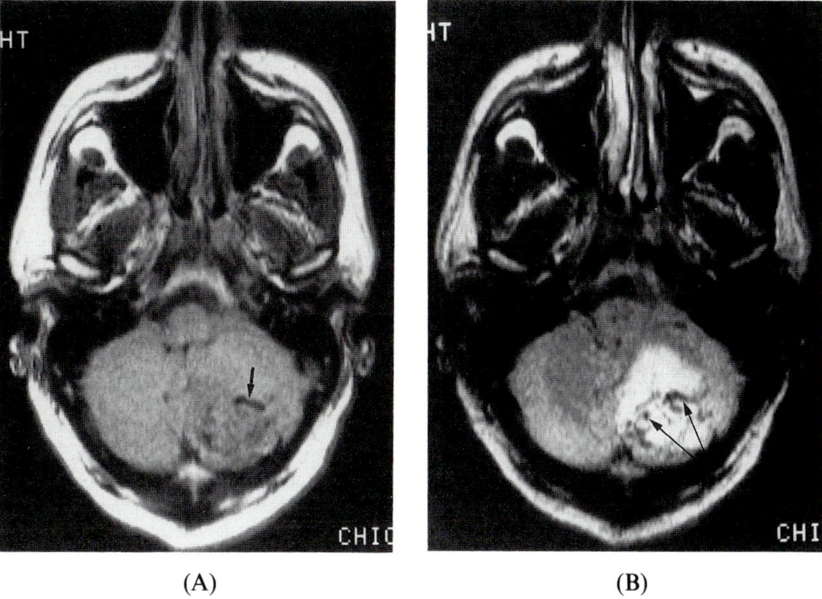

(A)   (B)

Figure 13. *LEFT CEREBELLAR HEMANGIOBLASTOMA. (A) Axial T1 weighted MR acquisition shows heterogenous largely iso-intense mass in the left cerebellar hemisphere containing several flow voids representing large vessels (arrow) (B) T2 weighted axial acquisition shows high signal intensity of tumor with residual serpiginous low intensity areas representing vascularity (arrows).*

B.   *Solid mass with central cystic area.* In this type the cyst is of low intensity on T1WI and high on T2WI compared to gray matter. The solid component is isointense to gray matter on T1WI and hyperintense on T2WI. The solid component of the tumor enhances markedly on post contrast scan. The cystic areas do not enhance.

C.   *Solid tumor without a cystic component.* These range from 4 mm to 2.5 cm in diameter and are iso or hypointense on T1WI and hyperintense on T2WI. Marked enhancement occurs in most of these lesions.

Abnormal vascularity (flow voids) are seen at MR in the large tumors but not in those less than 1 cm [33]. Hemorrhage is demon-

31

strated in some of each of the morphologic types. In some cases, a fluid-fluid level can be seen [33]. Hemorrhage may be spontaneous or secondary to surgery [33]. The same authors report that one case of medullary hemangioblastoma had an associated cervical syrinx.

References

1. Simpson JA, Weiner ESC. The Oxford English Dictionary 2nd edn. Oxford, Clarendon Press, 1989;I:651.
2. Gardeur D, Palmieri A, Mashaly R. Cranial computed tomography in the phakomatoses. Neuroradiology 1983;25:293-304.
3. Braffman BH, Bilaniuk LT, Zimmerman RA. MR of central nervous system neoplasia of the phakomatoses. Semin Roentgenol 1990;24:198-217.
4. Aoki S, Barkovich AJ, Nishimura K, et al. Neurofibromatosis types 1 and 2: cranial MR findings. Radiology 1989;172:527-534.
5. National Institutes of Health Consensus Development. Neurofibromatosis. Arch Neurol 1988;45:575-578.
6. Hurst RW, Newman SA, Cail WS. Multifocal intracranial MR abnormalities in neurofibromatosis. AJNR 1988;9:293-296.
7. Bognanno JR, Edwards MK, Lee TA, et al. Cranial MR imaging in neurofibromatosis. AJNR 1988;9:461-468.
8. Lubs ML, Bauer MS, Formas ME, Djokic B. Lisch nodules in neurofibromatosis type I. N Engl J Med 1991;324:1264-1266.
9. Mirowitz SA, Sartor K, Gado M. High intensity basal ganglia lesions on T1 weighted MR images in neurofibromatosis. AJNR 1989;10:1159-1163.
10. Binet EF, Kieffer SA, Martin SH, et al. Orbital dysplasia in neurofibromatosis. Radiology 1969;93:829-833.
11. Deans WR, Bloch S, Leibrock L, et al. Arteriovenous fistula in patients with neurofibromatosis. Radiology 1982;144:103-107.
12. Kim T, Foust RJ, Mojtahedi S. MR imaging of asymptomatic brainstem and spinal cord lesions in sisters with neurofibromatosis. AJNR 1989;10:S71-S72.
13. Riccardi VM. Von Recklinghausen neurofibromatosis, N Engl J Med 1981;305:1617-1627.
14. Cammarata CA, Deveikis JP, Schellinger D, et al. Neuroradiology case of the day. Case 1: neurofibromatosis 2. AJR 1990;154:13-37.
15. Lee BCP, Gawler J. Tuberous sclerosis. Radiology 1978;127:403-407.
16. Fryer ARE, Chalmers A, Connor JM, et al. Evidence that the gene for tuberous sclerosis is on chromosome 9. Lancet 1987;1:659-61.
17. Legge M, Sauerbrei E, MacDonald A. Intracranial tuberous sclerosis in infancy. Radiology 1984;153:667-668.
18. Monaghan HP, Krafchik BR, MacGregor DL, et al. Tuberous sclerosis complex in children. Am J Dis Child 1981;135:912-917.
19. McMurdo Jr. SK, Moore SG, Brant-Zawadzki M, et al. MR imaging of intracranial tuberous sclerosis. AJNR 1987;8:77-72.
20. Roach ES, Williams DP, Laster W. Magnetic resonance imaging in tuberous sclerosis. Arch Neurol 1987;44:301-303.
21. Richardson Jr. EP. Tuberous sclerosis another success for magnetic resonance imaging. Mayo Clin Proc 1989;64:371-373.

22. Iwasaki S, Nakagawa H, Kibhikawa K, et al. MR and CT of tuberous sclerosis: linear abnormalities in the cerebral white matter. AJNR 1990;11:1029-1034.
23. Hatfield M, Muraki A, Wollman R, et al. Isolated frontal lobe calcification in Sturge-Weber syndrome. AJNR 1988;9:203-204.
24. Cerosoli M, Campanile S, Campanile A, et al. Unusual findings in Sturge-Weber syndrome. AJNR 1989;10:S85.
25. Wasenko JJ, Rosenbloom SA, Duchesneau PM, et al. The Sturge-Weber syndrome: comparison of MR and CT characteristics. AJNR 1990;11:131-134.
26. Elster AD, Chen MYM. MR imaging of Sturge-Weber syndrome: role of gadopentetate dimeglumine and gradient-echo techniques. AJNR 1990;11:685-689.
27. Lipski S, Brunelle F, Aicardi J, et al. Gd-DOTA-enhanced MR imaging in two cases of Sturge-Weber syndrome. AJNR 1990;11:690-692.
28. Sato Y, Waziri M, Smith W, et al. Hippel-Lindau disease: MR imaging. Radiology 1988;166:241-246.
29. Case records of the Massachusetts General Hospital, N Engl J Med 1991;324:1119-1127.
30. Bachmann K, Markwalder R, Seiler RW. Supratentorial hemangioblastoma. Acta Neurochir 1978;44:173-177.
31. Jeffreys RV. Supratentorial hemangioblastoma. Acta Neurochir 1974;31:55-65.
32. Wylie IG, Jeffreys RV, Maclaine MRCP. Cerebral hemangioblastoma. Brit J Radiol 1973;46:472-476.
33. Lee SR, Sanches J, Mark AS, et al. Posterior fossa hemangioblastomas: MR imaging. Radiology 1989;171:463-468.
34. Fill WL, Lamiell JM, Polk NO. The radiographic manifestations of von Hippel-Lindau disease. Radiology 1979;133:289-295.
35. Wirtala AO, Loop JW. Association of an enlarged tentorial artery with cerebellar hemangioblastoma. Radiology 1970;96:67-68.
36. Wolpert SM. The neuroradiology of hemangioblastomas of the cerebellum. AJR 1970;110:56-66.
37. Jamieson KG, Yelland JDN, Merry GS. Hemangioblastomas of the hindbrain: a report of 18 cases. Aust N.Z. J. Surg. 1974;44:254-257.
38. Seeger JF, Burke DP, Knake JE, Gabrielsen TO. Computed tomographic and angiographic evaluation of hemangioblastomas. Radiology 1981;138:65-73.
39. Baleriaux-Waha D, Retif J, Noterman, et al. CT scanning for the diagnosis of the cerebellar and spinal lesions of von Hippel-Lindau's disease. Neuroradiology 1978,14:241-244.

Intracranial Neoplasms

Anne G. Osborn

Department of Radiology, University of Utah, Salt Lake City, Utah, USA

Introduction

The urge to classify or group things, a basic human impulse, has with brain neoplasms (as with many other lesions) produced more on-going controversy than consensus. While any scheme presented for categorizing CNS neoplasms has its share of detractors, in general the original system proposed by Bailey and Cushing in the 1920s has, with some modifications, remained the most widely used classification of brain neoplasms. The Bailey-Cushing system is conceptually based on supposed histogenesis or "cell of origin." While the shortcomings of this approach are numerous and both immunological and ultrastructural techniques have greatly expanded our identification of specific cell types comprising CNS neoplasms, the imaging features of brain neoplasms and their radiologic-pathologic correlations will be presented using the modified Bailey-Cushing approach delineated in Okazaki's recent text, *Fundamentals of Neuropathology* (where appropriate, classification of individual brain neoplasms according to the 1991 World Health Organization (WHO) system will also be identified). Nevertheless, a detailed discussion will focus on the most frequent types of primary intracranial neoplasms, i.e., glial neoplasms.

Origin of Intracranial Neoplasms by Cell Type

With the possible exception of the neuron itself, any of the following cell types (or precursors thereof) can give rise to primary CNS neoplasms.

A. Neurons. Mature neurons do not divide and therefore do not have derivative CNS neoplasms. The only actively dividing neural tissue that could be considered as belonging to the CNS is the olfactory mucosa, which gives rise to olfactory neuroblastomas (esthesioneuroblastoma).

B. Glial cells. These outnumber the trillion neurons by 5-10 times and comprise over half the CNS by volume. Numerous types of glial (sometimes termed "neuroglial") cells exist; some of the more important are:
    - protoplasmic astrocyte
    - fibrous astrocyte
    - oligodendrocyte
    - pendymal cells
    - choroid plexus (modified ependyma)

C. Nerve sheath
    - Schwann cells
    - Fibroblasts (exiting spinal roots, cutaneous nerves)

D. Mesenchymal tissue
    - Meninges
    - Blood vessels
    - Bone

E. Lymphocytes, leukocytes

F. Germ cells

G. Pituitary and pineal glands

CNS Neoplasms: General Classification and Incidence

A. Primary neoplasms (70-75% of intracranial neoplasms)
    - Glial neoplasms (40-50% of primary brain neoplasms)
    - Nonglial neoplasms
    - neoplasms of primitive bipotential precursors and nerve cells (examples: medulloblastoma, primitive neuro-ectodermal neoplasm or "PNET")
    - nerve sheath neoplasms (schwannoma)
    - mesenchymal neoplasms (examples: meningioma, hemangioblastoma)
    - lymphoreticular neoplasms (lymphoma, leukemia, neoplastic-like disorders such as histiocytosis)

- neoplasms of maldevelopmental origin (examples: dermoid/epidermoid; germ cell neoplasms like germinoma, teratoma)
- phakomatoses

B. Metastatic neoplasms (25-30% of intracranial neoplasms)

CNS Neoplasms: Age, Location

A. < 15 years of age (15-20% of all intracranial neoplasms)
- CNS neoplasms second most common pediatric neoplasm (#1 = leukemia)
- 50-70% of all pediatric brain neoplasms are infratentorial (in children under 2, two-thirds are supratentorial)
- Metastases rare

B. > 15 years of age (adult)
- 70% supratentorial
- Metastases common

Glial Neoplasms

These arise from neuroglial cells (astrocytes, oligodendrocytes, ependymal cells and choroid plexus). Time does not permit exhaustive consideration of each of these neoplasms but some basic concepts are outlined below.

Astrocytoma, General

A. Incidence
- 40-50% of all primary CNS neoplasms are gliomas
- 70% of gliomas are astrocytomas
- 50% of astrocytomas are glioblastoma multiforme (the most malignant variety of astrocytoma)

B. Common types of astrocytoma
- Fibrillary (common in adults)
- Pilocytic (common in children and young adults)
- Subependymal giant cell (most common in tuberous sclerosis)
- Protoplasmic (about 1% of astrocytomas)

C. Grading astrocytoma
    1. Traditional (Kernohan)
        - Grade 1 (anaplasia minimal to absent)
        - Grade 2 (early anaplastic changes in roughly half of cells)
        - Grade 3 (anaplastic astrocytoma)
        - Grade 4 (glioblastoma multiforme)
    2. 1991 World Health Organization classification groups astrocytomas into three categories:
        - Low-grade ("benign" or well-differentiated) astrocytoma
        - Anaplastic astrocytoma
        - Glioblastoma multiforme

Low Grade Astrocytoma ("Benign" Astrocytoma)

A. Incidence: 25-30% of astrocytomas
B. Age: these are generally neoplasms of younger patients
    - Childhood
    - Adults from 20-40 y
C. Location: proportional to amount of white matter present
D. Pathology: most of these are fibrillary astrocytomas
    - No necrosis
    - No neovascularity; hemorrhage rare; edema uncommon
    - Often cystic
    - 15-20% calcify
    - Usually focal but occasionally diffusely infiltrating
E. Imaging
    - CT: typically well-delineated low density mass with no enhancement (Fig. 1). If diffusely infiltrating, scans may show only nonspecific, low density white matter disease (Fig. 2A).
    - MR: Well-defined, iso/hypointense on T1WI, hyperintense on T2WI; hemorrhage, signal heterogeneity uncommon. Little mass effect or edema. If diffusely infiltrating, confluent white matter foci of increased signal on T2W1 associated with mild mass effect (Fig. 2B).
F. Survival: 3-10 y

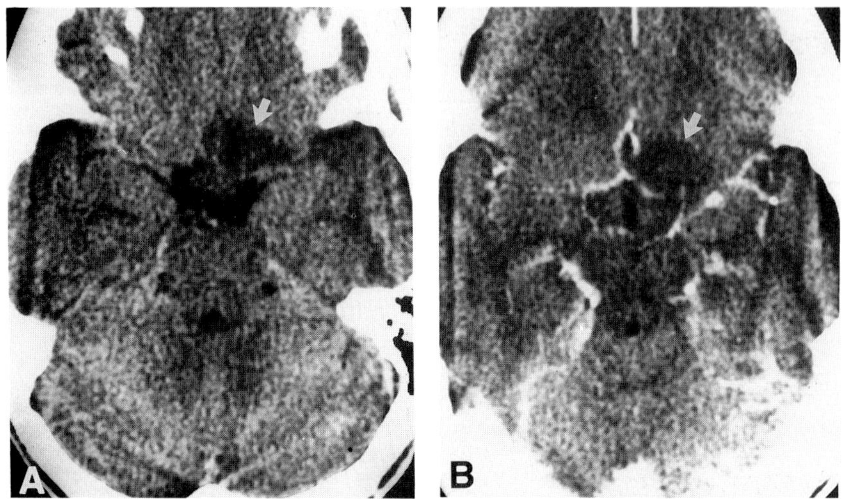

Figure 1. *FOCAL LOW GRADE ("BENIGN") ASTROCYTOMA. Axial CT scans without (A) and with (B) contrast enhancement in a 27-year-old male who has been followed for 9 years with a low grade posterior frontal lobe astrocytoma (arrow). Well-delineated low density mass without enhancement following contrast is the most typical appearance for benign (grade I) fibrillary astrocytoma.*

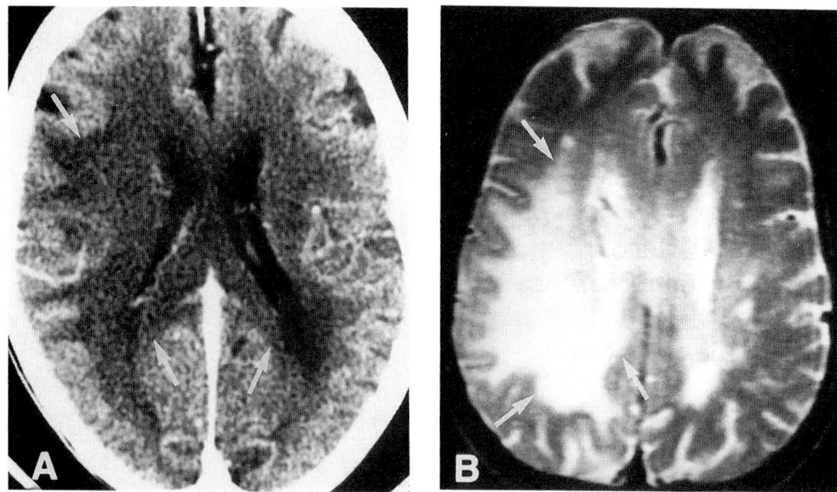

Figure 2. *DIFFUSE LOW-GRADE ("BENIGN") ASTROCYTOMA. Axial post-contrast CT scan (A) and T2-weighted MR scan (B) in a patient with biopsy-proven diffusely infiltrating astrocytoma. The neoplasm (arrows) is poorly marginated and has mild mass effect (shown by slight compression of the adjacent lateral ventricle). (Case courtesy of T. Burt, Boise, Idaho).*

Anaplastic ("Malignant") Astrocytoma

A. Incidence: 25-30% of astrocytomas
B. Age: mostly > 40 y
C. Location: proportional to amount of white matter
D. Pathology: most are fibrillary astrocytomas (often overlap at either end with low-grade astrocytoma, glioblastoma)
E. Imaging
   - Varies from relatively well defined (Fig. 3) to poorly delineated (Fig. 4)
   - More mass effect
   - More contrast enhancement
   - More heterogeneity on both CT, MR
F. Survival: 2-3 y

Glioblastoma Multiforme (GBM)

A. Incidence: 50% of astrocytomas
B. Age: 5th-7th decades (single most powerful predictive factor of histology as well as survival is age at diagnosis; the older the patient, in general the more malignant the astrocytoma and the worse the prognosis)
C. Location: supratentorial cerebral hemispheres (posterior fossa GBM rare)
D. Pathology: characterized by necrosis, hemorrhage (Fig. 5)
E. Imaging (Fig. 6): more mass effect, vasogenic edema, heterogeneity, enhancement. N.B. - in GBM, viable neoplasm cells can almost always be found in edematous areas *outside* the region of contrast enhancement.

Juvenile Pilocytic Astrocytoma

A. Neoplasm of children, young adults; often (but not always) associated with neurofibromatosis
B. Pathology: pilocytic ("hairlike") astrocytes
C. Location: tend to occur around third, fourth ventricles
   - optic chiasm/hypothalamus most common
   - cerebellar vermis next
   - cerebellar hemispheres
   - less common: cerebral hemispheres

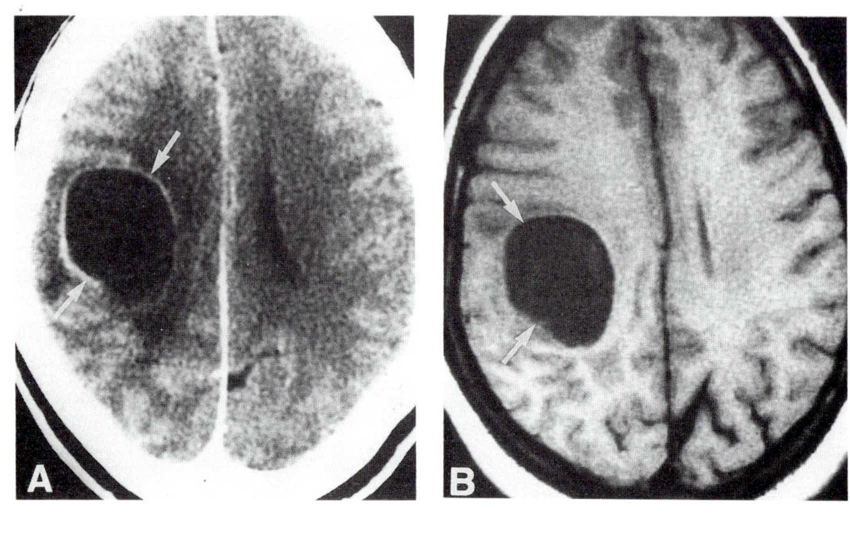

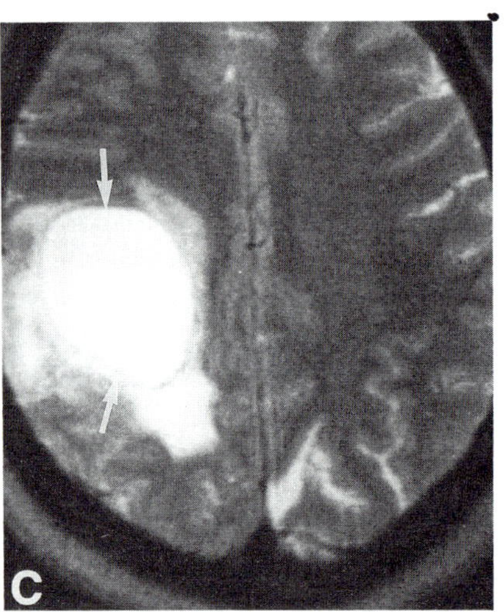

Figure 3. *FOCAL MALIGNANT ASTROCYTOMA. Post-contrast CT scan shows a relatively well-delineated cystic mass with rim enhancement (arrows). Axial T1 (B) and T2-weighted MR scans show the lesion (arrows) is well-marginated but has moderate mass effect and surrounding edema (note effacement of adjacent sulci, abnormal signal around the neoplasm). Malignant astrocytoma (grade II on Kernhan scale).*

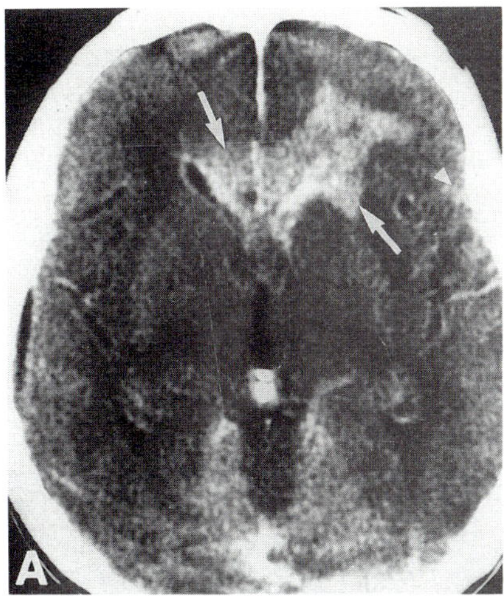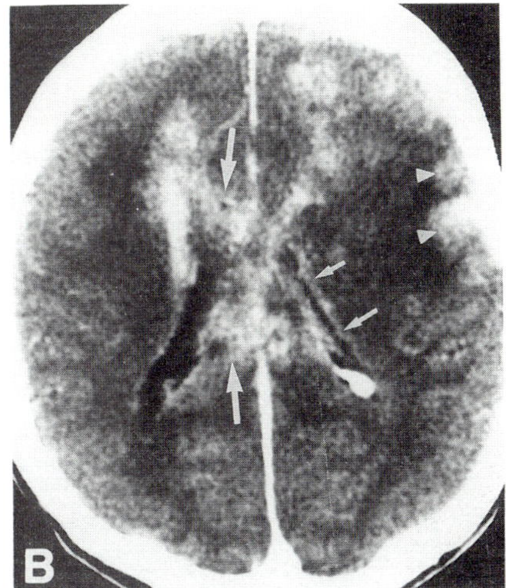

Figure 4. *DIFFUSE ANAPLASTIC ("MALIGNANT" OR GRADE III) ASTROCYTOMA. Axial post-contrast CT scans in a patient with highly anaplastic (grade III) astrocytoma. The bilateral contrast-enhancing neoplasm infiltrates diffusely along white matter tracts (large arrows). Note subependymal neoplasm spread (small arrows) as well as subarachnoid metastases (arrowheads).*

D. Imaging (Fig. 7)
- sharply marginated, well-delineated
- edema rare
- cyst formation common (with mural nodule)
- Ca^{++} occasionally
- CT: iso/hypodense, marked enhancement
- MR: iso/hypointense on T1WI, hyperintense on T2WI, enhancement following contrast

Subependymal Giant Cell Astrocytoma

Mostly found in patients with tuberous sclerosis (see congenital malformations) (Fig. 8).

Nonastrocytic Glial Neoplasms

These are neoplasms that arise from oligodendroglial cells as well as ependyma and modified ependyma (choroid plexus).

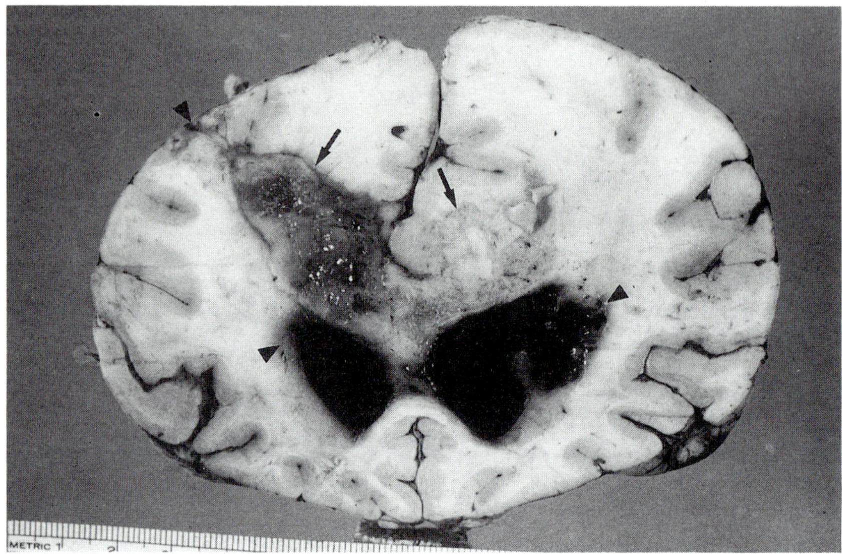

Figure 5. *GLIOBLASTOMA MULTIFORME (PATHOLOGY). Gross pathology, coronal section, of glioblastoma multiforme. Note hemorrhagic, necrotic neoplasm with infiltration along the white matter of the corpus callosum (small arrows). Subependymal and subarachnoid neoplasm spread (arrowheads) can also be identified.*

Oligodendroglioma

A. Incidence: 5% of all primary brain neoplasms
B. Adults vs. children = 8:1; peak age 35-40 y
C. Location: 85% supratentorial, mostly hemispheric
   - Often cortical, subcortical
   - Intraventricular rare
   - Frontal lobe most common

Figure 6. *GLIOBLASTOMA MULTIFORME (GRADE IV ASTROCY-TOMA). Axial pre- (A) and post-contrast (B) CT scans in a patient with glioblastoma multiforme. The heterogeneous mass (A, arrows) shows some foci of contrast enhancement (B, arrows). Note marked adjacent edema, mass effect. Pre-contrast axial T1 (C) MR scan shows the very heterogeneous mass (arrows) contains blood degradation products. Post-contrast T1-weighted scan (D) shows both nodular and rim enhancement (arrows). T2-weighted scan demonstrates both the blood degradation products within the neoplasm from recent hemorrhage (large arrows) as well as marked surrounding edema (small arrows).*

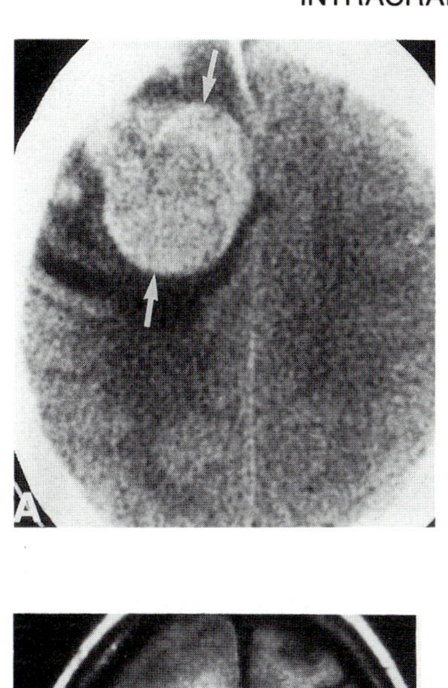
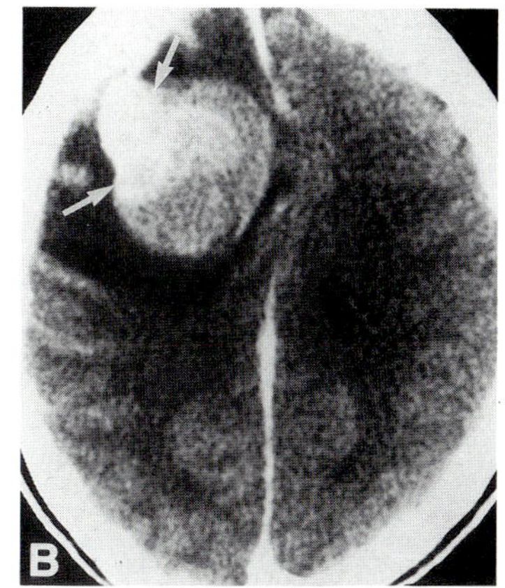
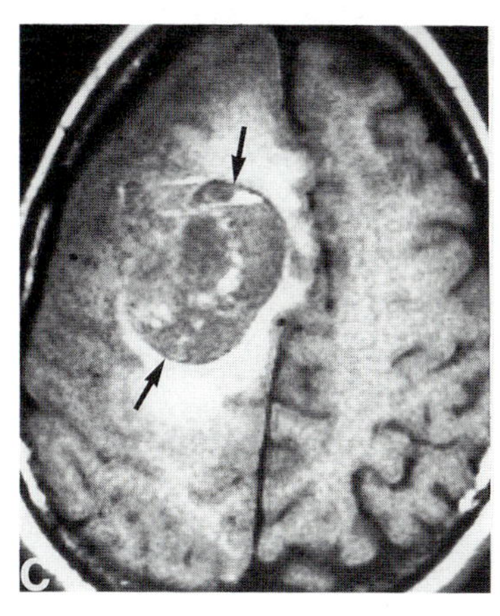
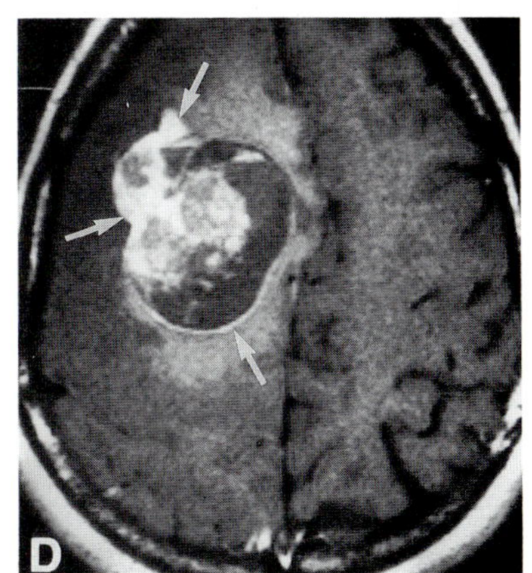
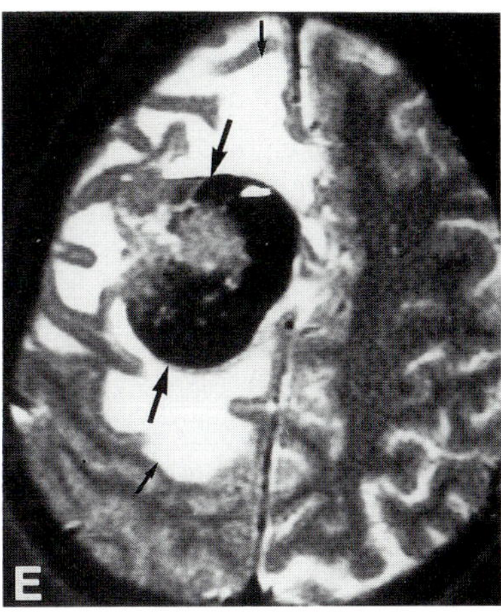

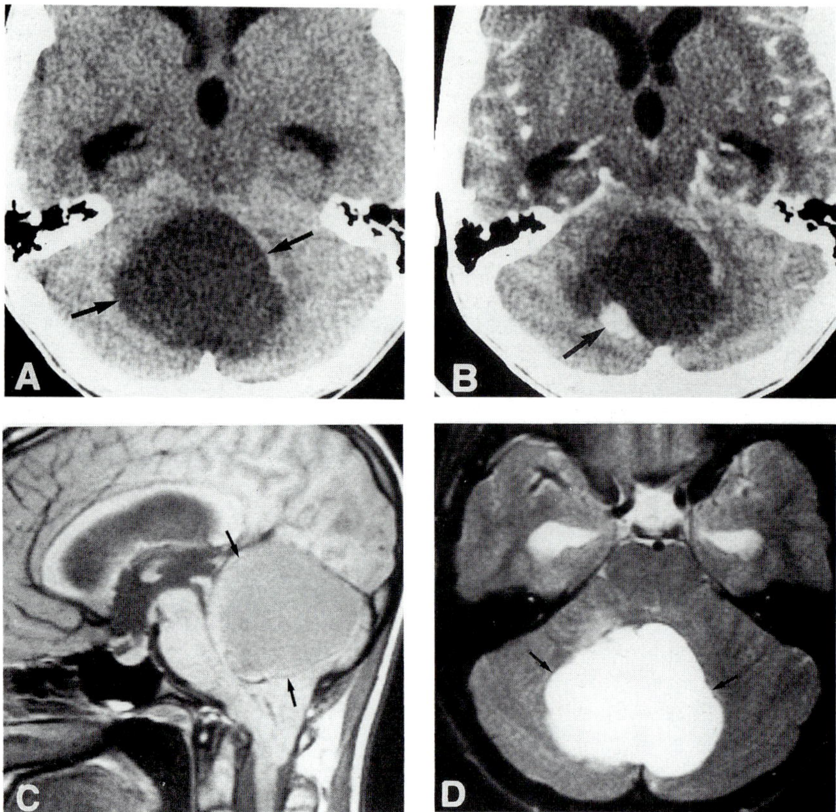

Figure 7. *PILOCYTIC ASTROCYTOMA. Axial pre-* (A) *and post-contrast* (B) *CT scans in a patient with cystic cerebellar astrocytoma. The well-delineated cyst* (A, *arrows) has an enhancing mural nodule* (B, *arrow). Sagittal T1* (C) *and axial T2-weighted* (D) *MR scans show the lesion has a well-defined wall (arrows).*

D. Pathology
- Well-defined, circumscribed, globular
- Hemorrhage, cyst formation rare
- Ca^{++} in > 70%
- Nearly 50% considered "mixed" (i.e., some astrocytic elements)

E. Imaging (Fig. 9)
- Heterogeneous mass, usually partially calcified, variable enhancement on CT
- Edema in < one-third

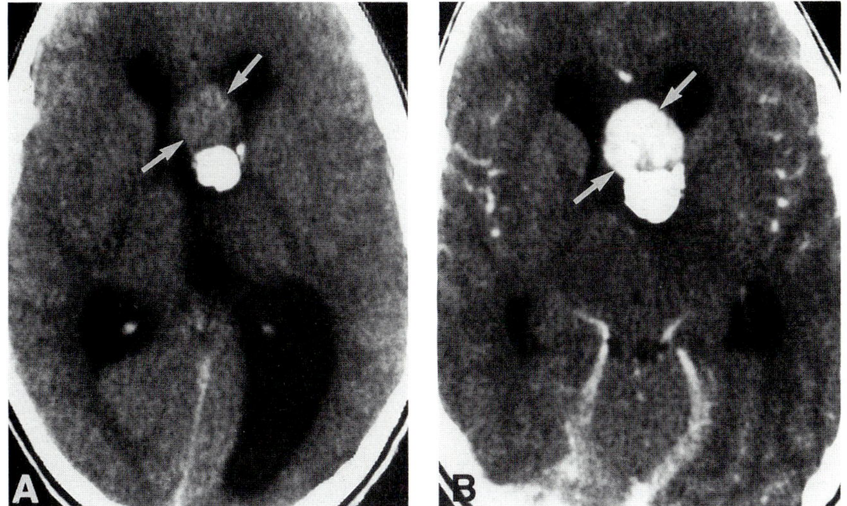

Figure 8. *GIANT CELL ASTROCYTOMA. Axial CT scan without (A) and with (B) contrast in a 12-year-old male with no skin abnormalities. Partially calcified mass at the foramen of Monro (A, arrows) shows strong enhancement (B, arrows) following contrast. No other lesions were identified. Giant cell astrocytoma without tuberous sclerosis. (Case courtesy R. Jahnke, Albuquerque, New Mexico).*

- MR: mixed iso/hypointense on T1WI, hyperintense on T2WI, variable enhancement
- Neoplasms often extend to or involve cortex

Ependymoma

A. Incidence: 5% of intracranial neoplasms (but are third most common intracranial neoplasm in children)
B. Age
- Childhood, adolescents; (50% < 5 y); second, much smaller peak in adults 30-40 y
- Middle-aged, elderly: subependymoma (only about one-third of these are symptomatic; the majority are incidental finding at autopsy)
C. Location
- 60-70% infratentorial (mostly children); 70% from fourth ventricle; often extend into cerebellopontine angle, vallecula (Fig. 10)

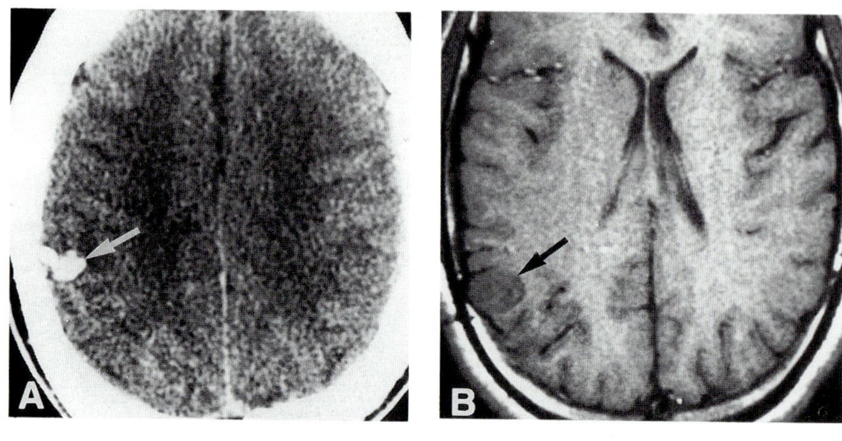

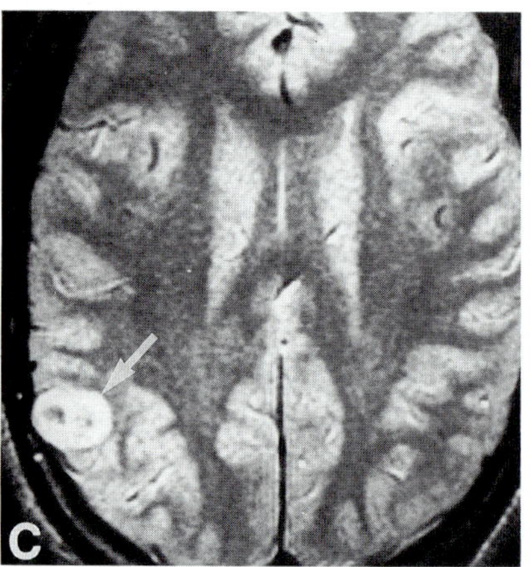

Figure 9. *OLIGODENDROGLIOMA. Axial nonenhanced CT scan (A) in a 31-year-old male with seizures shows a solitary right parietal calcific focus (arrow). No change was noted following contrast administration. Axial T1-weighted (B) and balanced or "proton density" (C) MR scan show a well-delineated mass (arrows) at the gray-white junction. Note slight erosion of the overlying calvarium indicating presence of a slowly growing lesion. Oligodendroglioma was found at surgery.*

- 30-40% supratentorial (often extraventricular); distributed evenly throughout all age groups

D. Pathology
- Most are slow-growing with low mitotic index. Malignancy rare. A variant, subependymoma, is often

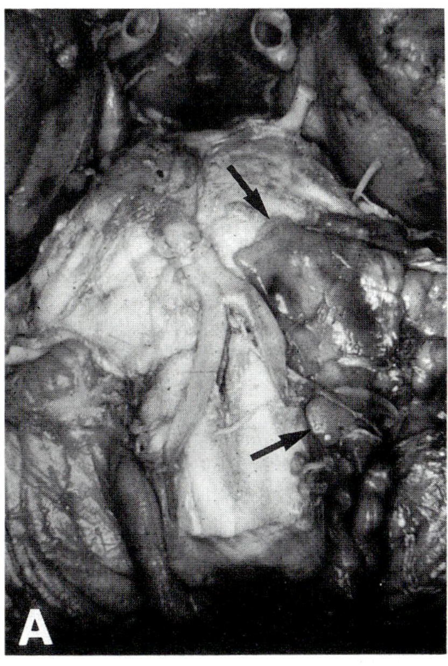

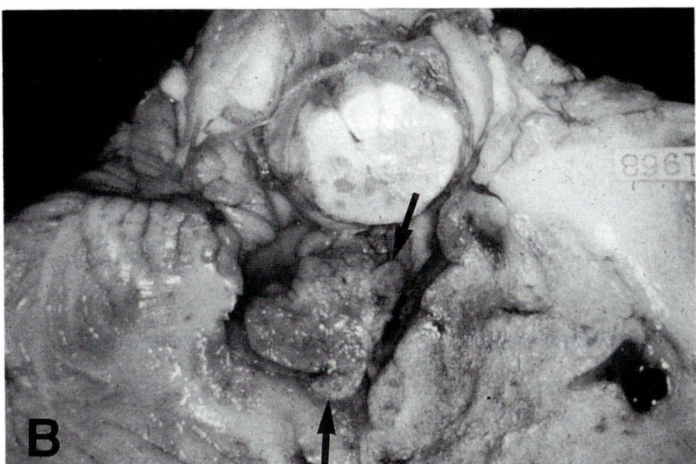

Figure 10. *EPENDYMOMA (PATHOLOGY). Gross pathology of a fourth ventricular ependymoma as seen from front* (A) *and base* (B) *views. The "plastic" nature of this neoplasm is nicely illustrated by lateral extension into the cerebellopontine angles* (A, arrows) *and a separate inferior extension through the vallecula into the cisterna magna* (B, arrows). *(Courtesy Armed Forces Institute of Pathology, Washington, D.C.).*

found at autopsy in older adults and is most frequent in the caudal fourth ventricle.

- Ca^{++} in 50%
- Cysts frequent; hemorrhage relatively uncommon (0-13%)

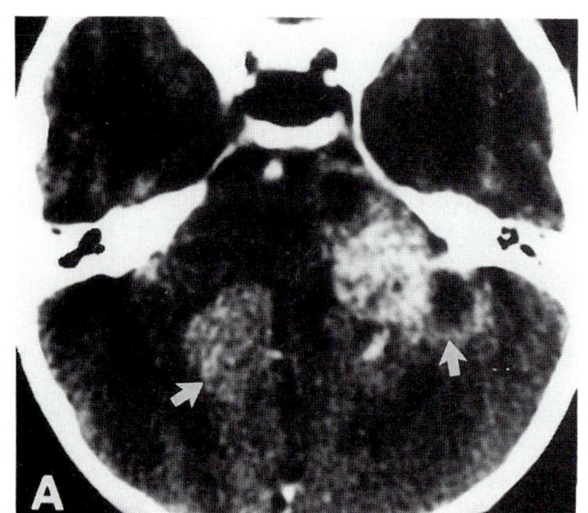
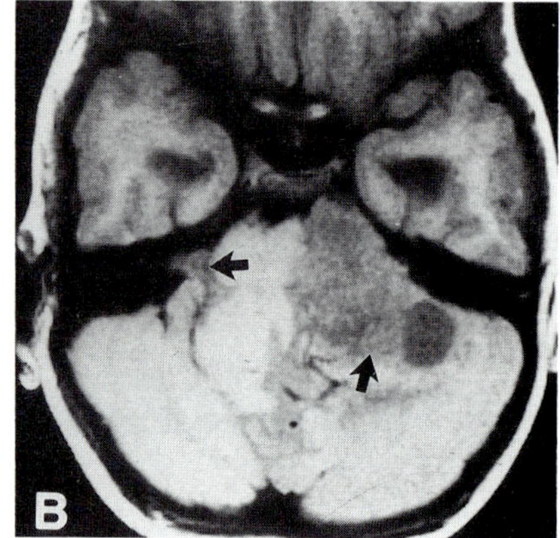

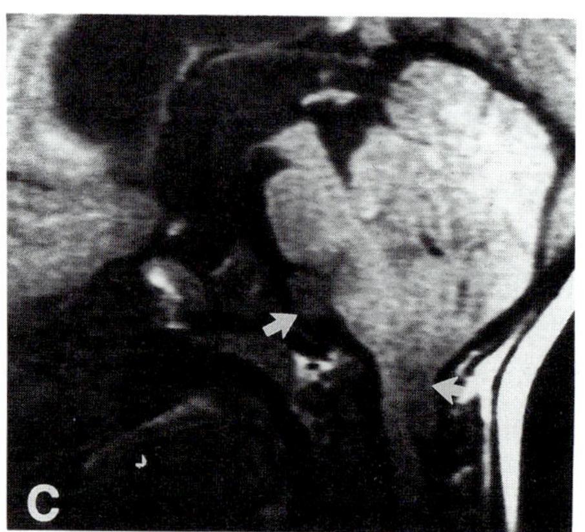

Figure 11. *EPENDYMOMA. Axial post-contrast CT scan (A) and axial (B), sagittal (C), T1-weighted MR scans show a large mass that extends from the fourth ventricle into the crebellopontine angles and cisterna magna (arrows). This ependymoma has the "plastic" configuration characteristic of these lesions.*

E.   Imaging (Fig. 11):
- CT: most common = mostly isodense (NECT), calcified (50%) partially cystic midline posterior fossa mass, variable enhancement. Often extends laterally into cerebellopontine angles, posteriorly into vallecula. Supratentorial ependymoma often periventricular or parenchymal, not intraventricular, less often calcified, may be indistinguishable radiographically from astrocytoma.
- MR: typical=solid fourth ventricular mass, nonspecific heterogeneous signal with propensity to spread via foramina of Magendie, Luschka ("plastic" configuration)

F.   Survival: despite low mitotic index, most of these recur and have relatively poor outcomes (25-50% 5 year survival)

Choroid Plexus Neoplasms

A.   Incidence: 0.5% of all intracranial neoplasms; 2-3% of gliomas. Most are choroid plexus papillomas (CPP).

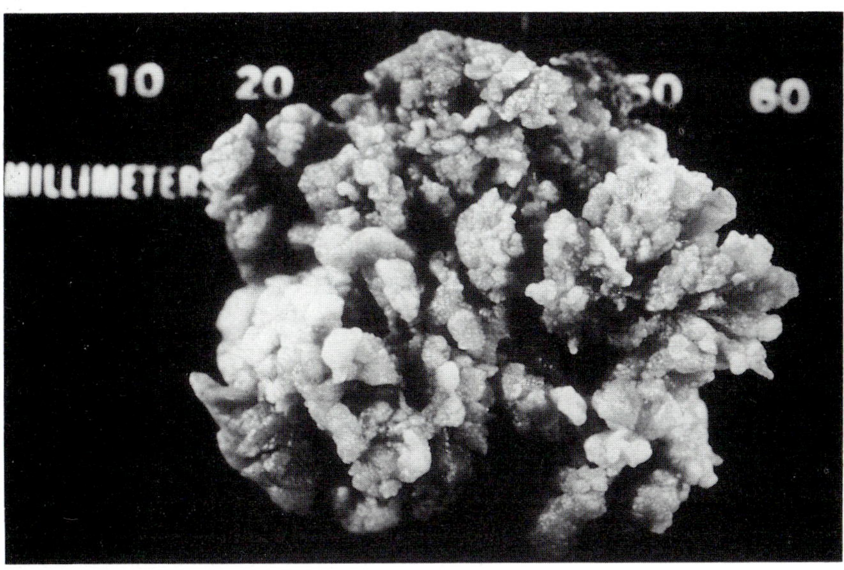

Figure 12. *CHOROID PLEXUS PAPILLOMA (PATHOLOGY). Gross pathologic specimen from a resected choroid plexus papilloma. Note the frond-like papillary projections from the mass. (Case courtesy of Armed Forces Institute of Pathology, Washington, D.C.).*

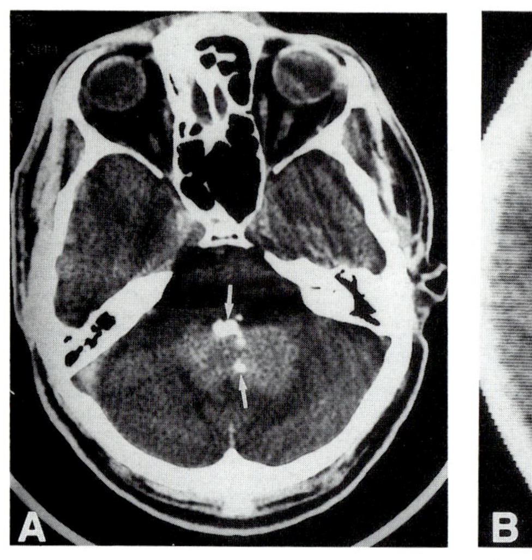
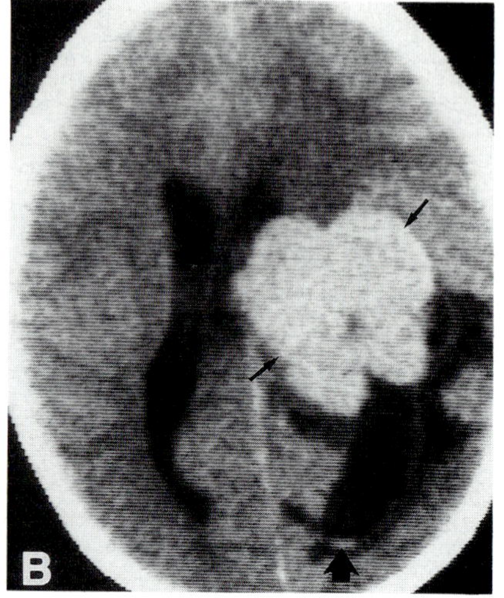
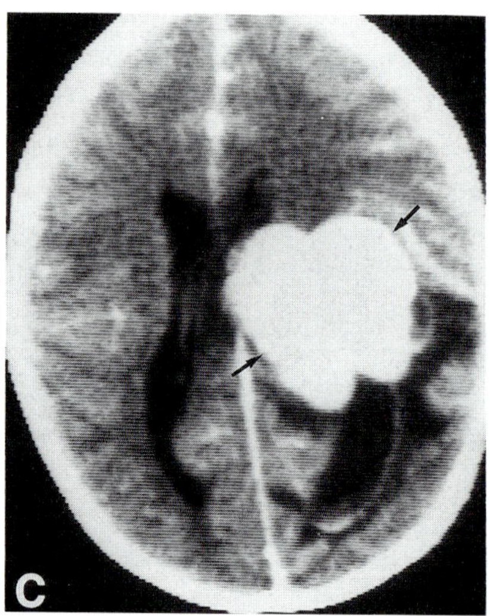

Figure 13. *CHOROID PLEXUS NEOPLASMS: CT. (A) Axial post-contrast CT scan in a patient with a fourth ventricular choroid plexus papilloma. Note the hyperdense mass has calcific foci (arrows). (B, C). Axial pre- (A) and post-contrast (B) CT scans in a patient with choroid plexus carcinoma (small arrows). Note presence of a small blood-cerebrospinal fluid level in the occipital horn of the left lateral ventricle (B, large arrow). Chronic hemorrhage may account for diffuse ventricular enlargement rather than "overproduction" hydrocephalus.*

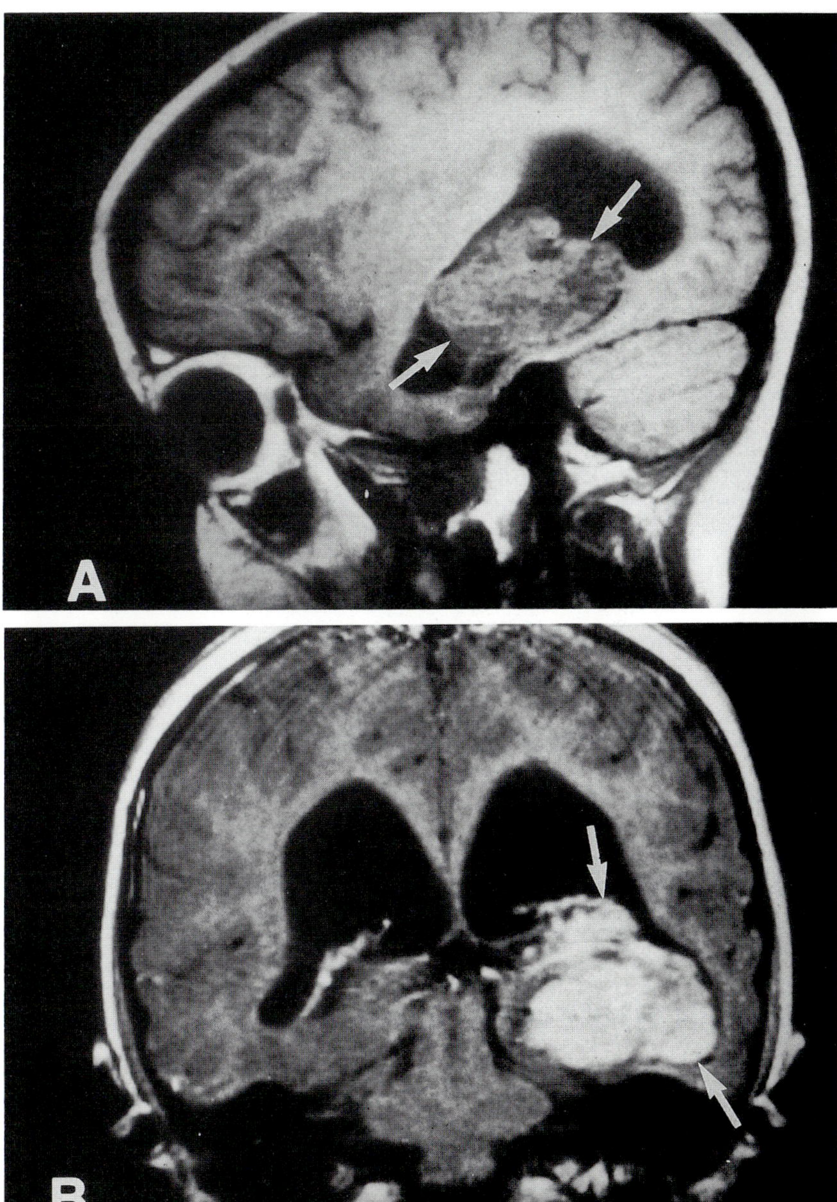

Figure 14. *CHOROID PLEXUS NEOPLASMS: MR. Sagittal pre-contrast* (A) *and coronal post-contrast* (B) *T1-weighted MR scan show a lobulated, strongly enhancing mass that arises from the choroid plexus within the atrium of the left lateral ventricle (arrows). Choroid plexus papilloma. (Case courtesy of L. Monsein, Baltimore, MD).*

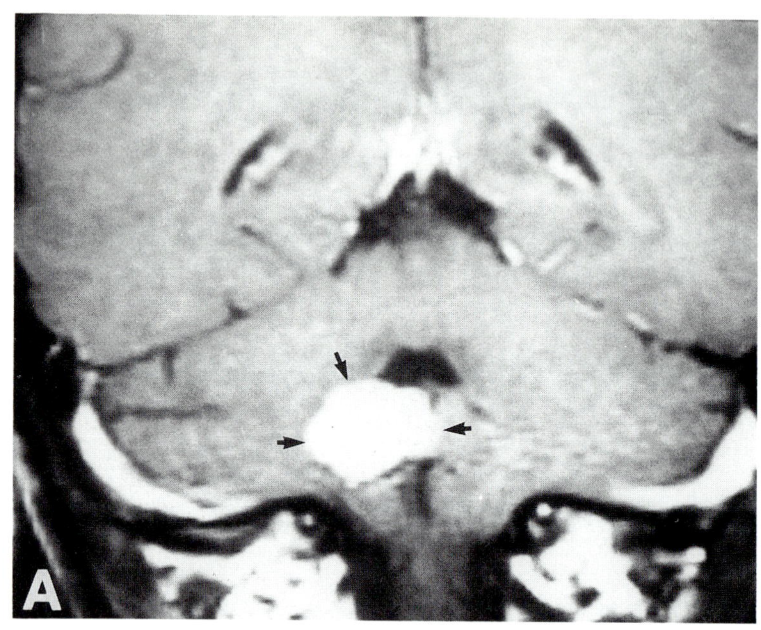

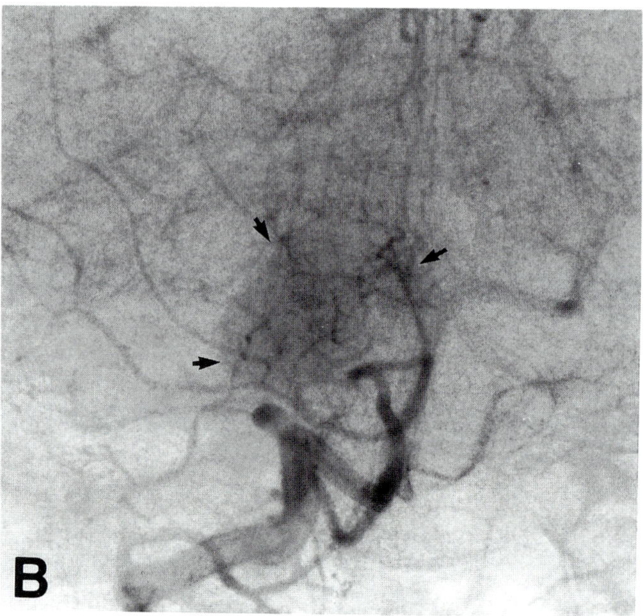

Figure 15. *CHOROID PLEXUS NEOPLASMS: ANGIOGRAPHY.* (A) *Coronal post-contrast T1-weighted MR scan in a 30-year-old female with a right sixth nerve palsy shows a strongly enhancing mass in the right lateral recess of the fourth ventricle (arrows). (B) Selective right vertebral angiogram, late arterial phase, AP view shows a dense vascular neoplasm stain (arrows) corresponding to the mass seen in (A). Choroid plexus papilloma. (Case courtesy J. Jones, Ogden, UT).*

B. Age
- Childhood (50-80% < 5 y; 40% < 1y)
- Adults (uncommon)

C. Location
- Childhood CPPs = at least 70% in atria of lateral ventricles; 10% third ventricle
- Adults = fourth ventricle

D. Pathology (Fig. 12)
- Histologically benign; only 10% malignant
- Reddish cauliflower-like mass
- Cystic degeneration
- Hydrocephalus (etiology controversial; "overproduction" of CSF vs. communicating hydrocephalus secondary to hemorrhage, etc.)
- Implantation and CSF seeding can occur with both benign and malignant choroid plexus neoplasms

E. Imaging
- CT (Fig. 13): well-marginated, smooth or lobulated iso-dense intraventricular mass, strong relatively uniform enhancement. Ca^{++} in 25-80%
- MR (Fig. 14): often intermediate intensity on both T1 and T2WI, areas of signal void. Calcification, old hemorrhage common. Extension outside ventricle suggests possibility of choroid plexus carcinoma but is not diagnostic of malignancy (papillomas may occasionally have extraventricular extension as well).
- Angiography (Fig. 15): Finely reticulated, dense vascular stain that persists into the venous phase is common. Arteriovenous shunting may be present.

References

1. Lee, YY, Van Tassel P. Intracranial oligodendrogliomas: imaging findings in 35 untreated cases. AJNR 1989;10:119-127.
2. Lee YY, Van Tassel P, Bruner JM, et al. Juvenile pilocytic astrocytomas: CT and MR characteristics. AJR 1989;152:1263-1270.
3. Coates TL, Hinshaw DB Jr, Peckman N, et al. Pediatric choroid plexus neoplasms: MR, CT and pathologic correlation. Radiology 1989;173:81-88.
4. Ellenbogen RG, Winston KR, Kupsky WJ. Neoplasms of the choroid plexus in children. Neurosurgery 1989;28:327-335.
5. Dean BL, Drayer BP, Bird CR, et al. Gliomas: classificaton with MR imaging. Radiology 1990;174:411-415.

6. Spoto GP, Press GA, Hesselink JR, Solomon M. Intracranial ependymoma and subependymoma: MR manifestations. AJNR 1990;11:83-91.

7. Jelinek J. Smirniotopoulos JJ, Paresi JE, Kanger M. Lateral ventricular neoplasms of the brain. AJNR 1990;11:567-574.

8. Atlas SW. Adult supratentorial neoplasms. Sem Roentgenol 1990;25:130-154.

9. Gusnard DA. Cerebellar neoplasms in children. Sem Roentgenol 1990;25:263-278.

10. Okazaki H. Neoplastic and related lesions. In: Fundamentals of Neuropathology, Igaku-Shoin, New York, 1989;203-273.

White Matter Disease

Michael S. Huckman
*Rush-Presbyterian University and St. Luke's Medical Center,
Chicago, Illinois, USA*

Introduction

White matter diseases are either demyelinating or dysmyelinating, that is there is either destruction of myelin and subsequent inflammatory reaction (demyelination) or there is a metabolic defect of production and maintenance of abnormal myelin dysmyelination). White matter diseases have a multitude of etiologies, presentations and pathologic mechanisms. It is rarely possible to make a definitive diagnosis of a specific white matter disease by imaging alone since; in most of these diseases there are certain common threads. On the CT scan there is usually hypodensity and on the MR scan there is usually high signal on proton density and T2-weighted scans in areas where white matter is normally found.

Anatomy and Composition of White Matter

White matter contains myelinated axons. It makes up the two-named tracts (i.e. the spino-thalamic tract), the lemnisci, peduncles, fasciculi, and commissures that connect the hemispheres. The largest commissure is the corpus callosum and the other large white matter structures that are normally visible on CT and MR scans are the internal and external capsules, the anterior commissure, and the cerebral and cerebellar peduncles. The largest areas of white matter surround the bodies of the lateral ventricles in each cerebral hemisphere, lie above the level of the corpus callosum and are referred to as the right and left centrum semiovale or collectively as the centrum ovale.

According to Brooks et al. [1], gray matter contains 8% more oxygen, 8% less carbon, more water, and less lipid than does white matter. It is apparently these differences in chemical composition that account for the contrast between gray and white matter that can be appreciated on CT and MR imaging studies.

Imaging of Normal Gray and White Matter

The ability of CT or MR to image white matter diseases depends on their ability to maximize the contrast between the two tissues. CT values for gray matter range from 31 to 39 Hounsfield (H) units and for white matter from 23 to 32 H [2]. The greater photoelectric absorption of gray matter is probably due to the greater water content and lower lipid content compared to white matter [1]. Therefore, white matter on the CT scan appears hypodense compared to gray matter and hyperdense compared to cerebrospinal fluid (Fig. 1).

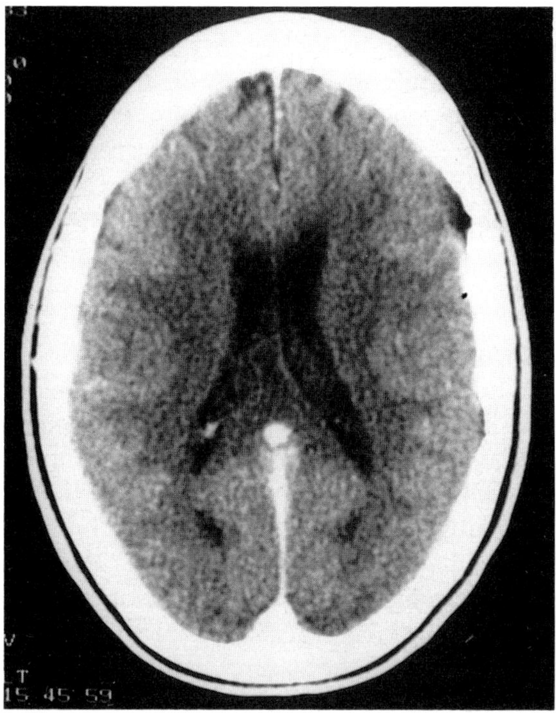

Figure 1. *NORMAL CT OF THE BRAIN. Normal post contrast CT scan with central white matter appearing less dense than surrounding gray matter.*

MR relaxation times of gray and white matter can be reliably and reproducibly measured in vivo [3]. The T1 value of cortical gray matter is approximately 701 msec compared to 419 msec for sub-cortical white matter. The T1 of cerebrospinal fluid is approximately 2719 msec. The T2 of cortical gray matter is 60 and subcortical white matter has a T2 of 53. Cerebrospinal fluid has a T2 of 166. The proton density of gray matter is approximately 1.2 times that of white matter [3]. T2 weighted and proton density sequences are the most useful spin echo sequences in differentiating gray and white matter on the normal scan (Fig. 2) and therefore most useful in detecting white matter abnormalities.

Curnes et al. [4] point out the importance of recognizing that, on T2 weighted sequences, extremely low signal in the basal ganglia, which has been attributed to heavy iron concentration [5], is not the explanation of the low signal seen in the major white

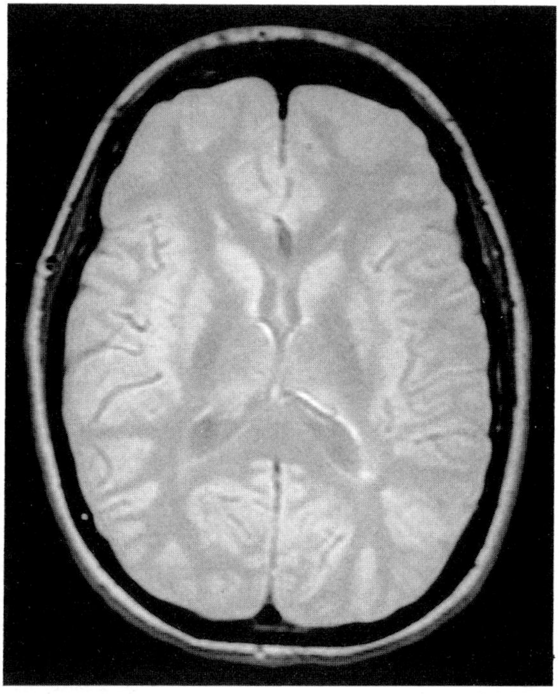

Figure 2. *NORMAL BRAIN MR. Normal proton density MR scan showing low intensity white matter in internal and external capsules, corpus callosum and frontal and occipital lobes.*

matter tracts. In the latter setting, the short T2 reflects heavy myelination and fiber density and not iron deposition. These areas are distinguishable from areas of iron deposition by the fact that, unlike iron deposition, they appear as high signal on T1 weighted sequences, and they can be seen with regularity in all normal patients over three years of age [4].

The Normal Pattern of Myelination

The process of myelination is one in which the water content of the white matter of the brain decreases and its lipid content increases. The process begins during gestation. However, up to age 8 months, there is a reversal of the usual adult pattern of gray matter-white matter contrast seen on the T2 weighted MR scan. Dietrich et al. remarked that "It is important that radiologists are familiar with this pattern and recognize it as a normal phenomenon so as not to confuse this infantile appearance with dysmyelinating or demyelinating disease, edema or other pathologic process. This appearance and its gradual reversion to the adult pattern correlates with an initially greater water content of unmyelinated white matter, followed by subsequent water loss occurring during the myelination process, as myelin is relatively hydrophobic" [6].

The normal sequence and pattern of myelination has been the subject of a number of studies. Dietrich et al. [6] described three patterns of gray-white differentiation on the MR scan; the infantile, the isointense, and the early adult. On T2 weighted spin echo MR scans, they assigned grades of signal intensity from 0 to 10 (0 = the intensity of air, and 10 = the intensity of subcutaneous fat) to various areas of known gray and white matter. Subjects were normal infants and children ranging in age from 4 days to 36 months. The *infantile pattern* (Fig. 3) was seen from 6 days to 6 months. In this pattern, white matter is two grades or more lighter than gray matter. In the *isointense pattern*, seen from 8-12 months of age, the gray and white matter differ in intensity by less than two grades. In the 10-31 month age group, the *early adult pattern* (Fig. 4) prevails in which the gray matter is two or more grades lighter than white matter.

Another study by Barkovich et al. [7] determined that for any given location, myelination is generally recognizable on T1 weighted sequences before it is seen on T2 weighted images. They further

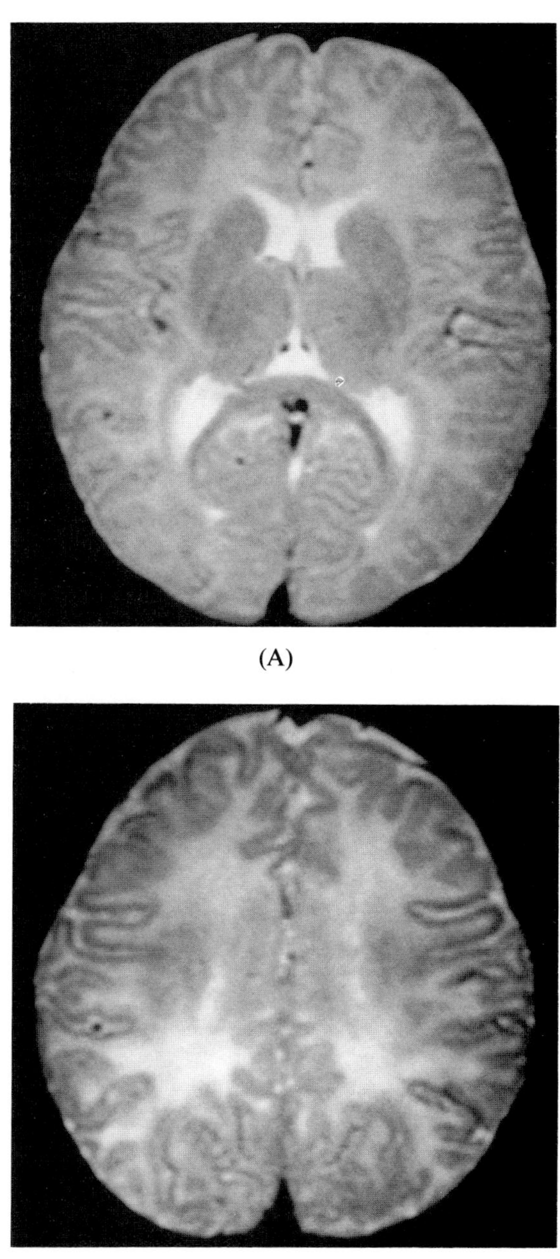

(A)

(B)

Figure 3 (A, B). *BRAIN OF NORMAL 5-MONTH-OLD CHILD. Normal proton density MR scan in a 5-month-old child demonstrating "infantile pattern."*

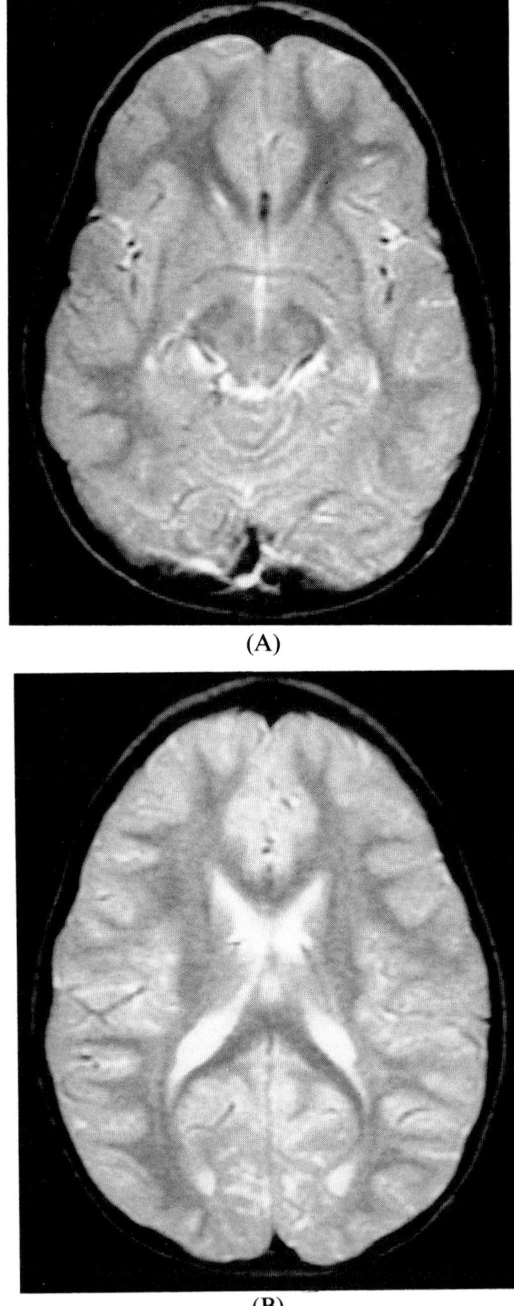

(A)

(B)

Figure 4 (A, B). *BRAIN OF NORMAL THREE YEAR OLD. T2 weighted MR scan showing early adult pattern of myelination in a normal three year old.*

noted that myelination proceeded from caudal to cephalad and from dorsal to ventral. This article lists myelination milestones on T1 and T2 weighted sequences for a number of brain locations using a 1.5 Tesla MR scanner. Several examples are: *Cerebellar white matter* is recognized as myelinated on T1 weighted image at 4 months and on T2 weighed image at 5 months; *Central occipital white matter* is myelinated on T1 weighted image at 5 months and on T2 weighted image at 14 months; the *Genu of the corpus callosum* shows myelination at 6 and 8 months for T1 and T2 weighted sequences respectively. They further state that the white matter in the areas around the trigones of the lateral ventricles may not myelinate in some normal patients until the age of 10 years. Therefore, one must not necessarily consider the isolated finding of high signal intensity in the peritrigonal area as abnormal in young children [7].

Stricker et al. [8] studied the development of myelination of the cerebellum by MR. In addition to recognizing normal MR milestones, they observed that the known milestones of myelination of the cerebellum, seen in pathologic studies, occur approximately six months before similar findings are seen on MR scan.

Imaging of Specific White Matter Diseases

Multiple Sclerosis (Pathology and Physiology)

MR alone is unable to make a definitive diagnosis of a white matter disease. However, it may provide strong confirmatory evidence in the presence of appropriate clinical and laboratory findings, and it may serve to rule out a demyelinating disease by recognizing the presence on a scan of its clinical imitators. Multiple sclerosis is the most common of the primary demyelinating diseases, and has a variety of radiographic appearances which must be distinguished from the diseases which mimic it clinically and on CT and MR scan.

Two excellent articles review the current theories of the epidemiology, pathology, etiology, and clinical findings in multiple sclerosis [9,10] and according to them, the disease is due to destruction of the myelin sheath with preservation of axons. It is believed that hydrolytic enzymes in macrophages are responsible for the myelin dissolution. A perivenular inflammatory reaction occurs with invasion of the white matter by macrophages, plasma cells and lymphocytes. This is followed by gliosis, which forms astrocytic plaques. Oligodendrocytes proliferate at the periphery of the plaque, and immunoglobulins are deposited within the plaque. Plaques are scattered throughout the central nervous system with a predilection for the periventricular white matter, brain stem, spinal cord (especially the cervical portion), and the optic nerves. It is these scattered plaques that give the disease its name. The presence of increased IgG levels in the cerebrospinal fluid, along with oligoclonal Ig bands, and the similarity of the pathologic lesions to those of a number of experimentally induced viral central nervous system diseases, suggests that an exogenous agent, presumably a virus, triggers the demyelination.

Clinical Course and Diagnosis of Multiple Sclerosis

The clinical course of the disease was recently summarized by McFarlin and McFarland [11]. According to them, the disease usually begins between the second and fifth decades. Sensory, visual, and motor dysfunctions are common, and 60% of patients have exacerbations and remissions. The most common symptoms are blurred vision, diplopia, vertigo, paresthesias, urinary retention and urgency, fecal incontinence, and impotence, whereas the most common signs are impaired visual acuity, nystagmus, asymmetric brisk tendon reflexes, positive Babinski signs, and absent abdominal reflexes [12]. The course is variable and may be terminal within months or may be slowly progressive. With each exacerbation and remission, there is greater permanent neurologic dysfunction.

The Poser Committee [13] has established strict criteria for the diagnosis of multiple sclerosis. Generally, diagnosis requires demonstration of two or more white matter lesions and two or more attacks. The Committee lists criteria to define age of onset, a lesion, an attack, a remission, and clinical and paraclinical and laboratory evidence of disease.

In 1986, the National Multiple Sclerosis Society stated its position on the role of MR in the diagnosis of multiple sclerosis [14]. According to that document, it was felt that MR could confirm dissemination of lesions in time and space. It further stated that a negative MR scan did not rule out multiple sclerosis, nor can MR make a diagnosis of multiple sclerosis without clinical confirmation.

Finally, it stated that a diagnosis of multiple sclerosis could be made solely on clinical grounds.

CT Imaging in Multiple Sclerosis

The imaging of multiple sclerosis is considered in the Poser Committee criteria as "paraclinical evidence" of the disease [13]. The CT scan shows three basic kinds of lesions: A) *white matter lesion*, B) *ventricular dilatation* and C) *cortical sulcus enlargement* [15]. The most common are white matter abnormalities and can be found in 74% of abnormal scans. They present as areas of decreased white matter density, usually around the bodies of the lateral ventricles and/or in the centrum semiovale (Fig. 5). While MR scanning is able to detect lesions in the brainstem, peduncles, medulla and spinal cord, the fact that these areas are small and surrounded by dense bone gives rise to beam-hardening artifact,

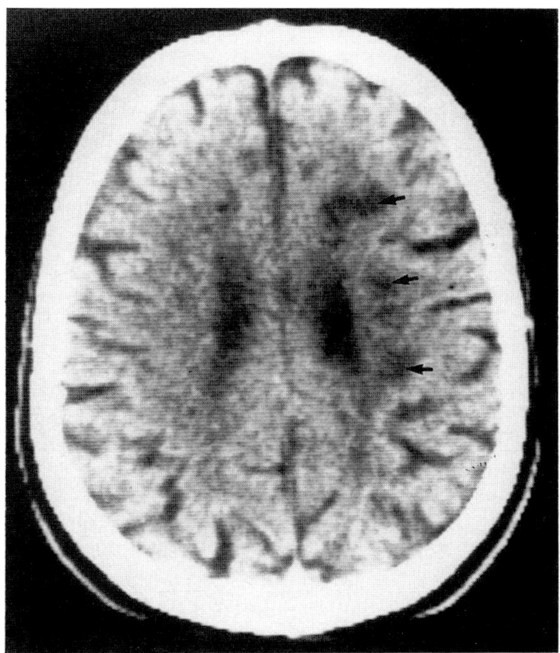

Figure 5. *MULTIPLE SCLEROSIS. Non-contrast CT scan in a patient with multiple sclerosis. Low density lesions surrounding body of left lateral ventricle represent placques (arrows).*

which makes it difficult to appreciate these latter lesions on CT scan. White matter lesions are single or multiple and may range in size from 5 mm to 72 mm [15]. Approximately one third of patients with CT detectable white matter lesions will demonstrate enhancement of at least one lesion following iodinated contrast enhancement (Fig. 6). This indicates disruption of the blood brain barrier, and is presumed to be secondary to the perivenular inflammatory reaction. Not only is post-contrast CT scanning able to detect more lesions than non-contrast CT [15], but when the dose of iodine is doubled from 40 to 80 grams, there is a further increase in the sensitivity of CT to these lesions [16,17].

There is no definite correlation between enhancement of lesions and activity of the disease, although sporadic case reports claim enhancement does reflect activity of the disease and its diminution on serial scans is a useful barometer [18]. Once an area has enhanced the degree of enhancement tends to decrease with time. High dose oral corticosteroid treatment has been reported to signi-

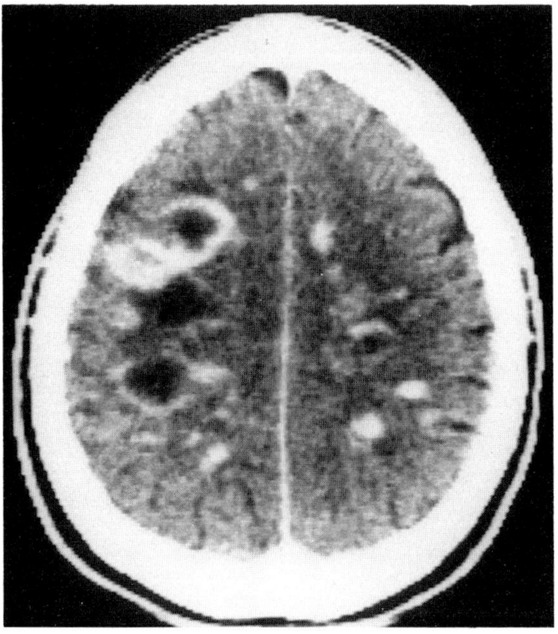

Figure 6. *MULTIPLE SCLEROSIS. Double dose delayed post contrast CT scan in a patient with acute exacerbation of multiple sclerosis. Multiple enhancing lesions are seen throughout the centrum ovale.*

ficantly but incompletely reduce enhancement of multiple sclerosis plaques, and low doses were shown to be less effective. The authors of this study [19] speculated that the enhancement in the multiple sclerosis lesions is due to focal edema associated with the demyelinating lesion and that the steroid treatment diminishes the edema.

Ventricular dilatation may also be seen with CT and is present in 20-57% of abnormal scans in multiple sclerosis [20]. While this finding did not correlate with the number of lesions present, it tended to be more marked in patients with a longer duration of disease. Rao et al. [20] evaluated the relationship between cerebral ventricular size and neuropsychological impairment. They found that there was strong evidence that cognitive dysfunction was related to ventricular enlargement. They also found that the width of the third ventricle was the best indicator of the intellectual and memory dysfunction. Enlarged cortical sulci were seen to be present on 32% of abnormal scans.

MR Scanning in Multiple Sclerosis

MR scanning in multiple sclerosis demonstrates plaques as areas of high signal intensity on proton density and T2 weighted sequences and often as low or high intensity lesions on T1 weighted images. Lesions may be single or multiple and according to Price et al. [21] give a "lumpy-bumpy" appearance to the ependymal surface of the lateral ventricle, which may serve to distinguish these lesions from infarcts. According to a study by Horowitz et al. [22], 86% of 59 patients showed oval shaped hyperintense lesions oriented with their long axes perpendicular to the antero-posterior axis of the brain on proton density and T2 weighted scans. They attribute this to the fact that demyelination in multiple sclerosis is perivenular and the blood vessels in the periventricular white matter are oriented perpendicular to the ventricular wall. Pathologists refer to this pattern of demyelination as a "Dawson's finger." Horowitz et al. believe that this oval lesion seen on MR (Fig. 7) is the imaging correlate of the "Dawson's finger." MS may present as large cystic lesions scattered throughout white matter but the associated periventricular lesions should suggest the diagnosis of MS. There may be giant plaques of MS (Fig. 8) which have the appearance of tumor. However, they may be differentiated from tumor by their

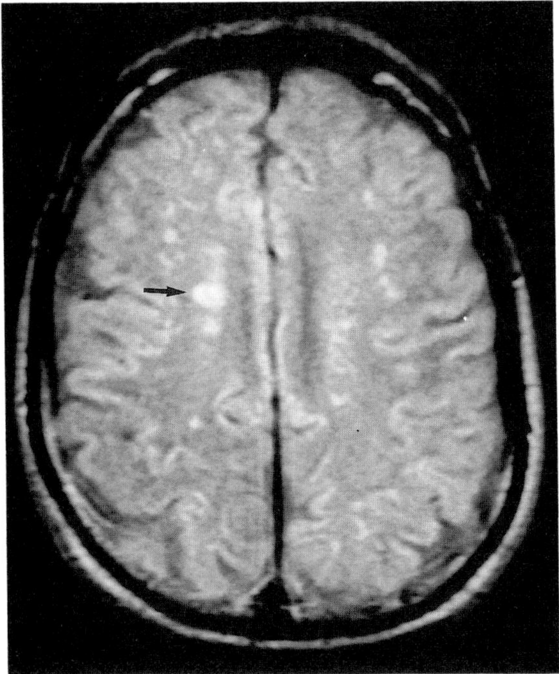

Figure 7. *MULTIPLE SCLEROSIS. Proton density MR scan in a patient with multiple sclerosis. Note the oval-shaped periventricular high intensity lesion (arrow) oriented with its long axis perpendicular to the anteroposterior axis of the brain.*

lack of mass effect and their dramatic response to steroids. Lymphoma may be difficult to differentiate from a giant plaque because of its tendency to lie adjacent to ventricular surfaces (Fig. 9) and its prompt response to steroids.

The proximity of MS lesions to the ventricles often raises a problem since the plaques may be identical in intensity to the cerebrospinal fluid. However, the use of two echoes on the long TR sequence usually allows for differentiation of the plaques from CSF on the shorter TE acquisition where the plaques tend to be brighter than the CSF. The proximity of MS plaques to bone is a problem in the CT imaging of brainstem and cerebellar lesions. However, the MR image is not degraded by the bone-hardening artifact, and therefore it is more sensitive than CT in identifying these lesions [23]. This is of particular importance in the imaging of adolescent patients with MS since Osborn et al. [24] have shown frequent occurrence of infratentorial lesions in these individuals.

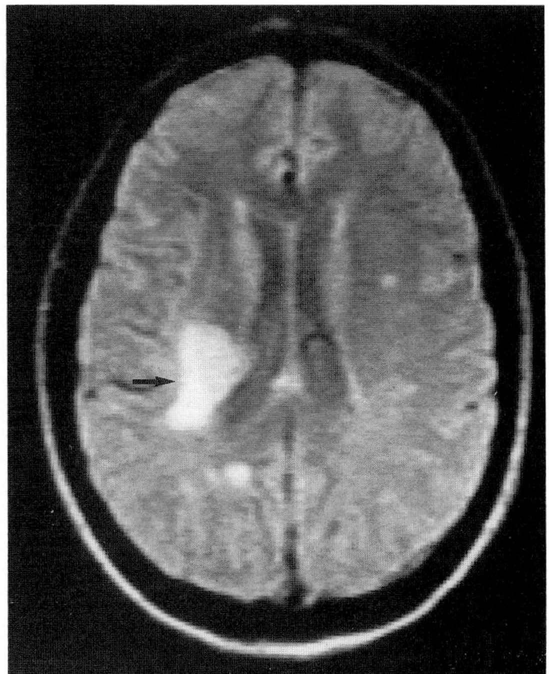

Figure 8. *MULTIPLE SCLEROSIS WITH GIANT PLACQUE. Proton density MR scan in a patient with multiple sclerosis. Note the high intensity giant periventricular placque adjacent to the atrium of the right lateral ventricular (arrow).*

There is considerable difference of opinion about the role of gadolinium-DTPA in the imaging of MS. Some feel that enhancement of MS plaques with paramagnetic contrast materials is a feature of new and active lesions that is detectable for up to 3 months [25]. Larson et al. [26] showed that enhancement of MS lesions in the cervical spinal cord was seen in patients with active disease but not in patients with stable disease. They also reported that decrease in enhancement paralleled decrease in the severity of clinical signs and symptoms. Grossman et al. showed enhancement in 13 of 14 patients in whom clinical activity had changed within 4 weeks of the study [27]. They also showed that the 3 minute post-injection short TR-short TE scan was most effective in detecting enhancement. It is probably safe to conclude that enhancement indicates blood brain barrier breakdown, but as yet there is no clear relationship between this phenomenon and the clinical severity of the disease. Poser et al. [28] reported that alteration of the blood-

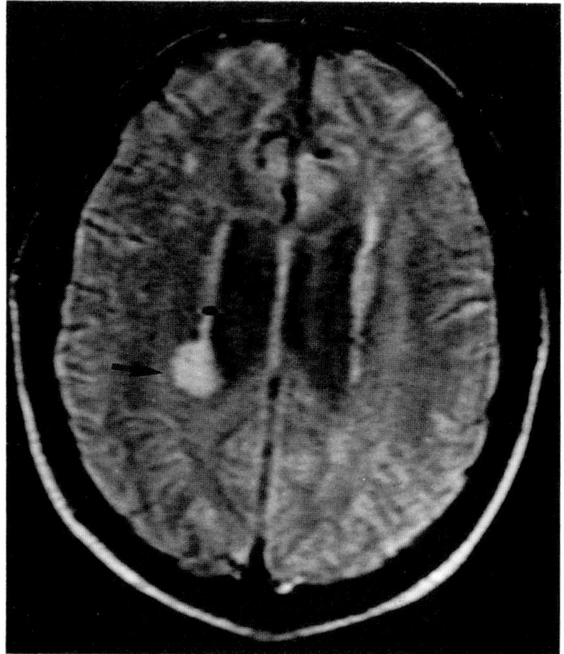

Figure 9. *LYMPHOMA. Proton density MR scan in a patient with lymphoma. The periventricular lesion (arrow) resembles a giant placque of multiple sclerosis.*

brain barrier in acute MS is not necessarily followed by a plaque if the case is vigorously treated with steroids early in the course of the disease.

Because of sagittal imaging, MR nicely demonstrates the atrophic changes in the corpus callosum, cerebellar vermis, and cervical spinal cord that may occur with MS. Simon et al. [29] showed the normal mid-sagittal area of the corpus callosum to be 601 sq mm and significantly less than that for patients with MS (Fig. 10). They also found this callosal atrophy to be proportional to the number of high intensity periventricular lesions. The cerebellar vermis (Fig. 11) and cervical cord (Fig. 12) may also show significant atrophy. Forty percent of MS patients will show callosal atrophy and 55% will show high intensity lesions in the corpus callosum on T2 weighted images.

Drayer et al. [30] have reported decreased signal in the thalamus and putamen in patients with long standing MS, particularly on T2 weighted images (Fig. 13). This is felt to represent the presence of

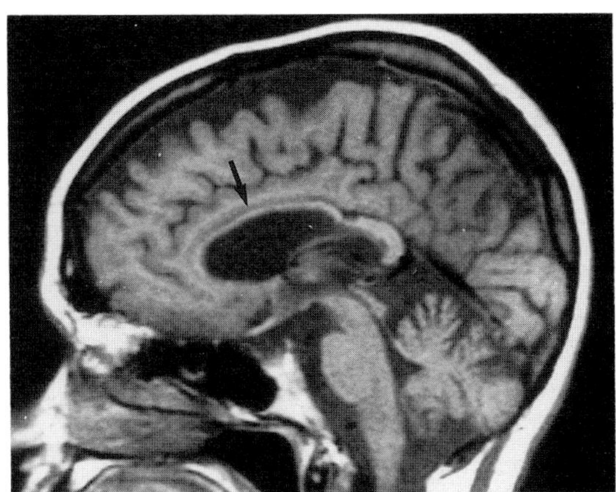

Figure 10. *MULTIPLE SCLEROSIS WITH CORPUS CALLOSUM ATROPHY. T1 weighted sagittal MR scan in a patient with multiple sclerosis. Note severe thinning of the corpus callosum (arrow), cerebral cortical atrophy, and cerebellar vermian atrophy.*

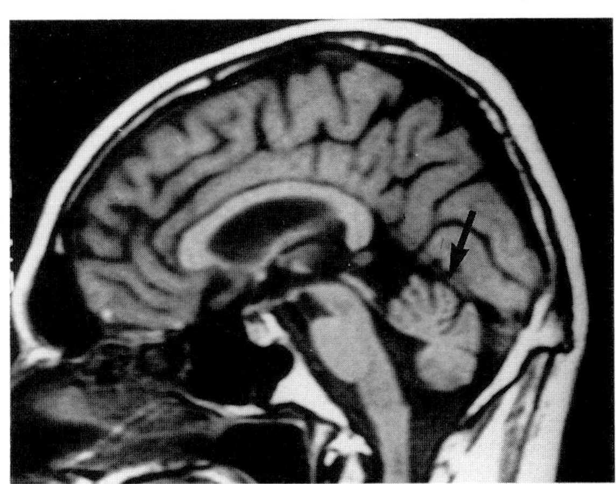

Figure 11. *MULTIPLE SCLEROSIS WITH CEREBELLAR ATROPHY. T1 weighted sagittal MR acquisition in a young woman with multiple sclerosis. Note significant atrophy of the cerebellar vermis (arrow).*

iron in macrophages. It may also be seen in other demyelinating and dysmyelinating diseases.

MS lesions in the spinal cord may occur with or without demonstrable brain lesions (Fig. 14). The cord may swell and tumor is a serious differential consideration. However, unlike tumors,

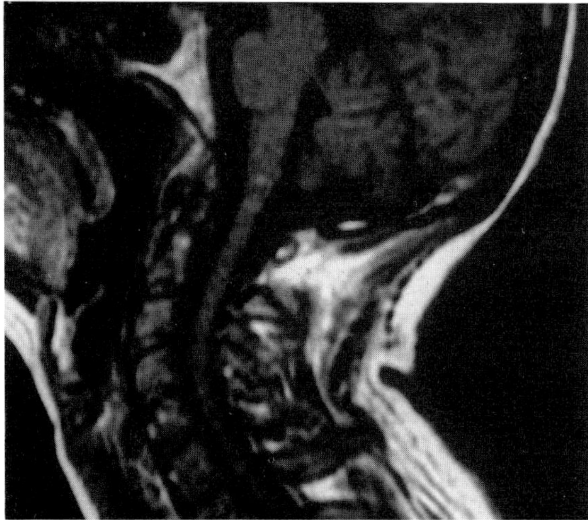

Figure 12. *MULTIPLE SCLEROSIS WITH CORD ATROPHY. T1 weighted sagittal MR acquisition in a patient with multiple sclerosis. Note the severe atrophy of the cerebellar vermis and cervical spinal cord.*

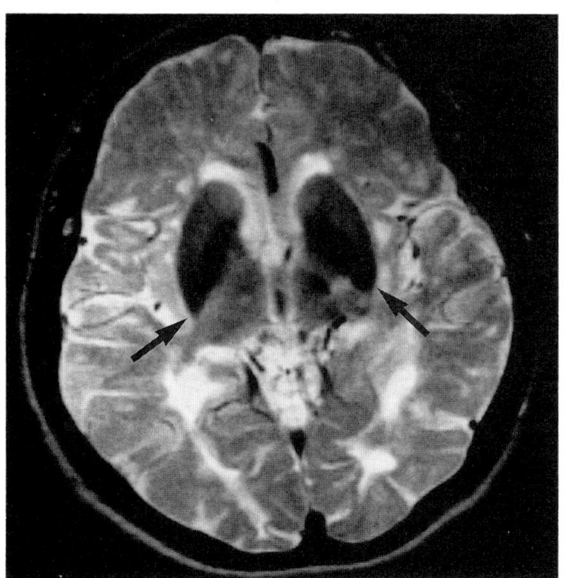

Figure 13. *MULTIPLE SCLEROSIS AND BASAL GANGLIA. Multiple sclerosis with low intensity in basal ganglia T2 weighted MR scan in a patient with multiple sclerosis. Note the extremely low intensity signal within both basal ganglia (arrows). This is felt to represent the presence of iron in macrophages.*

70

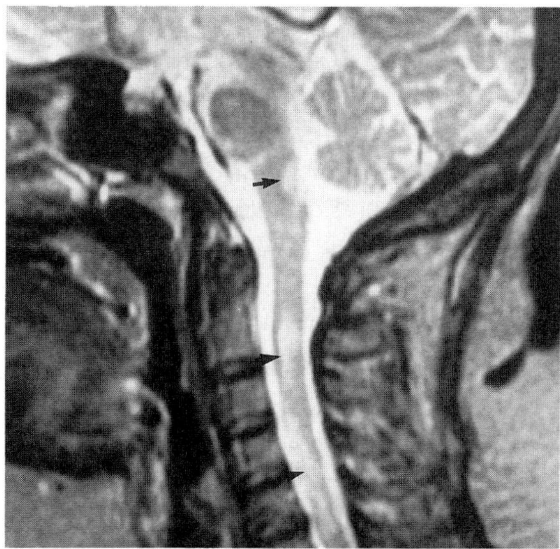

Figure 14. *MULTIPLE SCLEROSIS OF CERVICAL CORD. T2 weighted sagittal MR scan of the cervical spine in a patient with acute multiple sclerosis. Note the presence of multiple high intensity lesions within the cervical cord and medulla (arrows).*

these lesions rarely show enhancement after Gd-DTPA administration. Lesions may be in gray or white matter in the cord and usually appear eccentric on axial section. Forty percent of MS patients have demonstrable cord lesions.

Optic neuritis is often the first sign of MS. Short T1 inversion recovery (STIR) sequences will suppress the signal from orbital fat [32], often enabling the identification of a high signal lesion in the optic nerve in this abnormality. Tien et al. [33] were able to demonstrate optic neuritis using a fat suppression post-contrast technique.

Accuracy of CT vs MR in Multiple Sclerosis

There is little doubt that MR is considerably more sensitive to the detection of demyelination and therefore is superior to CT as a screening technique in multiple sclerosis. Jackson et al. [34] showed that MR detected lesions in 76% of 32 patients with definite MS and double dose delay CT only detected lesions in 60%. Shelton et al. [35] showed that MR was positive in 85% of patients with definite MS, and CT was positive in 25% of similar patients. They also observed that MR was always positive when CT was positive. Gebarski et al. [36] also confirmed the superiority of MR and showed that CT only detected the largest of the lesions. Kirshner et al. [23] evaluated 35 MS patients and correlated severity of disease on MR with the clinical severity and found no correlation, probably because lesion location rather than lesion number and size seems to be a more important factor. This particular study demonstrated 15 lesions in the brainstem with MR, none of which were seen on CT. Conversely, the study of Edwards et al. [37] showed a strong correlation of MR findings and clinical severity by two rating methods and significant correlation with a third method of clinical rating.

The Mayo Clinic group [38] also confirmed superiority of MR over CT in detection of lesions (80% vs. 29% respectively). The number of lesions detected on MR correlated with a longer duration of the disease, and a pattern of confluent periventricular signal around the lateral ventricle was associated with a greater duration of MS and greater patient disability findings later borne out by the study of Uhlenbrock et al. [39]. The latter study showed no correlation with cerebrospinal fluid findings nor with visual evoked potential findings, but the Mayo clinic study did show that MR was positive in their 109 MS patients more often than was any single evoked potential study [38]. Probably the most convincing study of the value of MR in the diagnosis of MS comes from the Medical College of Wisconsin [40] where the MR scans of 92 patients with MS, 100 healthy volunteers, 60 patients with Alzheimer disease, and eight patients with unspecified dementia were evaluated by two neuroradiologists without the aid of demographic information and again after knowing the age and sex of the patients. A case was considered as MS if it had multiple oblong or ovoid foci of high signal intensity on T2 weighted spin-echo sequences. The "specificity" (proportion of subjects without MS who were classified as negative) was 95-90% depending on whether questionable cases were classified as positive or negative. Sensitivity of diagnosis ranged from 68% to 80% and improved to 80% and 83% when demographic information was supplied. The authors did remark that 2-4% of healthy subjects have periventricular high intensity abnormalities that cannot be differentiated from MS on the basis of current MR imaging criteria.

The "Five Red Flags" of Multiple Sclerosis

Many diseases mimic MS in their clinical symptoms. Examples are tentorial edge meningioma (Fig. 15) and Chiari I malformation (Fig. 16), lesions which can present with multiple cranial nerve findings and other neurologic signs and symptoms with temporal and spatial patterns suggestive of MS. Rudick et al. [41] have described the "Five Red Flags" of MS, clinical features, which if present, should cast doubt on the diagnosis of multiple sclerosis. They are:

- Absence of eye findings
- Absence of clinical remission
- Localized disease
- Atypical clinical features
- Absence of CSF abnormalities

Diseases that Mimic the CT and MR Appearance of Multiple Sclerosis

A number of diseases may mimic the appearance of MS on CT and MR scan. These were summarized in a recent paper [42] and some

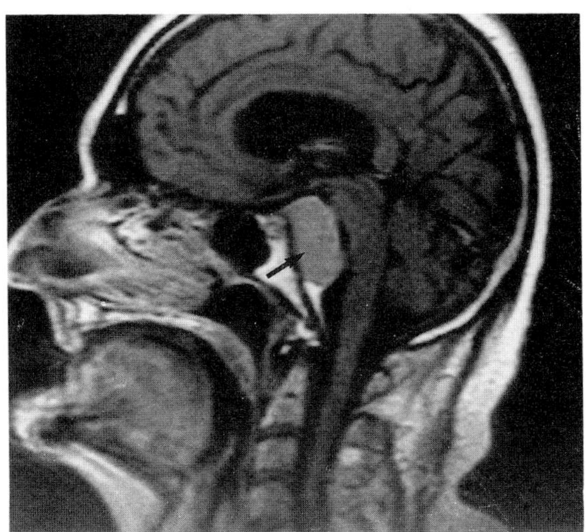

Figure 15. *CLIVUS MENINGIOMA. T1 weighted sagittal post contrast MR scan showing a large enhancing meningioma (arrow) of the clivus. Symptoms of this lesion often mimic those of multiple sclerosis.*

are listed below:

Multiple Sclerosis
Infarction
- Thromboembolic infarcts
- Lacunes
- Binswanger disease
- Vasculitis
- Moya-moya disease
- Venous thrombosis
Demyelination
- Acquired immune deficiency syndrome
- Acute disseminated encephalomyelitis
- Progressive multifocal leukoencephalopathy
- Inherited white matter disease
- Post-radiation therapy

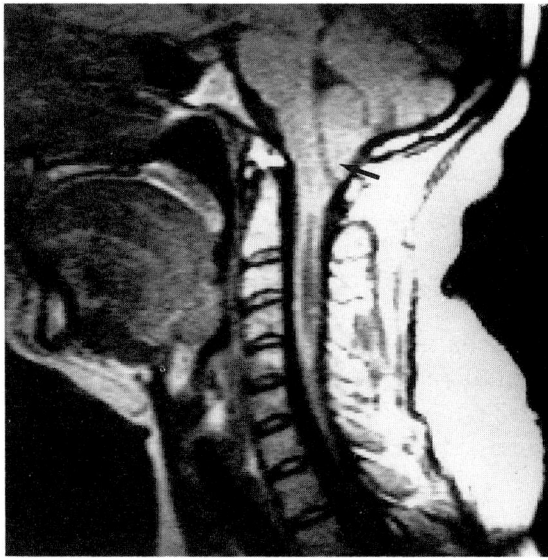

Figure 16. *CHIARI 1 MALFORMATION - TONSILLAR ECTOPIA. T1 weighted sagittal MR acquisition demonstrating the cerebellar tonsil (arrow) to lie well below the foramen magnum. Also present is a related syrinx in the cervical cord. This is a Chiari 1 malformation, the symptoms of which may often mimic those of multiple sclerosis.*

Neoplasm
- CSF borne tumor spread
- Primary CNS lymphoma

Hydrocephalus with CSF interstitial edema
Normal elderly, especially if hypertensive
Unidentified bright objects

Some of these and a few not mentioned by Kapila and Whitaker will be discussed below.

Lymphomatoid Granulomatosis

The lesions of this disease may mimic MS by being focal and peri-ventricular [43]. The disease is a systemic necrotizing vasculitis which predominates in females with onset usually between 45 and 50 years of age. In addition to the nervous system, the disease may affect the skin, GU, GI, and respiratory systems. There may be peripheral and cranial neuropathies, seizures, aphasia and ataxia. Cranial and peripheral nerves are infiltrated by perivascular lymphocytes and vascular thromboses and vasculitis may ensue. Lesions may be single or multiple, have gliosis, edema and blood brain barrier breakdown, and possibly mass effect. The edema causes high signal intensity on long TR MR sequences. The multi-system involvement should distinguish this disease from MS.

Phakomatoses

Some phakomas and heterotopias may mimic the CT and MR appearances of MS. Neurofibromatosis (Von Recklinghausen disease) is often characterized by heterotopias or hamartomas which are not detectable on CT but which appear as foci of high signal on long TR sequences on MR [44]. The external stigmata of the phakomatoses should distinguish them from MS. Heterotopias may appear on MR as areas of increased periventricular signal, but the intensity of the signal is usually less than that of the MS plaque on proton density MR scan.

Inflammatory Disease

Infectious diseases may be misidentified as MS on the MR scan. Lyme disease is due to a tick-borne spirochete and may present

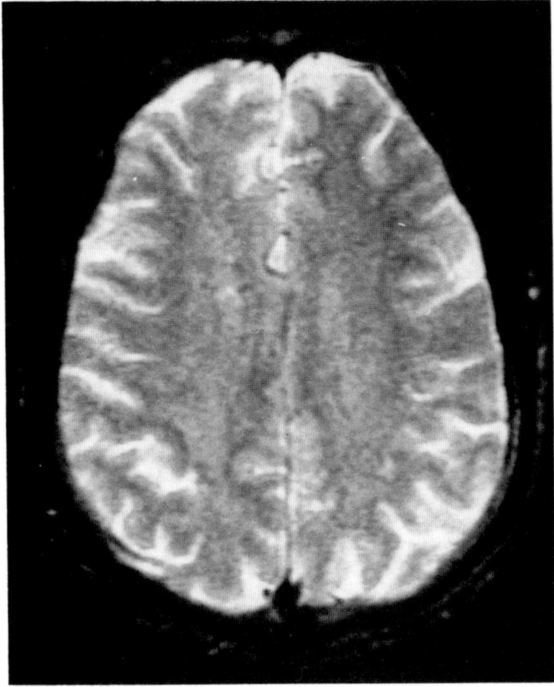

Figure 17. *AIDS ENCEPHALOPATHY. T2 weighted MR scan in a patient with AIDS. Note the "myelin pallor" in the centrum ovale.*

with neurologic symptoms such as optic neuritis, chronic encephalopathy, polyneuropathy, and leukoencephalitis [45]. Lesions may be present in the brainstem and throughout white matter on MR scan [45,47]. The presence of CSF antibody to the spirochete should distinguish this disease from MS.

A hereditary sensorimotor disease which occurs in members of the Navajo Amerindian Tribe may have CNS abnormalities which have the appearance of a leukoencephalopathy on long TR sequences. The diagnosis is made by the detection of corneal scarring, acral mutilation, and a positive sural nerve biopsy. The disease is referred to as "Navajo neuropathy", and the CNS findings are felt to be due to demyelination (48).

Sjögrens syndrome may show multifocal cerebral involvement with seizures and dementia. These periventricular lesions represent an immune vasculopathy with mononuclear infiltrates around vessels and subsequent infarcts. The disease is distinguished from

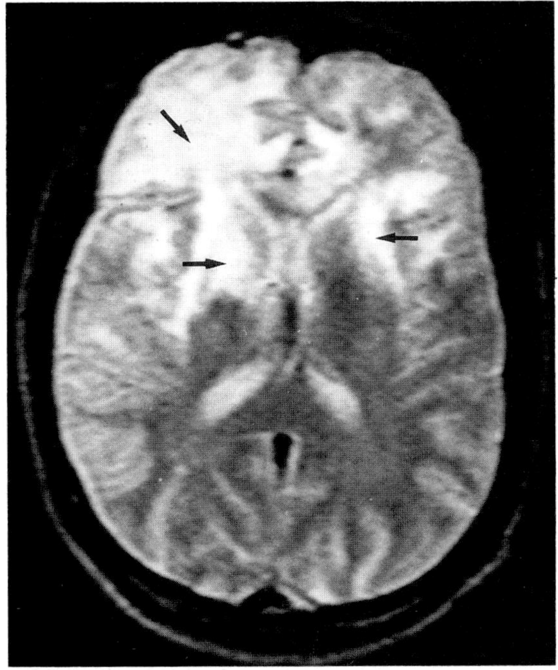

Figure 18. *AIDS AND PML. T2 weighted axial MR in a patient with AIDS and progressive multifocal leukoencephalopathy. Note high signal intensity in frontal and subcortical white matter (arrows).*

MS by the presence of xerostomia and xerophthalmia (49).

Acquired immune deficiency syndrome (AIDS) has direct and indirect effects on the CNS. The direct effects are due to invasion of neural elements by the HIV virus which results in a myelin pallor in the central cerebral white matter. On imaging studies, there is brain atrophy. Demyelination and vacuolation of white matter tracts accompanying severe HIV infection causes hypoattenuation on CT and hyperintensity on long TR MR sequences, especially in sub-insular and peritrigonal white matter areas [50,51] (Fig. 17). Imaging may detect the indirect effects of AIDS such as opportunistic infection like toxoplasmosis, cryptococcosis and tuberculosis, or progressive multifocal leukoencephalopathy (PML), or lymphoma. All of these may involve white matter and fall into the radiographic differential diagnosis of MS. Most of the opportunistic infections and lymphomas that complicate AIDS will show some degree of lesion enhancement with paramagnetic contrast materials.

PML is due to a papova virus and is seen in 1-5% of AIDS patients. The disease has personality change, memory loss, and cognitive defects. CT shows non-enhancing low density lesions in white matter, and MR shows multiple asymmetric hyperintense foci in white matter on T2 weighted scan (Fig. 18) [51]. However, PML may have a purely periventricular location on MR. Mark and Atlas reported that PML may involve gray matter in 50% of patients [52]. The history of immunodepression should distinguish this disease from MS.

Sarcoidosis may present with high intensity periventricular lesions on T2 weighted MR scan. These may be indistinguishable form the lesions of MS [53]. The symptoms in the two diseases may be identical, even down to the optic neuritis which may occur in both. Sarcoidosis has more of a predilection for the meninges [54] than the parenchyma, and these meningeal lesions are likely to enhance on post contrast MR studies.

Iatrogenic Demyelination

Patients with meningeal carcinomatosis, lymphoma, or leukemia may be treated with intrathecal methotrexate (MTX). While there is therapeutic benefit, such treatment has a morbidity of its own. This topic is reviewed in a paper by Ebner et al. [55]. MTX is lipid soluble but normally does not cross the blood brain barrier, However, it may cause chemical arachnoiditis, motor dysfunction, and a disseminated necrotizing leukoencephalopathy (DNL). The combination of radiation therapy and MTX treatment increases the likelihood that neurotoxicity will occur. CT shows diffuse white matter lucency, and, on MR scan, there will be diffuse white matter hyperintensity on T2 weighted acquisition. However, post contrast CT or MR usually do not show any enhancement of the abnormal white matter, although there may be enhancement of the condition under treatment such as a lymphoma or meningeal carcinomatosis [56]. It is not surprising that the CT and MR appearance of DNL and the changes of radiation therapy alone should resemble MS, since the pathologic changes are basically due to endothelial injury in small vessels with confluent foci of demyelination, astrocyte hypertrophy, loss of oligodendroglia, axonal swelling and edema [55,57].

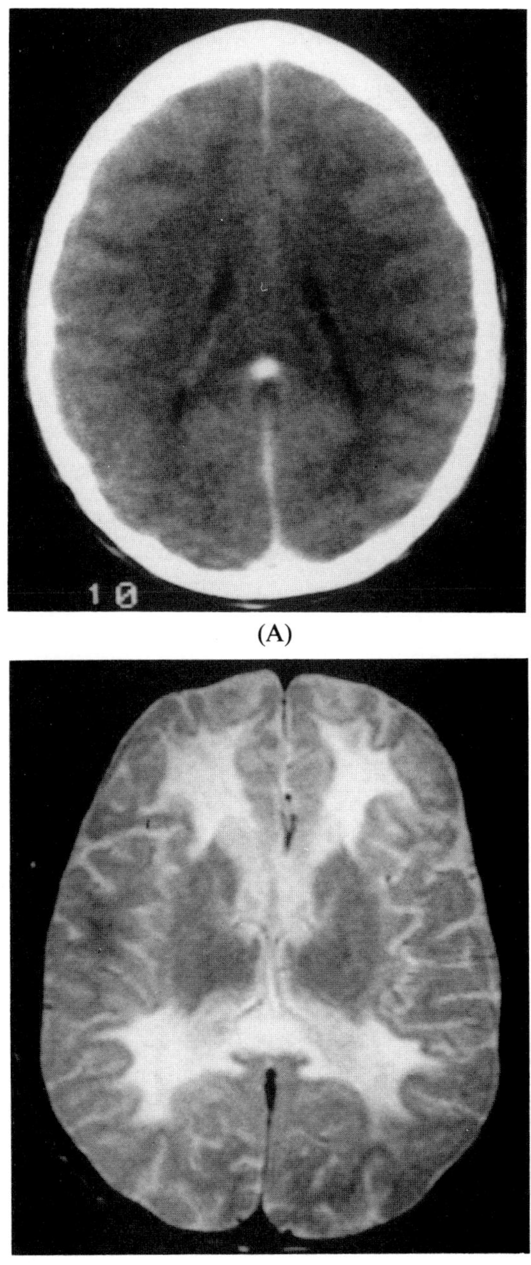

(A)

(B)

Figure 19. *ADRENOLEUKODYSTROPHY. (A) CT scan in an eight-year-old boy with adrenoleukodystrophy. Note symmetrical low density surrounding the lateral ventricles. (B) T2 weighted MR scan in the same child shows symmetrical high signal intensity in cerebral white matter.*

Metabolic Diseases and Leukodystrophies

Leukodystrophies are diseases where demyelination occurs as a result of the production and maintenance of abnormal myelin. Adrenoleukodystrophy (ALD) is a genetic disorder with progressive central demyelination and adrenal cortical insufficiency. Patients show increased levels of saturated unbranched very-long-chain fatty acids because of impaired ability to degrade these substances. This degradation normally is done by a subcellular organelle, the peroxisome, and therefore, this is classified as a "peroxisomal disorder" [58].

On CT, the typical lesions are symmetrical areas of low density surrounding the lateral ventricles (Fig. 19), often with peripheral contrast enhancement. The extension of these lesions is usually anterior and may progressively involve the corpus callosum [59].

On MR, similar areas show the characteristic picture of demyelination [60]. There is high signal intensity on T2 weighted image in the areas where there is low density on CT (Fig. 19). As in multiple sclerosis, there may be low signal intensity in the basal ganglia in severe cases.

Canavan disease is a lethal neurodegenerative disorder of infancy. There is a deficiency of the enzyme aspartoacylase which results in an increase in n-acetylaspartic acid in plasma and urine. CT and MR scans show white matter disease, sometimes sparing the external and internal capsules, the corpus callosum, and deep white matter. The radiographic findings may be abnormal in the face of a normal clinical picture and the biochemical test results make the diagnosis [61,62].

Phenylketonuria (PKU) is due either to a deficiency of phenylalanine hydroxylase or one of its co-factors. The result is the accumulation of phenylalanine which results in white matter disease manifested on MR by symmetric high signal intensity of white matter in the posterior cerebral hemispheres [63,64,65].

References

1. Brooks RA, Di Chiro G, Keller MR. Explanation of cerebral white-gray contrast in computed tomography. J Comput Assist Tomogr 1980;4:489-491.
2. Arimitsu T, Di Chiro G, Brooks RA, Smith PB. White-gray matter differentiation in computed tomography. J Comput Assist Tomogr 1977;1:437-442.

3. Kjos BO, Ehman RL, Brant-Zawadzki, et al. Reproducibility of relaxation times and spin density calculated from routine MR imaging sequences: Clinical Study of the CNS. AJNR 1985;6:271-276.

4. Curnes JT, Burger PC, Djang WT, et al. MR imaging of compact white matter pathways. AJNR 1988;9:1061-1068.

5. Drayer BP, Burger P, Darwin R, et al. Magnetic resonance imaging of brain iron. AJNR 1986;7:373-380.

6. Dietrich RB, Bradley WG, Zaragoza EJ, et al. MR evaluation of early myelination patterns in normal and developmentally delayed infants. AJNR 1988;9:69-76.

7. Barkovich AJ, Kjos BO, Jackson DE, Norman D. Normal maturation of the neonatal and infant brain: MR imaging at 1.5T. Radiology 1988;166:173-180.

8. Stricker T, Martin E, Boesch C. Development of the human cerebellum observed with high-field-strength MR imaging. Radiology 1990;177:431-435.

9. Rodriguez M. Multiple sclerosis: basic concepts and hypothesis. Mayo Clin Proc 1989;64:570-576.

10. Goodman A, McFarlin DE. Multiple sclerosis. Curr Neurol 1987;7:91-128.

11. McFarlin DE, McFarland HF. Multiple sclerosis (first of two parts). N Engl J Med 1982;307:1183-1188.

12. Hart RG, Sherman DG. The diagnosis of multiple sclerosis. JAMA 1982;247:498-503.

13. Poser CM, Paty DW, Scheinberg LS, et al. New diagnostic criteria for multiple sclerosis: guidelines for research protocols. Ann Neurol 1983;227-231.

14. National Multiple Sclerosis Society Working Group on Neuro-Imaging for the Medical Advisory Board. Use of magnetic resonance imaging in the diagnosis of multiple sclerosis. Magn Res Med 1986;3:821-822.

15. Hershey LA, Gado MH, Trotter JL. Computerized tomography in the diagnostic evaluation of multiple sclerosis. Ann Neurol 1979;5:32-39.

16. Vineula FV, Fox AJ, Debrun GM, et al. New perspectives in CT of MS. AJNR 1982;3:277-281.

17. Sears S, McCammon A, Bigelow R, Hayman LA. Maximizing the harvest of contrast enhancing lesions in MS. Neurology 1982;32:815-820.

18. Morariu, MA, Wilkins DE, Patel S. Multiple sclerosis and serial computerized tomography: delayed contrast enhancement of acute early lesions. Arch Neurol 1980;37:189-190.

19. Troiano RA, Hafstein MP, Zito G, et al. The effect of oral corticosteroid dosage on CT enhancing multiple sclerosis plaques. J Neurol Sci 1985;70:67-72.

20. Rao SM, Glatt S, Hammeke TA, et al. Chronic progressive multiple sclerosis: relationship between cerebral ventricular size and neuropsychological impairment. Arch Neurol 1985;42:678-682.

21. Price AC, Runge VM, Kirshner HS, et al. Improved CT diagnosis of multiple sclerosis after magnetic resonance imaging evaluation (abs). AJNR 1984;5:678-679.

22. Horowitz AL, Kaplan RD, Grewe G, et al. The ovoid lesion: a new MR observation in patients with multiple sclerosis. AJNR 1989;10:303-305.

23. Kirshner HS, Tsai SI, Runge VM, Price AC. Magnetic resonance imaging and other techniques in the diagnosis of multiple sclerosis. Arch Neurol 1985;42:859-863.

24. Osborn AG, Harnsberger HR, Smoker WRK, et al. Multiple sclerosis in adolescents: CT and MR findings. AJNR 1990;11:489-494.

25. Miller DH, Rudge P, Johnson G, et al. Serial gadolinium enhanced magnetic resonance imaging in multiple sclerosis. Brain 1988;11:927-939.

26. Larsson EM, Holtas S, Nilsson O. Gd-DTPA-enhanced MR of suspected spinal multiple sclerosis. AJNR 1989;10:1071-1076.

27. Grossman RI, Braffman BH, Brorson JR, et al. Multiple sclerosis: serial study of gadolinium-enhanced MR imaging. Radiology 1988;169:117-122.

28. Poser CM, Kleefield J, O'Reilly GV, Jolesz F. Neuroimaging and the lesion of multiple sclerosis. AJNR 1987;8:549-552.
29. Simon JH, Schiffer RB, Ruddick RA, Herndon RM. Quantitative determination of MS-induced corpus callosum atrophy in vivo using MR imaging. AJNR 1987;8:599-604.
30. Drayer B, Burger P, Hurwitz B, et al. Reduced signal intensity on MR images of thalamus and putamen in multiple sclerosis: increased iron content? AJNR 1987;8:413-419.
31. Maravilla KR, Weinreb JC, Sus R, Nunnally RL. Magnetic resonance demonstration of multiple sclerosis plaques in the cervical cord. AJNR 1984;5:685-689.
32. Hendrix LE, Kneeland JB, Haughton VM, et al. MR imaging of optic nerve lesions: value of gadopentetate dimeglumine and fat-suppression technique. AJNR 1990;11:749-754.
33. Tien, RD, Chu PK, Hasselink JR, Szumowski J. Intra- and paraorbital lesions: value of fat-suppression MR imaging with paramagnetic contrast enhancement. AJNR 1991;12:245-253.
34. Jackson JA, Leake DR, Schneiders NJ, et al. Magnetic resonance imaging in multiple sclerosis. AJNR 1985;6:171-176.
35. Sheldon JJ, Siddharthan R, Tobias J, et al. MR imaging of multiple sclerosis: comparison with clinical and CT examinations in 74 patients. AJNR 1985;6:683-690.
36. Gebarski SS, Gabrielsen TO, Gilman S, et al. The initial diagnosis of multiple sclerosis: clinical impact of magnetic resonance imaging. Ann Neurol 1985;17:469-474.
37. Edwards MK, Farlow MR, Stevens JC. Multiple sclerosis: MRI and clinical correlation. AJNR 1986;7:595-598.
38. Stewart JM, Houser OW, Baker HL, et al. Magnetic resonance imaging and clinical relationships in multiple sclerosis. Mayo Clin Proc 1987;62:174-184.
39. Uhlenbrock D, Seidel D, Gehlen W, et al. MR imaging in MS: comparison with clinical, CSF, and visual evoked-potential findings. AJNR 1988;9:59-67.
40. Yetkin FZ, Haughton VM, Papke RA, et al. Multiple sclerosis: specificity of MR for diagnosis. Radiology 1991;178:447-451.
41. Rudick RA, Schiffer RB, Schwetz KM, Herndon RM. Multiple sclerosis: the problem of incorrect diagnosis. Arch Neurol 1986;43:578-583.
42. Kapila A, Whitaker JN. Cranial magnetic resonance imaging in multiple sclerosis. Ala J Med Sci 1987;24:290-300.
43. Smith AS, Huang TE, Weinstein MA. Periventricular involvement in CNS lymphomatoid granulomatosis; MR demonstration. J Comput Assist Tomogr 1990;14:291-293.
44. Bognanno JR, Edwards MK, Lee TA, et al. Cranial MR imaging in neurofibromatosis. AJNR 1988;9:461-468.
45. Logigian EL, Kaplan RF, Steere AC. Chronic neurologic manifestations of lyme disease. N Engl J Med 1990;323:1438-44.
46. Fernandez RE, Rothberg M, Ferencz G, Wujack D. Lyme disease of the CNS: MR imaging findings in 14 cases. AJNR 1990;11:479-481.
47. Rafto SE, Milton WJ, Galetta SL, Grossman RI. Biopsy-confirmed CNS lyme disease: MR appearance at 1.5T. AJNR 1990;11:482-484.
48. Williams KD, Drayer BP, Johnsen SD, Johnson PC. MR imaging of leukoencephalopathy associated with Navajo neuropathy. AJNR 1990;11:400-402.
49. Alexander EL, Provost TT, Stevens MB, et al. Neurologic complications of Sjogren's syndrome. Medicine 1982;61:247-257.
50. Chrysikopoulos HS, Press GA, Grafe MR, et al. Encephalitis caused by human immunodeficiency virus: CT and MR imaging manifestations with clinical and pathologic correlation. Radiology 1990;175:185-191.

51. Flowers CH, Mafee MF, Crowell R, et al. Encephalopathy in AIDS patients: evaluation with MR imaging. AJNR 1990;11:1235-1245.

52. Mark AS, Atlas SW. Progressive multifocal leukoencephalopathy in patients with AIDS: appearance on MR images. Radiology 1989;173:517-520.

53. Smith AS, Meisler DM, Weinstein MA, et al. High-signal periventricular lesions in patients with sarcoidosis: neurosarcoidosis or multiple sclerosis? AJNR 1989;10:485-490.

54. Sherman JL, Stern BJ. Sarcoidosis of the CNS: comparison of unenhanced and enhanced MR images. AJNR 1990;11:915-923.

55. Ebner F, Ranner G, Slavc I, et al. MR findings in methotrexate-induced CNS abnormalities. AJNR 1989;10:959-964.

56. Peylan-Ramu N, Poplack DG, Pizzo PA, et al. Abnormal CT scans of the brain in asymptomatic children with acute lymphocytic leukemia after prophalatic treatment of the central nervous system with radiation and intrathecal chemotherapy. N Engl J Med 1978;298:815-818.

57. Dooms GC, Hecht S, Brant-Zawadzki M, et al. Brain radiation lesions: MR imaging. Radiology 1986;158:149-155.

58. Moser HW, Moser AE, Singh I, O'Neill BP. Adrenoleukodystrophy: survey of 303 cases: biochemistry, diagnosis, and therapy. Ann Neurol 1984;16:628-641.

59. Aubourg P Diebler C. Adrenoleukodystrophy - its diverse CT appearances and an evolutive or phenotypic variant: the leukodystrophy without adrenal insufficiency. Neuroradiology 1982;24:33-42.

60. Van der Knaap MS, Valk J. MR of adrenoleukodystrophy: histopathologic correlations. AJNR 1989;10:S12-S14.

61. Brismar J, Brismar G, Gascon G, Ozand P. Canavan disease: CT and MR imaging of the brain. AJNR 1990;11:805-810.

62. McAdams HP, Geyer CA, Done SL, et al. CT and MR imaging of Canavan disease. AJNR 1990;11:397-399.

63. Brismar J, Aqeel A, Gascon G, Ozand P. Malignant hyperphenylalaninemia: CT and MR of the brain. AJNR 1990;11:135-138.

64. Pearsen KD, Gean-Marton AD, Levy HL, Davis KR. Phenylketonuria: MR imaging of the brain with clinical correlation. Radiology 1990;177:437-440.

65. Shaw DWW, Weinberger E, Maravilla KR. Cranial MR in phenylketonuria. J Comput Assist Tomogr 1990;14:458-460.

Radiology of Head Injuries

Ian Isherwood
University of Manchester, Manchester, England

"In patients who have been injured the role of Radiology is to assist in diagnosing - whilst doing no harm - the type and severity of the injury."   McRae.

Introduction

Head injuries consist of a heterogeneous group of conditions, many being of minor character. Serious accidental head injuries are usually the result of road traffic accidents. Head injuries account for half of all road traffic accident deaths [1].

The most effective way to prevent head injuries is to prevent accidents. Seat belt legislation in the U.K. resulted in a 25% reduction in the number of car accident patients requiring admission to hospital, with a 25% reduction in deaths. Studies have also shown that wearing a helmet reduces the incidence of head injury in motorcyclists. Both seat belts and helmets, however, may give rise to an increase in the number of cervical spine injuries. Other important causes of head injury which may be influenced by preventive measures include sports injuries, particularly horse riding, golf and boxing.

Head injuries may occur alone or may be part of a complex of multiple injuries, or may be even the consequence of previous and existing disease. The aims of clinical management in all circumstances are to anticipate the complications which may lead to secondary brain damage, to optimize the conditions for recovery and to expedite rehabilitation of the patient back into the community.

A widespread acceptance of the Glasgow Coma Scale [2] has

made it possible to quantify head injuries and compare groups of patients one with another. It has also made it possible to use clear terminology which can be applied to all head injury patients. "Coma" is defined as "not obeying commands, no verbal response and no eye opening." Such definitions are widely accepted and will be used in this discussion. Careful monitoring of head injured patients is important and achieved by a combination of careful clinical evaluation, imaging, electrophysiological markers and a variety of biochemical measurements [3]. Only imaging will be considered in this discussion.

Mechanisms and Classification of Head Injury

Principal mechanisms of brain damage following a blunt head injury are from brain compression, torsion stresses and axonal shearing. Brain may be damaged adjacent to the site of trauma (coup injury) or at a distance due to contrecoup impact of the brain with the skull or the rigid dural membrane. Typical sites of contrecoup injuries include the opposite hemisphere in lateral blows and the frontal and temporal lobes in antero-posterior trauma. The latter can be produced by a deceleration or "whiplash" injury without any evidence of direct blow to the cranium.

A useful anatomical classification of head injury is into extra-axial, intra-axial and vascular compartments. Extra-axial injuries include hemorrhage in the sub- or extra-dural space and dural tears resulting in leakage of cerebrospinal fluid into the paranasal or ear cavities. Intra-axial injuries include contusions, hemorrhage, axonal shearing, brain swelling and ischemia. Vascular injuries may be intra- or extra-cranial and result in intimal dissection or occlusion.

Management of Head Injuries

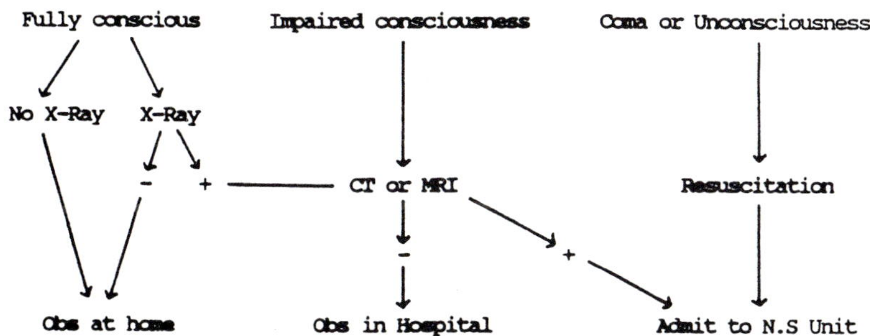

Morbidity and Mortality

The major killing factors following head injury are intra-cerebral hemorrhage, cerebral hypoxia and brain swelling [4].

Of patients who die 60% die before or soon after reaching hospital and 88% die during the first week. A third of those who die will both walk and talk before death. Of those patients who talk after injury and subsequently die 75% will have an intra-cranial hematoma.

Imaging

Radiology is vital in the effective management of head injuries. The imaging methods to be employed depend upon their availability, which may present either a socio-economic or a geographical problem. The methods include plain radiographs, Computed Tomography (CT), Magnetic Resonance Imaging (MRI), angiography and Ultrasound (US). The principal method of investigation in the developed world is CT, with increasing interest and emphasis on MRI. The role of the plain film in these circumstances is controversial. Where access to CT and MR is limited, and particularly in medically disadvantaged countries, the plain film is of considerable importance and even the traditional air ventriculogram may be employed.

Plain Films

The presence of a skull fracture increases the likelihood of a secondary complication, particularly intracranial hematoma and infection. Skull radiography can therefore have a valuable role in selecting patients for admission to hospital for observation or selection for CT where access is limited.

Severe head injuries

A severe head injury is defined as "coma for more than six hours after the injury." In these circumstances a fracture involving the vault or the base of the skull will be found in 75 to 80%. In this group of patients where the incidence of profuse white matter damage is high an extra-dural hematoma will be found in 90% and an acute sub-dural hematoma or intrasomal hematoma in 75%.

Mild uncomplicated head injuries admitted to hospital for observation

In this group a fracture of the skull will be found in 6 to 10%.

Mild uncomplicated head injury and sent home

Fracture incidence in this group is 1.5%.

In this last group skull radiography can be wasteful of resource and may not affect clinical management. Over 600,000 skull radiographs are performed annually in Accident and Emergency Departments of the UK at a cost of over £6,000,000. The risk of missing an intra-cranial hematoma in an uncomplicated head injury not requiring admission is estimated at 1 in 4,828. Clinical guidelines for referral of head injured patients to Radiology for plain skull radiographs are clearly necessary. The Royal College of Radiologists in the UK [5,6,7] have undertaken studies and provided appropriate guidelines. The indications for skull radiography after head injury include loss of consciousness, amnesia, neurological deficit, cerebro-spinal fluid leak, skull laceration and medico-legal reasons limited to road traffic accidents and criminal assault [8,9,10].

It is important to recognize that 50% of compound depressed fractures and 30 to 40% of intracranial hematomas will suffer no loss of consciousness. In the unconscious patient Accident and Emergency clinicians need to be alert to the possibility of coma from other causes with secondary head injury.

If skull radiography is to be carried out then quality control is paramount. Both radiographer and radiologist have an essential role in ensuring a good quality examination. Studies have demonstrated that over 50% of skull radiographs obtained in Accident and Emergency Units are diagnostically unsatisfactory. Very few of these (5 to 6%) are due to the patient's inability to cooperate.

Recommended radiographic projections

Three views are valuable:

a. brow up lateral with a horizontal beam. This projection is important not only for the detection of fluid levels but also the avoidance of neck rotation.

b. anteroposterior axial 30° tilt to the feet.

c. anteroposterior axial 20° tilt to the feet.

A lateral projection of the cervical spine should be obtained in all patients who are in coma and in all those who have clinical features which might suggest a cervical spine injury. The upper cervical spine should always be included in the standard brow up lateral projection.

Radiological features on the plain radiograph in acute head injury

Fractures

Linear

The margins of a linear fracture are well defined but not corticated and do not branch, though they may cross vascular markings. Angulation may occur. Linear fractures can extend into sutures and give rise to diastasis. A diastasis may be present without any obvious fracture. Vascular channels normally branch but the deep middle temporal artery, with a short linear groove in the squamous temporal bone, can be deceptive. Sutures have a zig zag pattern in adults and are corticated.

Fractures involving the skull base are less common and may be characterized clinically by bilateral periorbital hematomas or retro-auricular hematomas appearing or persisting after 24 to 48 hours. Fractures of the temporal bone are either vertical or horizontal and can give rise to ossicular dislocation. Fractures of the dorsum sella are rare and should not be confused with the spheno-occipital synchondrosis which fuses late in adolescence.

Depressed

Depressed fractures increase the risk of dural tear and potential intracranial infection. If a depressed fragment is en face it may appear only as a local area of increased density requiring tangential views for its elucidation.

Displacement of normal structures

Displacement of the calcified pineal is valuable as an indicator of a mass lesion. Rotational deformities of the brain produce secondary displacements of the calcified choroid plexuses.

Fluid levels

Fluid levels in the air sinuses or in the intracranial cavity indicate a fracture and dural tear (Fig. 1). Location of the spicule of bone responsible for the dural tear in the anterior fossa can sometimes be located by stereoscopy or by reformatted computed tomography (see below) (Fig. 2).

Intracranial air

An aerocoele indicates a fracture and dural tear.

Note: whilst most fractures heal within 2-3 years the inclusion of arachnoid in a non-healing fracture can give rise to a lepto meningeal cyst which expands with CSF pulsation giving rise to a "growing fracture". The cyst may be porencephalic, i.e. in communication

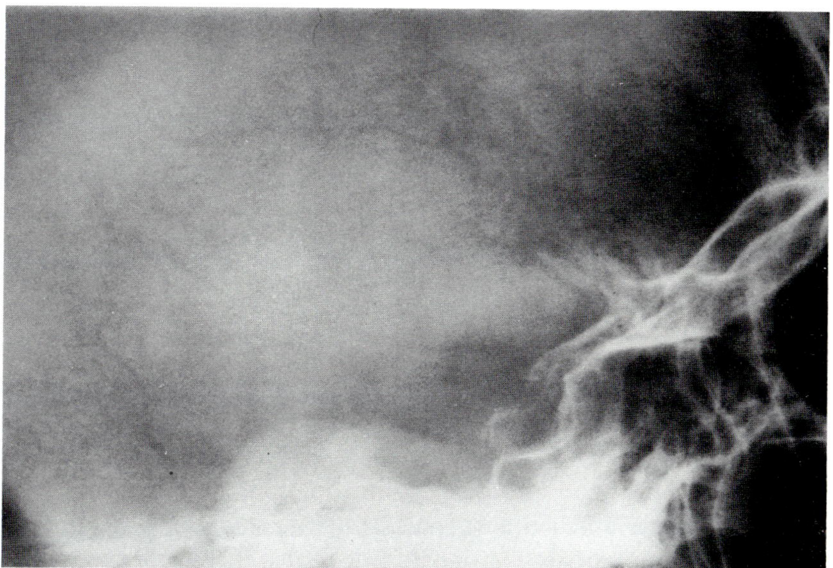

Figure 1. *Brow up lateral skull radiograph demonstrating fluid level in the sphenoidal air sinus.*

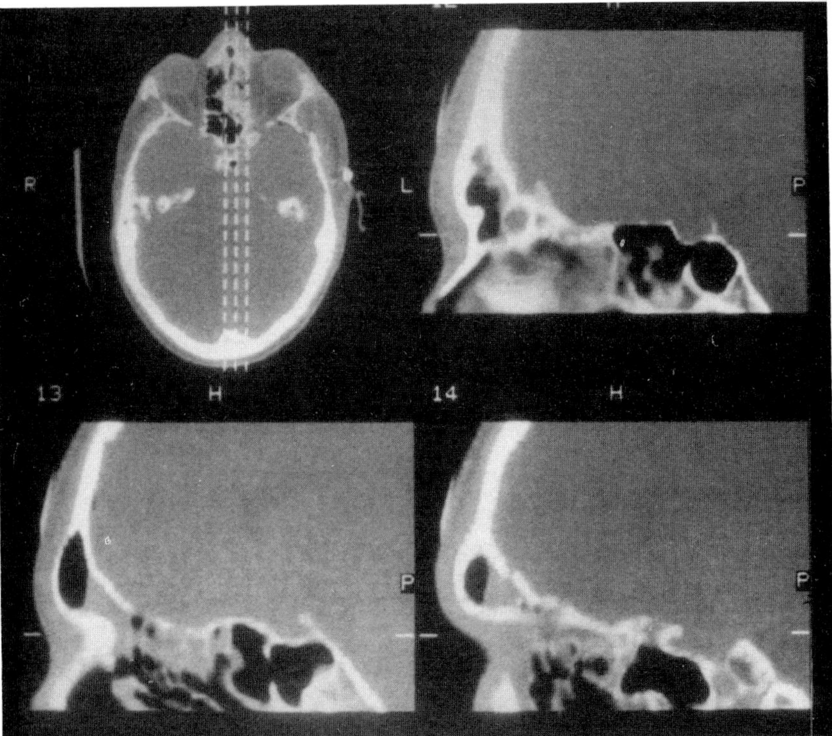

Figure 2. *Computed Tomography sagittal reformatted images demonstrating a comminuted fracture of the floor of the anterior cranial fossa. A fluid level is present in the frontal sinus.*

with the cerebral ventricles. A growing fracture is characterized by sclerotic or scolloped margins (Fig. 3).

Computed Tomography (CT)

The advent of CT in 1973 opened new opportunities for the investigation of head injuries and replaced the indirect technique of ventriculography. CT is now the most important modality for the investigation of head injuries, permitting direct visualisation of brain, meninges and skull [11,12,13]. The availability of general purpose scanners provides opportunities for the general radiologist as well as the neuroradiologist to investigate head injuries and to be involved in the management decisions.

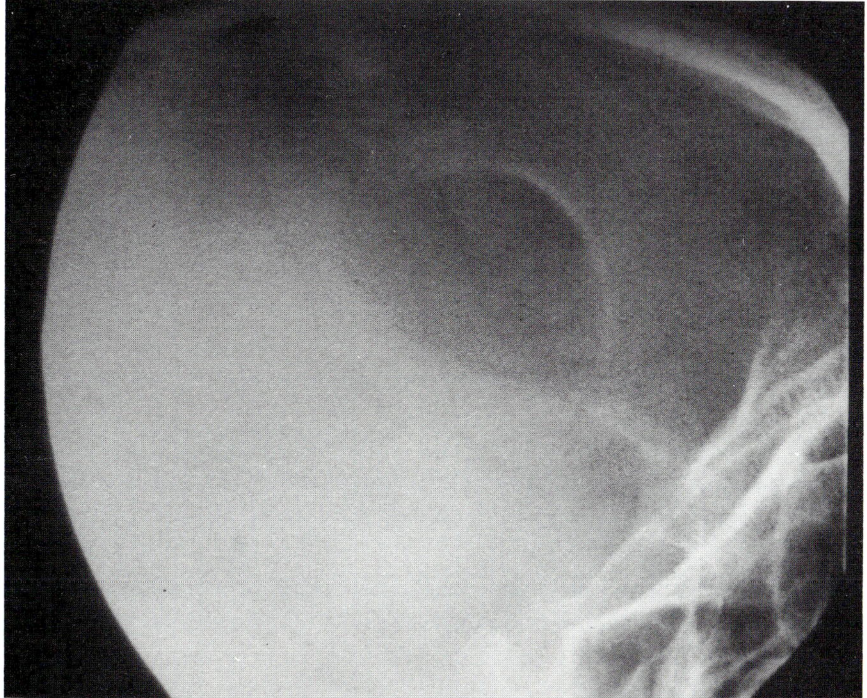

Figure 3. *"Growing fracture" due to inclusion of arachnoid in a non-healing fracture. Note the sclerotic margin anteriorly.*

The conventional technique of CT is to obtain contiguous 5-10 mm trans-axial sections from the foramen magnum to the skull vault. A dynamic scan technique can be employed with thinner sections (1.5-3 mm) and low radiographic factors (200-140 mAs) to enable alternative plane reformats to be obtained. Three-dimensional presentation of this data can be of value in the assessment of complex facial and skull base injuries [14]. A similar technique with special bone algorithms is valuable in the more detailed investigation of the petrous bones and ossicular chain.

CT features in acute head injury

Attenuation of X-rays is influenced by the atomic number and the electron density of tissue and the effective energy of the X-ray beam. Bone, calcium and iodinated contrast media contain high atomic number elements and therefore have a high attenuation. Fresh blood and hematoma also have high attenuation, i.e. high density [15,16], but due to the presence of the macromolecule hemoglobin which gives rise to a high electron density. There is insufficient high atomic number calcium or iron in blood to affect the attenuation. If the hematocrit is low or there is disseminated intravascular coagulation (DIC), a hematological abnormality resulting from pathological activation of the blood clotting enzymes within fresh blood, a hematoma may not be of high attenuation but instead, isodense or even lower density than surrounding brain. DIC occurs in 30-56% of patients who have head trauma and its presence is a significant risk factor for death. In normal circumstances a high attenuation of blood clot is observed during the first 48 hours. As hemoglobin is redistributed hematoma becomes isodense with its surroundings within 10-14 days and hypodense thereafter. Any recurrent bleeding will give rise to a mixed attenuation.

Extra Axial

All extra axial collections are characterized by displacement inwards of the gray white interface.

Subdural hematoma

Subdural hematoma is the commonest post-traumatic intracranial hemorrhage. It is normally of high attenuation and crescent shaped, usually over the hemisphere but may extend to a para falcine subtentorial or suboccipital location. There is usually a mid line displacement with ipsilateral ventricular compression and contralateral dilatation due to brain rotation (Fig. 4).

An acute isodense subdural hematoma is less common and may only be detectable by a mid line displacement (Fig. 5). Homogeneous enhancement may be obtained with intravenous contrast agents [17]. In general contrast enhancement in head injuries is unwise because of the risk of extravasation of hypermolar and chemotoxic material into neural tissue. If undertaken at all it should be with low volumes of low osmolar non-ionic contrast medium.

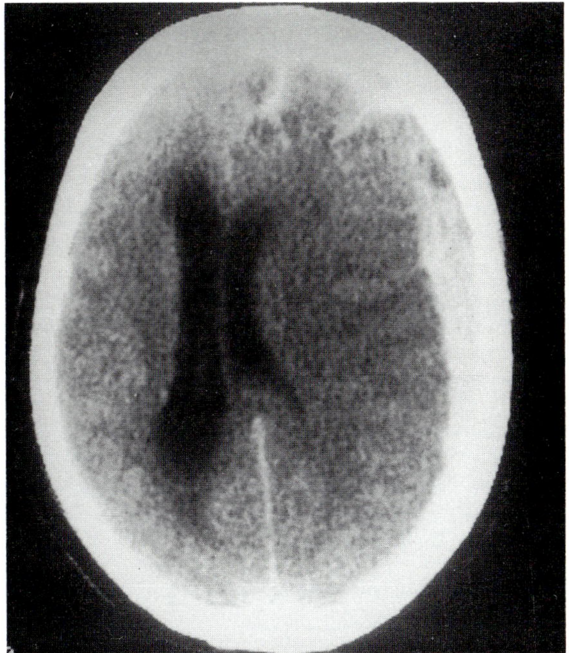

Figure 4. *Crescentic subdural hematoma of high attenuation with displacement of the gray/white interface and the mid-line.*

Bilateral isodense subdural hematomata can be difficult to detect in the absence of mid line displacement. A characteristic feature is bilateral symmetrical compression of the anterior cerebral ventricles which appear like "rabbit ears" (Fig. 6).

Chronic subdural hematomas are of low attenuation (Fig. 7) but may be altered by rebleeding to a mixed attenuation with the presence of fluid levels. "Silent" subdural hygromas occur frequently following head injuries [18]. They are crescentic extra cerebral collections extending over both hemispheres and involving the inter hemispheric fissure. Major cortical sulci are preserved. The mechanism is thought to be due to a tear in the arachnoid with a one way valve allowing CSF to enter the subdural space (Fig. 8).

Extradural hematoma

Extradural hematomas are normally of high attenuation and lenticular in shape. They are the direct result of tearing of meningeal

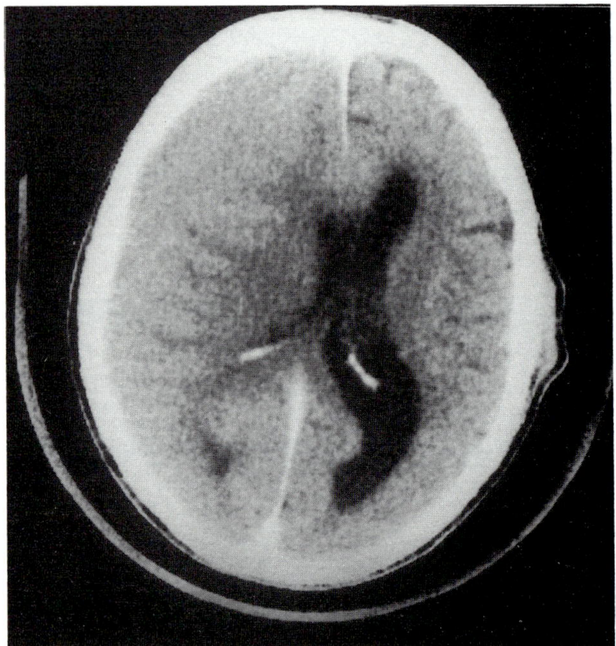

Figure 5. *Acute isodense subdural hematoma with mid-line displacement. Note the inward displacement of the gray/white interface.*

vessels. They are classically over the convexities but may be less easy to appreciate in the posterior fossa and the floor of the temporal fossa. They are almost always associated with a fracture. Extradural hematomas, by stripping the dura off the inner table of the skull vault, may give rise to a fibrotic and thickened dura which enhances with intravenous contrast. Ossification can occur in a relatively short time, e.g. 5-6 months.

Intra Axial

Contusions

Contusions or bruises are due to contact between the brain and the skull. They can appear at sites remote from blunt injury, i.e. contre-coup, or by deceleration effects. They are typically located in the frontal and temporal poles. They are of mixed attenuation due to high density blood and edema. They are subcortical and may involve white matter.

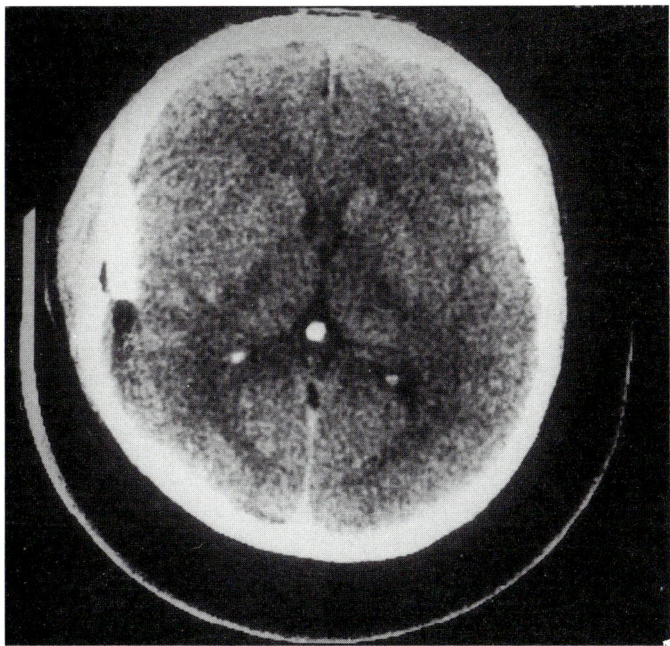

Figure 6. *Bilateral compression of the anterior cerebral ventricles (rabbit ears) due to bilateral isodense subdural hematomas at a higher level. Note depressed fracture on the right.*

Intracerebral hemorrhage

Intraparenchymal hemorrhage is due to blood vessel rupture and indistinguishable from spontaneous hemorrhage (Fig. 9). Indeed if no convincing clinical or radiological evidence of head injury can be detected angiography may be required to exclude a primary vascular lesion, e.g. angioma. Intracerebral hemorrhages are normally of high attenuation with surrounding low attenuation edema. They progress to iso- and subsequently hypodensity. Intracranial hemorrhages may be delayed, occuring secondary to a contusion, to resuscitation procedures, or post operatively.

"Shearing" injury

Severe brain deformity due to shearing forces can give rise to axial or axonal tears characteristically of the gray white interfaces [19,20].

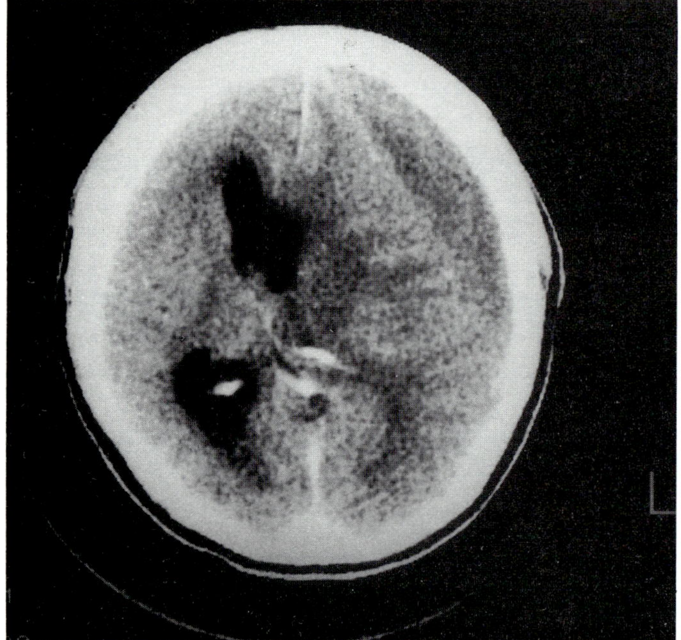

Figure 7. *Chronic subdural hematoma of low attenuation with mid-line displacement and rotation of the brain.*

Axonal tears are associated with ruptured blood vessels. Hematomas are therefore multiple from minor to those exerting mass effects at typical sites which include gray/white junction zones centrally and peripherally, the corpus callosum and the cerebral peduncles. Diffuse axonal injury is associated with a poor prognosis (Fig. 10) [21].

Intraventricular hemorrhage

Intraventricular hemorrhage is usually secondary to shearing and associated with a poor prognosis.

Subarachnoid hemorrhage

Subarachnoid hemorrhage is common particularly in infants and the elderly. It may be the only sign of head injury. When observed in a parafalcine location in infants non-accidental injury should be suspected [22].

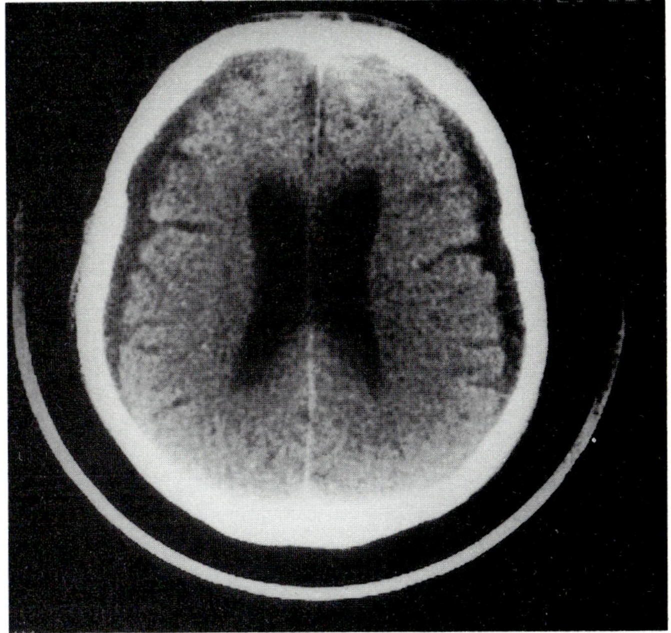

Figure 8. *Bilateral subdural hygromas. Cortical sulci well preserved.*

Brain swelling

Brain swelling is due to venous engorgement and edema. When generalized it gives rise to compression of the cerebral ventricles but small changes may be difficult to assess especially in children. Dilatation of the contralateral ventricle with mid line shift is due to brain rotation, raised intracranial pressure and tentorial herniation. Focal brain swelling is associated with zones of low attenuation and compartmental displacements.

Ischemia

A typical location of ischemia is in the occipital lobe due to posterior cerebral artery compression at the tentorium by herniated brain. Infarction is characterized by an area of low attenuation. Other areas of ischemia can be found at boundary zones between the anterior middle cerebral arteries and the middle and posterior cerebral arteries. The areas are often ill defined.

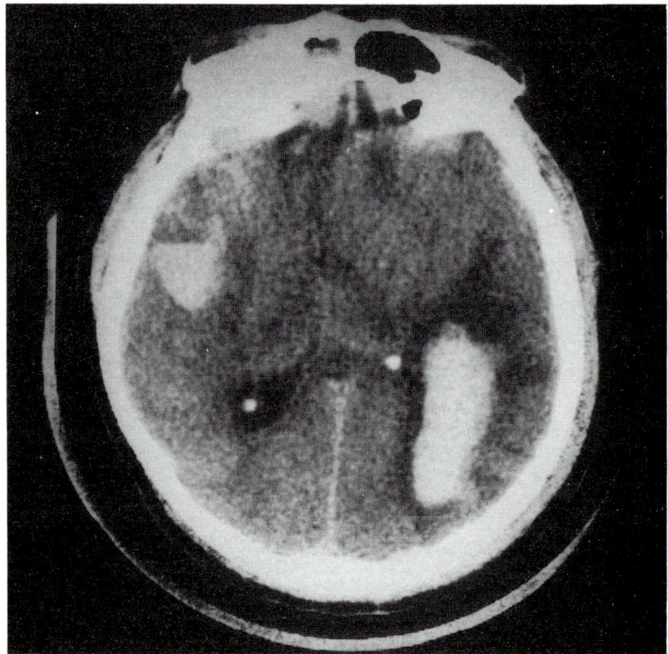

Figure 9. *Bilateral intracerebral hemorrhages. Note fluid level on the right.*

Brain Stem

Brain stem injuries are either (i) primary due to local or contrecoup injuries or to lateral herniation, or (ii) secondary following development of a supratentorial mass. The secondary damage is due to rotational and compressive forces giving rise to brain stem vascular damage (Fig. 11). These are the events which kill patients or give rise to serious disability and are sometimes preventable. Obliteration of the contralateral mesenchymal cisterns and contralateral temporal horn widening [23] due to transtentorial herniation may be detectable (Fig. 12).

Chronic sequel angle of head injuries

Gliosis

Gliosis occurs secondary to contusions and intracerebral hemorrhage and is characterised by areas of low attenuation at the site of these lesions (Fig. 13).

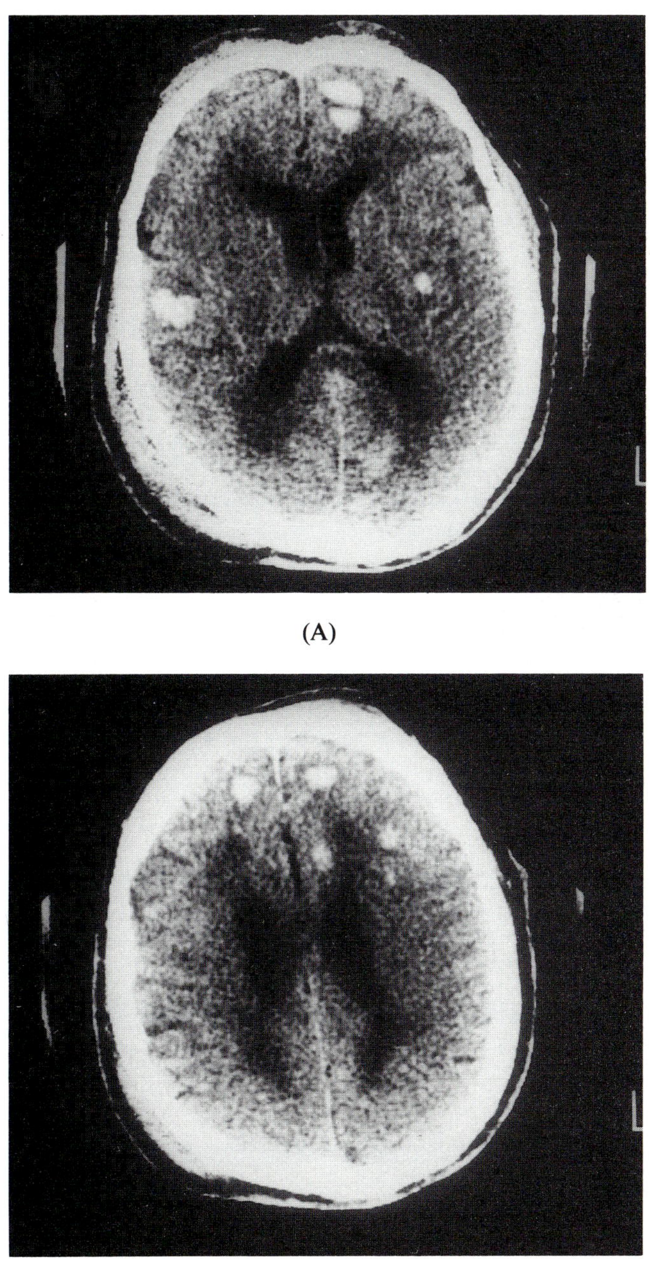

(A)

(B)

Figure 10. (A) *and* (B). *Diffuse axonal injury characterized by multiple hematomas at gray/white junction zones.*

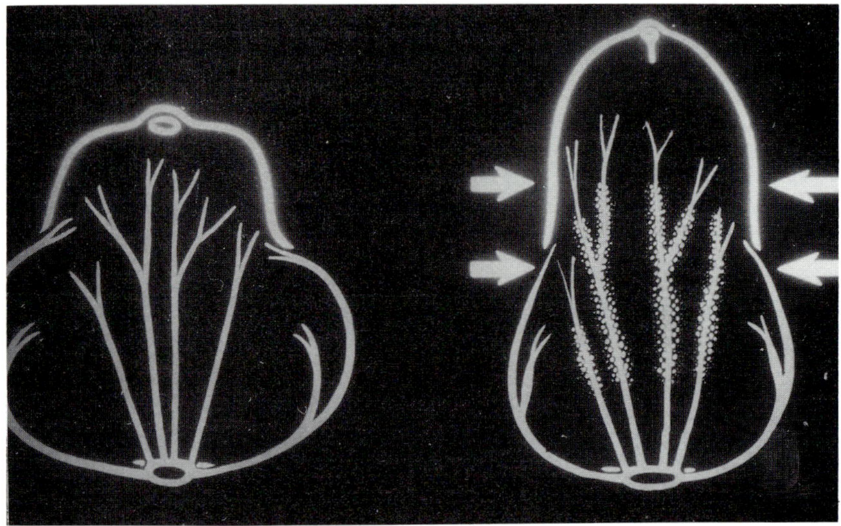

Figure 11. *Diagrammatic representation of tentorial compressive forces giving rise to rupture of brain stem blood vessels.*

Cerebral atrophy

Cerebral atrophy may commence within 4-6 months of a head injury and be progressive with ventricular dilatation and expanded cortical salcae.

Absorption mechanism defect

Dementia following head injury can be due to malabsorption of CSF. The cortical salci are usually absent due to adhesive arachnoiditis with associated dilatation of the cerebral ventricles. This so-called "normal pressure hydrocephalus" can be demonstrated by a reversal of CSF flow into the lateral ventricles with retention of subarachnoid water soluble contrast media or radionuclide for up to 48 hours.

Carotid cavernous fistulae

Carotid cavernous fistulae can occur with or without a basal fracture due to rupture of the carotid artery directly into the cavernous sinus [24]. Pulsating exophthalmos is usually ipsi- and unilateral but

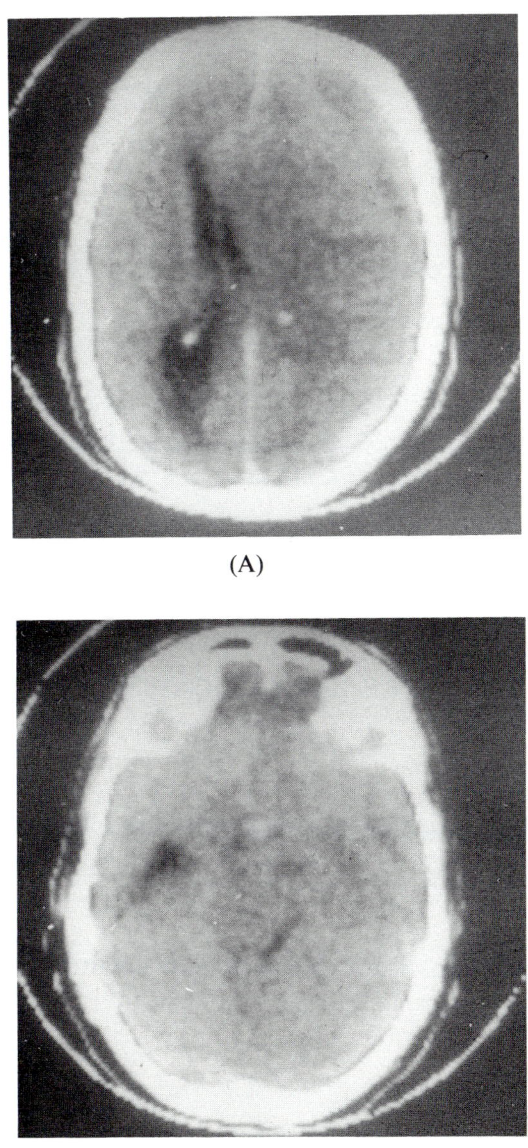

(A)

(B)

Figure 12. *Mixed attenuation subdural collection giving rise to (A) displacement and rotation of brain, (B) obliteration of the contralateral ambient cistern. Note dilatation of contralateral temple horn.*

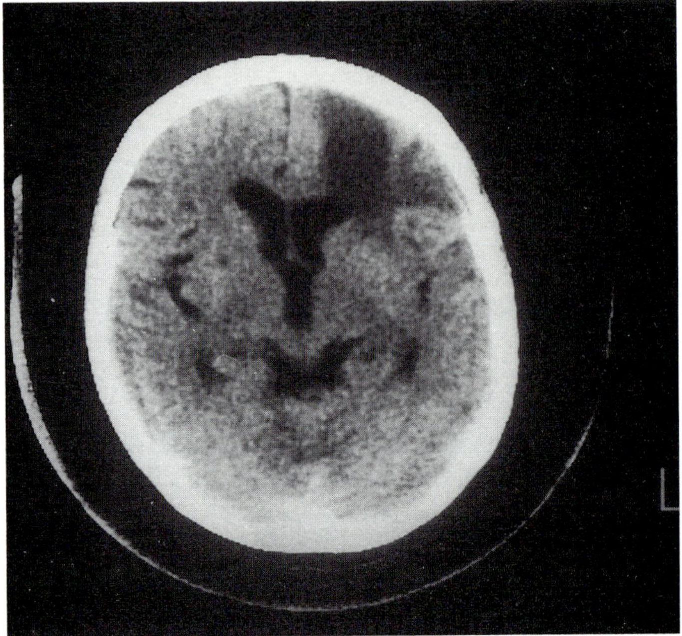

Figure 13. *Low attenuation gliosis secondary to frontal lobe intracerebral hemorrhage.*

may be contralateral or even bilateral. Pituitary and hypothalamic dysfunction may be associated features. Treatment is radiological by balloon embolization (Fig. 14).

Unilateral deafness

Dislocation of the ossicle can give rise to unilateral deafness. The appearance is a characteristic on high resolution thin section bone algorithm CT. The condition is eminently treatable.

Angiography

Intracranial cerebral angiography

Intracranial cerebral angiography for intracranial lesions has been largely superseded by CT. Mass lesions, both intra and extra-cerebral, can be located by typical vascular displacements or the

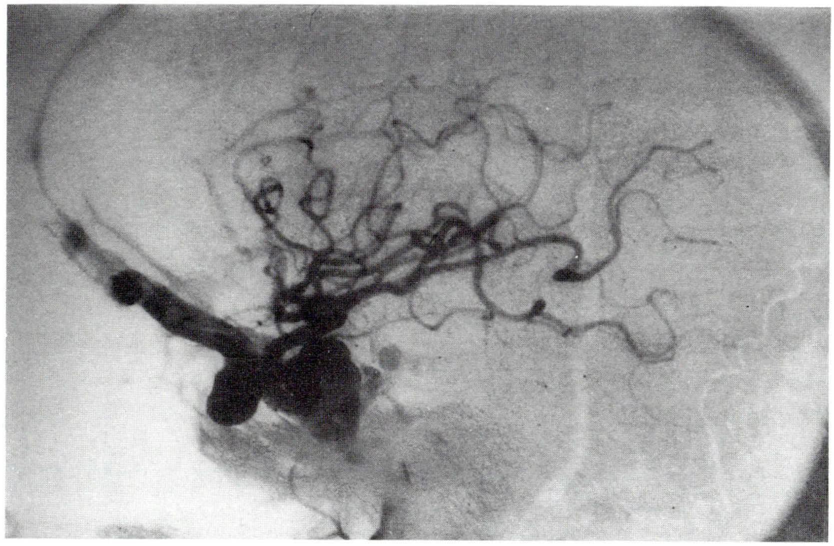

Figure 14. *Carotid cavernous fistula due to rupture of the carotid artery directly into the cavernous sinus with retrograde filling of the superior ophthalmic vein.*

presence of avascular zones. Pseudoaneurysms may reveal the source of the hemorrhage (Fig. 15).

Angiography is mandatory in the investigation of fistulae, e.g. carotid cavernous fistulae, in particular prior to balloon embolization.

Cervical

Both direct trauma to the neck and deceleration injuries can give rise to carotid artery damage with dissection or occlusion [25]. Pseudoaneurysms may also occur. The commonest sites of such injuries are those where the artery is subject to stress from adjacent structures such as the dura or the entry point into the petrous bone at the skull base (Fig. 16).

Magnetic resonance imaging

The role of Magnetic Resonance Imaging in the management of acute head injuries is still limited. This reflects both the availability

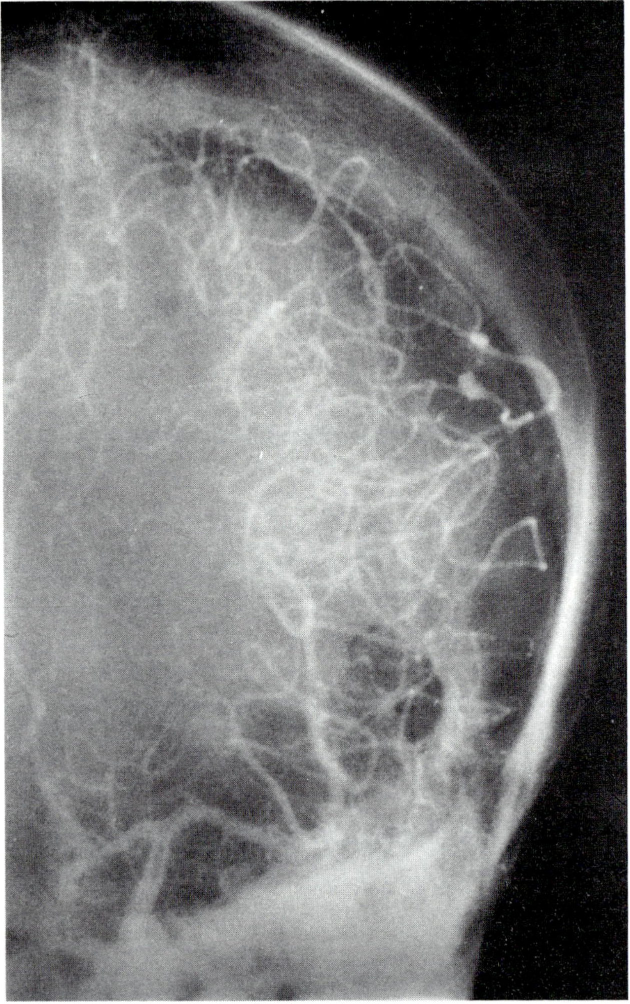

Figure 15. *Pseudoaneurysm on the medial aspect of an avascular subdural hematoma.*

of the facility and the problems related to provision of life support systems in a magnetic field [26,27,28,29].

Magnetic Resonance Imaging is concerned with determining the distribution of hydrogen in biological tissue. Hydrogen is found in great abundance in human tissue in both water and fat. Since hydrogen with a single proton at its nucleus is both electrically charged and spinning it creates its own magnetic field and is there-

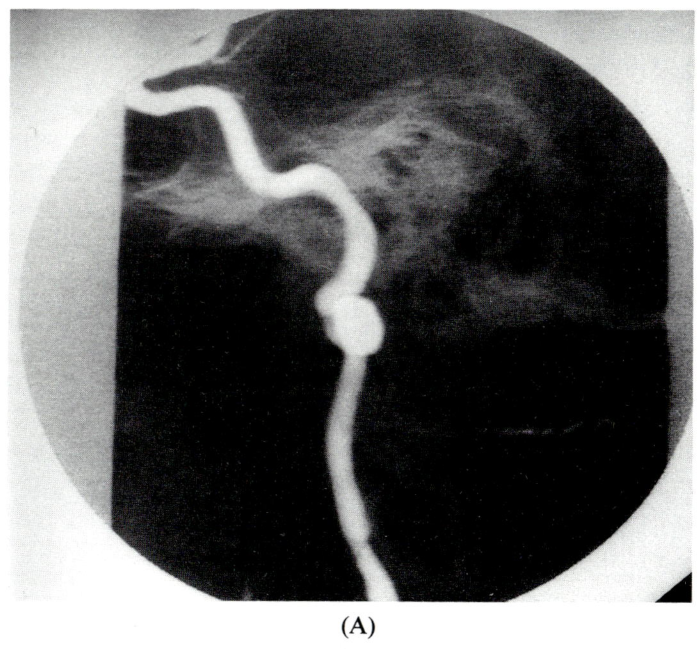

(A)

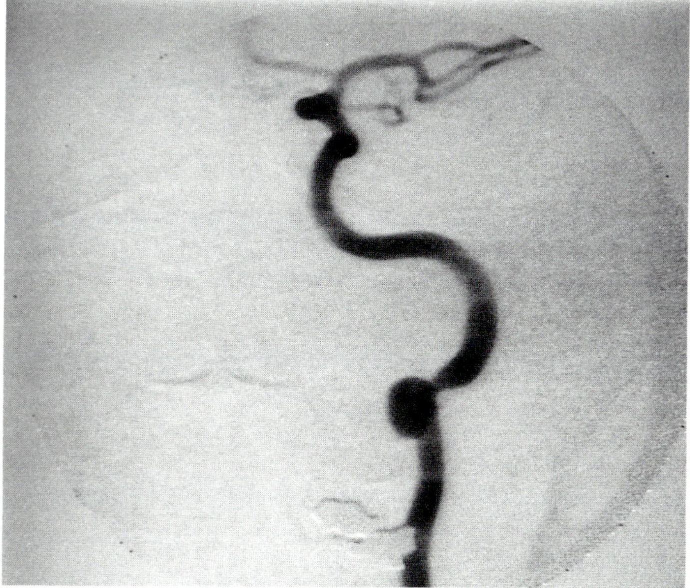

(B)

Figure 16. *Internal carotid artery dissection and pseudoaneurysm at the skull base due to a deceleration injury. (A) Conventional angiogram. (B) Digital subtraction.*

fore influenced by the large magnetic field of the imaging system into which it is placed. Radio frequency pulses are applied to perturb this influence briefly. Magnetic relocation of the hydrogen atoms provides a signal from which an image can be created. The speed with which magnetic relocation occurs is a function of two tissue parameters - the relaxation times T1 and T2. Other tissue parameters which influence the image include proton density, i.e. the number of hydrogen atoms present, blood flow, diffusion, perfusion and chemical shift, i.e. the difference in distribution of hydrogen between water and fat. Variations in the radiofrequency pulse applied to perturb the hydrogen atoms can produce profound changes in image contrast. Particular advantages of MRI are the lack of ionizing radiation and the facility to obtain thin sections in any plane, orthogonal or oblique. The principal disadvantages of MRI in the management of head injuries include the magnetic materials in life support systems and the limited access to a scarce facility.

MRI intrinsically is more sensitive than CT to the detection of soft tissue changes. The interpretation of MR images is more complex than CT because of the variations introduced by differing pulse sequences. Nevertheless the pathophysiological principles and the morphological changes to be anticipated in acute head injuries apply to both CT and MRI.

Contraindications to MRI include metallic foreign bodies, particularly aneurysm clips. Non-ferrous materials are helpful but may not eliminate magnetic effects entirely. Electrical implants, e.g. cochlea implants, are a contraindication, together with cardiac pacemakers.

Interpretation of MR images

On T1 weighted images the CSF and gray matter are dark whilst white matter is bright. On T2 weighted images CSF and grey matter are bright whilst white matter is dark. In proton density images both grey and white matter are bright and CSF is dark. T1 weighted images can be produced either by spin echo or inversion recovery sequences.

Intracranial hemorrhage

Whereas in CT the presence or absence of hemoglobin influences the attenuation values, in Magnetic Resonance Imaging the whole evolution and natural history of the hematoma can be studied in a characteristic sequence of signal intensity patterns [30,31].

● Very acute stage, i.e. first 1-2 hours

At this stage, signal intensities reflect an increased water and protein content. Signal intensity is decreased on T1 weighted and increased on T2 weighted images.

● Acute, i.e. 2-12 hours

Serum is absorbed and oxyhemoglobin is reduced to deoxyhemoglobin at a rate dependent on the local oxygen tension and pH. The hematoma is isointense on T1 weighted images and has a reduced signal intensity on T2 weighted images. At this stage the hematoma is surrounded by absorbed serum and vasogenic edema, represented by a low signal rim on T1 weighted images and a high signal rim on T2 weighted images.

● Sub-acute stage (3 days to 1 month)

Methemoglobin forms about day 3 but is established within 1 week to 1 month. It occurs first as a peripheral ring which extends inwards to involve the entire hematoma. The typical appearance is then that of high signal intensity on both T1 weighted and T2 weighted images (Fig. 17).

● Chronic hemorrhage (1 month onwards)

Hemoglobin is broken down at this stage by macrophages which sequester hemosiderin and persist indefinitely in the hematoma periphery. This is detectable as a ring of low or isointensity signal on T1 weighted images and a low signal on T2 weighted images (Fig. 18). During this time edema becomes less well demarcated and the hypo and hyperintensity of the edema on T1 and T2 weighted images resolves over 1-3 months. Reduction in edema and loss

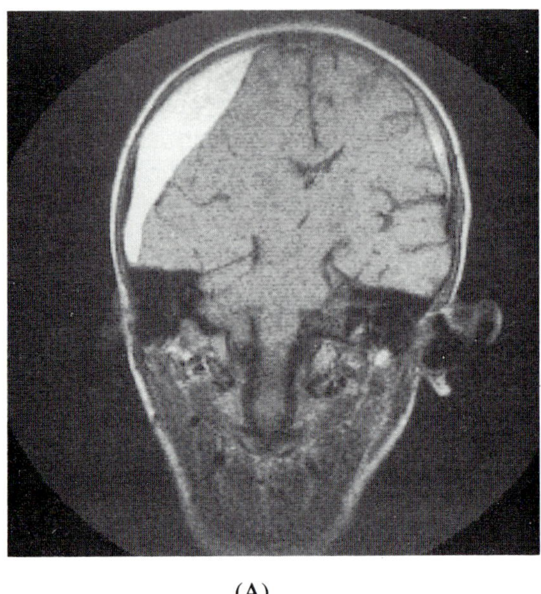

(A)

(B)

Figure 17. *Magnetic Resonance Imaging bilateral subdural hematomas. (A) T1 weighted image. (B) Coronal T2 weighted image. Note high signal on both sequences.*

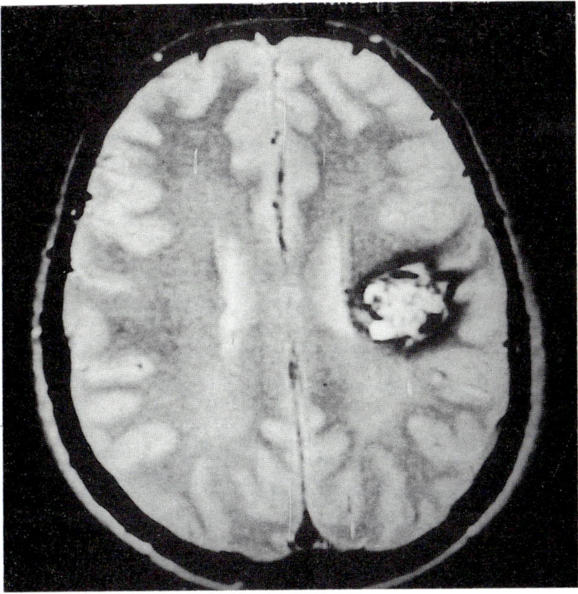

Figure 18. *Magnetic Resonance T2 weighted transverse section. Intracerebral hematoma with peripheral ring of low signal due to hemosiderin.*

of mass effect occurs within 1-3 months and gives rise to either gliosis and/or CSF filled cavities.

Subdural and extradural hematomas behave similarly, though their appearance may be modified by a decreased resorption of serum and varying degrees of liquefaction. Non-paramagnetic hemiochromes form instead of hemosiderin, giving a decreased signal intensity compared to that of the sub-acute stage. Direct alternative plane imaging is of particular value in demonstrating extracerebral collections.

Selected References

1. Hadley DM. Head Trauma. Contrast Imaging 1991;3:64-73.
2. Teasdale G, Jennett B. Assessment of coma and impaired consciousness: a practical side. Lancet 1974;ii:81-84.
3. Mendelow AD. Head injuries. Current Imaging in Neurology and Neurosurgey 1988;1:37-45.
4. Teasdale GM, Murray G, Anderson E, et al. Risks of acute intracranial haematoma in children and adults: implications for managing head injuries. Br Med J 1990;300:363-367.

5. Royal College of Radiologists. A study of the utilization of skull radiography in nine accident and emergency units in the UK. Lancet 1980;2:1234-1236.

6. Masters SI et al. Skull X-ray examination after head trauma: recommendations by a multidisciplinary panel and validation study. N Eng J Med 1987;316:84-91.

7. Fowkes FGR, Ennis WP, Evans RC, Roberts CJ, Williams LA. Admission guidelines for head injuries: Variance with clinical procedure in accident and emergency units in the UK. BJ Surg 1986;73:891-893.

8. Clarke JA, Adams JE. A critical appraisal of "out of hours" radiography in a major teaching hospital. BJR 1988;61:1100-1105.

9. Clarke JA, Adams JE. The Application of Clinical Guidelines for Skull Radiography in the Accident and Emergency Departments. Theory and Practice. Clin Rad 1990;41:152-155.

10. de Lacey G, McCabe M, Constant O, Welsh T, Spinks C, McNally E. Testing a policy for skull radiography (and admission) following mild head injury. Br J Radiol 1990;63:14-18.

11. Van Dongen K, Braakman R, Gelpke G. The prognostic value of computerised tomography in comatose head-injured patients. J Neurosurg 1984;59:951-957.

12. Teasdale E, Cardoso E, Galbraith S, Teasdale G. CT scan in severe diffuse head injury: physiological and clinical correlations. J Neurol Neurosurg Psychiatry 1984;47:600-603.

13. Zimmermann RA, Bilaniuk L, Dolinskas C. Computed tomography of acute intracranial haemorrhage contusion. Axial tomogr 1977;1:271-280.

14. Gillespie JE, Quayle, Barker J, Isherwood I. JDCT Reformations in the assessment of congenital and traumatic cranio-facial deformations. B.J. Oral. Maxillofacial Surgery, 1987;25:171-177.

15. Eisenberg HM, Gary HE, Aldrich EF, et al. Initial CT findings in 753 patients with severe head injury: A report from the NIH traumatic coma data bank. J Neurosurgery 1990;73:688-698.

16. Paterson OF, Esperson JO. How to distinguish between bleeding and coagulated and extradural haematomas on plain CT scanning. Neuroradiol 1984;26:285-292.

17. Boyko DB, Cooper DF, Grossman CB. Contrast enhanced CT of Acute Isodense Subdural Haematoma. AJNR 1991;12:341-343.

18. Masuzawa T, Kumagai M, Sato F, et al. CT evaluation of post traumatic subdural hygroma in young adults. Neuroradiology 1984;26:245-248.

19. Zimmermann RA, Bilaniuk LT, Generali T. Computed tomography of shearing injuries of the cerebral white matter. Radiology 1978;127:393-396.

20. Levi L, Guilbund JN, Lemburger A, Soustiel JF, Feinsod M. Diffuse axonal injury: analysis/100 patients with radiological signals. Neurosurgery 1990;27:429-432.

21. MacPherson P, Teasdale E, Dhaker S, Allardyce G, Galbraith S. The significance of traumatic haematoma in the region of the basal ganglia. J Neurol Neurosurg Psychiatry 1986;49:29-34.

22. Cohen RA, Kaufman RA, Myers PA, Towbin A. Cranial computed tomography in the abused child with head injury. Am J Neuroradiol 1985;6:883-888.

23. Stovring J. Contralateral temporal horn widening in unilateral supratentorial mass lesions: a diagnostic sign indicating tentorial herniation. J Comput Assist Tomogr 1977;1:319-323.

24. Corradino G, Wolf AL, Mirvis S, Joslyn J. Trauma of the clivus : classification and clinical features. Neurosurgery 1990;27:592-596.

25. Morgan MK, Besser M, Johnstone I, Chaseling R. Intracranial carotid artery injury in closed head trauma. J Neurosurg 1987;66:192-197.

26. Zimmerman RA, Bilaniuk LT, Hackncy DB, Goldberg HI, Grossman RI. Head injury: early results of comparing CT and high-field MR. Am J Neuroradiol 1986;1:757-764.

27. Jenkins A, Teasdale G, Hadley DM, MacPherson P, Rown JO. Brain lesions detected by magnetic resonance imaging in mild and severe head injuries. Lancet 1986;2:445-446.
28. Bydder GM, Steiner RE, Young IR. Low-field MR imaging of intra-cerebral haemorrhage. Radiol 1986;161:350.
29. Hadley DM, Teasdale GM, Jenkins A, et al. Magnetic resonance imaging in acute head injury. Clin Radiol 1988;39:131-139.
30. Gomori JM, Grossman RI. Head and neck haemorrhage. In: HY Kressel, ed. Magnetic resonance annual. New York, Raven Press 1987;71-112.
31. Winkler ML, Olsen WL, Mills TC, Kaufman L. Hemorrhagic and nonhemorrhagic brain lesions: evaluation with 0.35-T fast MR imaging. Radiology 1987;165:203-207.

Pituitary Gland and Parasellar Lesions: MRI Evaluation

Giuseppe Scotti
Servizio de Neuroradiologica, Ospedale San Raffaele, Milano, Italy

Introduction

Diagnosis of sellar and parasellar lesions has significantly changed with the advent of CT: plain films of the sella, polytomography and pneumoencephalography were completely abandoned in the seventies to the advantage of CT. MRI is now almost completely replacing CT.

This revolution is the result of the exquisite depiction of anatomy of the pituitary and of the sella region provided by MR [1,2].

In fact, understanding of the pathology of this region requires the knowledge of the complex anatomy of nervous, bony, vascular and meningeal systems and structures. The close relationship of all these components in less than 5 cubic centimeters explains why symptoms of lesions in this area involve neuroendocrine functions as well as vision, oculomotion, vascular supply of the brain, face sensitivity, complex behavioral patterns.

Not only can MRI visualize at the same time bone, endocrine and brain parenchyma, subarachnoid spaces and vessels, but it is also sensitive to functional changes due to endocrine activity. The different signal of the neurohypophysis, markedly hyperintense with respect to the adenohypophysis reflects the specific hormonal activity related to the production of vasopressin and oxytocin [3].

MRI Technique

Although MR has a much better contrast resolution than CT, the best spatial resolution offered by the machines must also be obtained.

The best signal to noise ratio obtained with high field super-conducting magnets (1.5T) thin slices (3 mm or less), matrix sizes 256 x 256, four acquisitions, field of view 16 cm.

Two orthogonal imaging planes, coronal and sagittal are sufficient for a complete and detailed demonstration of the anatomy of the region.

The pulse sequences that we use routinely for demonstration of the pituitary are T1W spin echo (short TR, short TE); T2W spin echo (long TR, long TE) may be used to better define the structural characteristics of large supra- of parasellar lesions. The use of Gd-DTPA however, provides most of the information regarding solid versus cystic components. 3DFT gradient echo images may represent a valid alternative to T1W SE.

Development and Normal Anatomy

Not only does the size of the pituitary change with age, as it may be expected, but also the signal intensity of the adenohypophysis varies in the first month of life. The pituitary gland is histologically composed of three different parts: anterior, intermediate and posterior lobes. While the intermediate lobe is physiologically irrelevant, anterior and posterior lobes are very active structures with, however, very different functions, reflected in their anatomy and also in signal characteristics.

The anterior lobe, or adenohypophysis, originates from an upward invagination of the Rathke's pouch and is of ectodermal origin. The posterior lobe, or neurohypophysis, is a downward extension of nervous structures from the hypothalamus. The neurohypophysis is directly connected to the hypothalamus through the pituitary stalk, and functions as a storage of antidiuretic hormones secreted in the hypothalamus and sent to the neuro-hypophysis through the pituitary stalk. The anterior lobe is an endocrine organ secreting hormones under stimulation from hypothalamus through releasing factors [4,5,6,7].

The pituitary gland is well seen in the coronal images and in the midline sagittal (Fig. 1); it is a small (about 0.5 gm in weight) ovoid structure with a shape varying with age. In young persons, particularly females, the superior margin is convex upward while in adults it is usually flat or concave. The dimensions vary from 12 mm in width, 8 mm in anteroposterior diameter and 3 to 8 mm in height.

In newborns also the anterior pituitary is hyperintense giving the pituitary gland a bright homogenous appearance. The hyperintensity of the anterior pituitary in the newborn is maximal in the first few days and rapidly decreases to become isointense to the brain parenchyma within 45 days from birth [8,9].

The precise reason for this hyperintensity is still controversial as that for the posterior pituitary. It could be due to the remarkable increase in protein synthetic activity of the newborn's pituitary.

In adults the two parts of the pituitary are easily recognizable on MR: the adenohypophysis is isointense while the neurohypophysis is hyperintense.

Above the pituitary gland and in front of the stalk lies the optic chiasm within the CSF of the suprasellar subarachnoid space.

Laterally to the pituitary are the two cavernous sinuses containing the cranial nerves III, IV, VI and the first branch of the V.

The cavernous sinus markedly enhances following intravenous administration of Gadolinium.

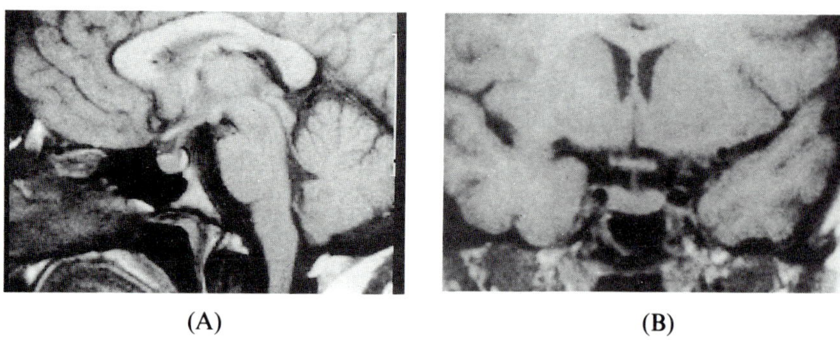

(A)   (B)

Figure 1. *NORMAL PITUITARY GLAND. (A) Sagittal view: the adenohypophysis is isointense, situated anteriorly to the crescentic hyperintense neurohypophysis. (B) Coronal view: the pituitary stalk is midline; the horizontal optic chiasm is well demonstrated.*

Pathology

Pituitary Hypoplasia and GH Deficiency

One of the most subtle and interesting "discoveries" of MR, hypoplasia of the pituitary with absent pituitary stalk, had been described in the past on the basis of CT findings but did not receive adequate attention [10,11]. A very common finding in pituitary dwarfs with GH deficiency, some authors considered the CT picture as representing an "empty sella" with secondary compression of the pituitary parenchyma and hormonal deficiency; for others, the presence of excessive CSF within the sella reflected primary hypoplasia of the pituitary gland, sometimes associated with anomalies of the pituitary stalk [12].

To verify with MR which of the two hypothesis was more correct and whether the "empty sella" could really be responsible for growth retardation in children, in 1987 we studied 5 consecutive children with GH deficiency. We found an anomaly of the pituitary stalk characterized by an ectopic higher position of the hyperintensity of the neurohypophysis, an absent stalk and an hypoplastic anterior lobe in all children [13] (Fig. 2). We concluded that empty sella was not a true or common entity in children, responsible for GH deficiency and that it was an epiphenomenon of a much more complex situation [14]. The same entity was described by two other groups; they proposed birth trauma as the cause of what they considered to be a transection of the stalk and

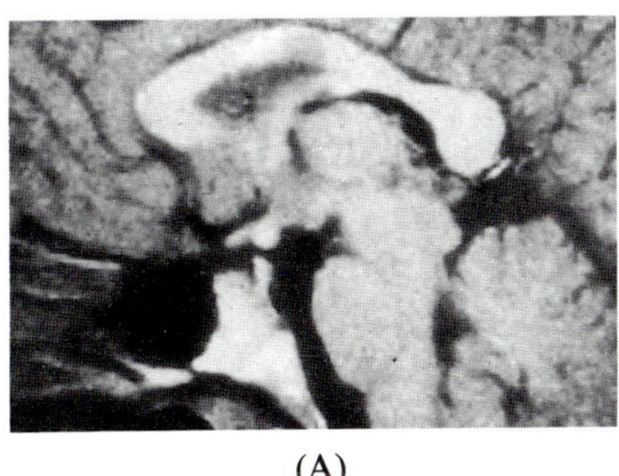
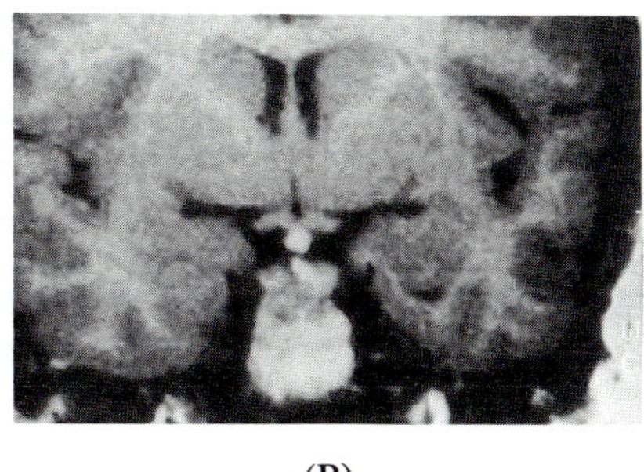

(A)   (B)

Figure 2. *DWARFISM. Ectopic posterior pituitary hyperintensity and absent stalk in a GH deficient dwarf. (A) Sagittal. (B) Coronal. The adenohypophysis is hypoplastic.*

separation from the anterior pituitary, due to the high number of abnormal or traumatic deliveries in these patients [15,16].

We think that this situation most likely represents an equivalent of a genetically determined disraphic state at the level of the fusion between neuroectoderm and Rathke's cleft ectoderm. The high proportion of patients with stalk abnormalities without traumatic delivery and vice versa, is in favor of this hypothesis as well as the high proportion of associated other midline anomalies. The high proportion of breech presentations could reflect endocrine abnormalities already present before birth, that could prevent a regular foetus presentation [17].

Diabetes Insipidus

Diabetes insipidus (DI) is a functional condition that may be idiopathic or caused by a variety of pathological situations, inflammatory or neoplastic. The most common cause of secondary diabetes insipidus is histiocytosis X.

In a study on 20 patients with clinical diagnosis of DI [18] we could not recognize the hyperintensity of the neurohypophysis in any patient (Fig. 3). In 7 patients morphological abnormalities of the hypothalamus and stalk were found suggesting a secondary DI, mainly due to histiocytosis. In the others the diagnosis was of primary DI. In two patients with psychogenic DI the hyperintensity of the neurohypophysis was normally present.

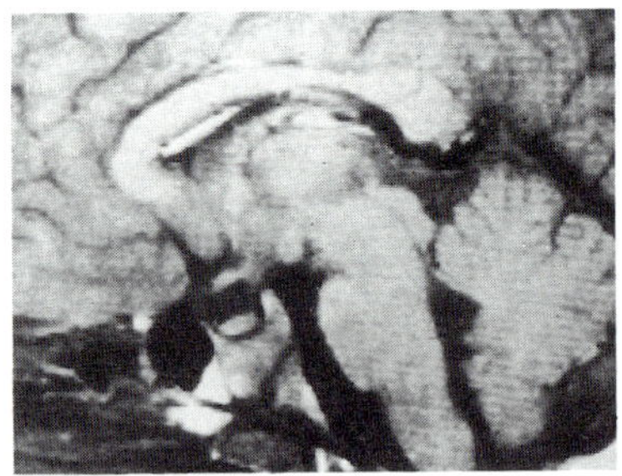

Figure 3. *IDIOPATHIC DIABETES INSIPIDUS. The hyperintensity of the posterior pituitary is not seen. No morphological or signal abnormalities are visible in the hypothalamus or pituitary stalk.*

Pituitary Adenomas

Pituitary adenomas may be classified according to different criteria; size, type of hormone secreted, histologic appearance. Classification by size is the most convenient to describe neuroradiological findings and to correlate them with the neurological symptoms. Tumors less than 10 mm in size are considered microadenomas; over 10 mm in size are called macroadenomas. The clinical presentation depends on the type of hormone secreted and nervous or vascular structures involved.

Microadenomas

Among microadenomas the most frequent tumor is the prolactinoma; MR is superior to CT in demonstrating these tumors [19,20, 21]. They usually present as small nodular areas of hyperintensity in T1WI and hyperintensity in T2WI, usually in a paramedian location (Fig. 4). Sometimes the nodule is hyperintense in T1WI reflecting previous intratumoral hemorrhage. If a nodule is not clearly defined on the basis of altered signal, indirect signs such as size of the pituitary, morphology of the superior margin, displacement of the stalk are less reliable. Differential diagnosis with other types of secreting microadenomas (ACTH, GH etc.) is impossible since there are no specific signal characteristics to distinguish the various types of adenomas from one another.

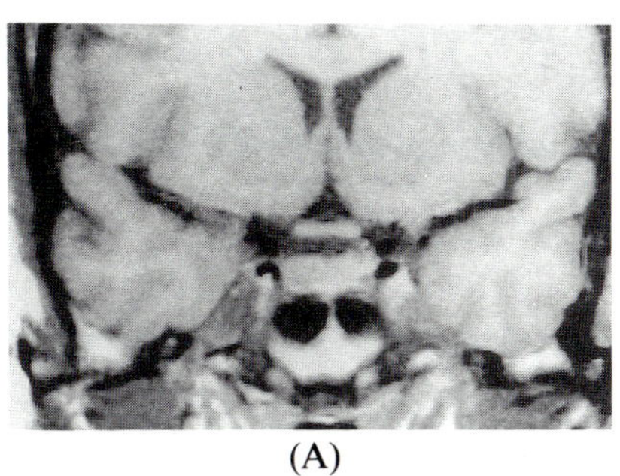
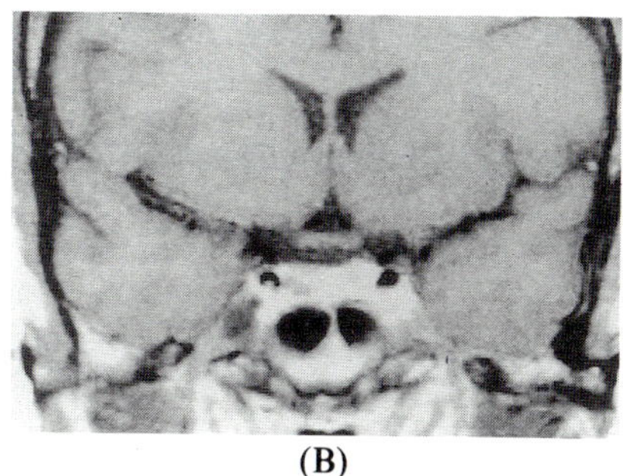

(A)   (B)

Figure 4. *PROLACTIN SECRETING MICROADENOMA. (A) T1W coronal view; a slightly hypointense nodule is appreciated in the right half of the pituitary gland. (B) After gadolinium injection the signal of the pituitary gland increases and the hypointense microadenoma is better appreciated.*

Gd-DTPA enhancement is not absolutely necessary but may increase the positive yield in patients with abnormal endocrine activity and ambiguous or negative plain MR study. The tumor nodule appears usually as an hypointense area within the enhancing pituitary parenchyma. In later phase, however, the tumor may enhance and become indistinguishable from the pituitary, or hyperintense with respect to the fading intensity of the pituitary [22].

Macroadenomas

Macroadenomas have similar signal characteristics and behavior as microadenomas (Fig. 5). The superb anatomical detail provided by MR allows a completely satisfactory typographical evaluation with clear demonstration of the relationship with optic chiasm, carotid vessels and cavernous sinus. Precise definition of cavernous sinus involvement is however difficult at a microscopic level.

Assessment of postoperative or post pharmacological treatment is easily and accurately performed [23]. Reduction of macroadenomas after surgery is not immediate: it takes about two to four weeks for the macroadenoma to shrink. After surgery the signal of the tumor however, changes drastically, usually following the presence of blood or surgical foreign material in the cavity (Fig. 6).

Craniopharyngioma

Craniopharyngiomas are thought to arise from epithelial remnants of Rathke's cleft, and develop both within or above the sella turcica. They are more frequent in children but also occur in adulthood around the sixth decade. They are hormonal inactive but may present with delayed growth, endocrine deficiency, and neurological signs such as visual field defects. They are frequently cystic and contain calcification.

The MR appearance varies according to the composition of the tumor [24]; the most classical aspect is that of an inhomogeneous mass with a cystic component hyperintense both in T1 and T2WI (Fig. 7). The solid component is usually isointense in T1 and hyperintense in T2. Calcification may be completely missed at MR and correlation with CT may be necessary. The parenchymatous portion and the capsule of the cyst usually enhance intensely following injection of contrast.

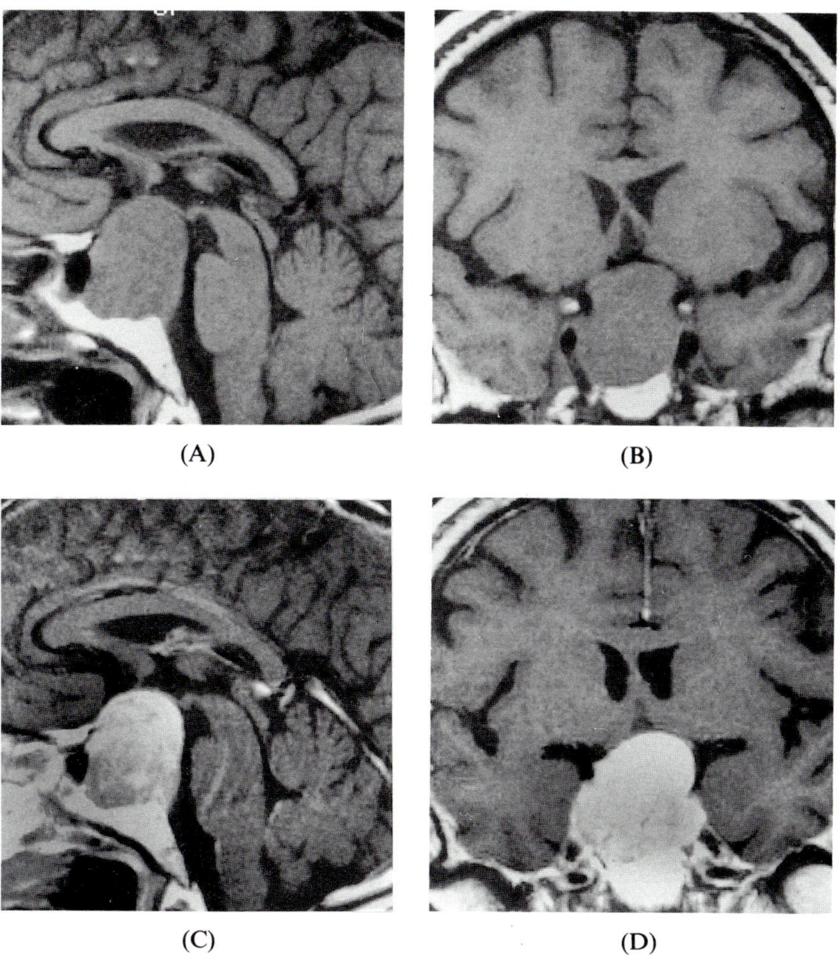

(A)   (B)

(C)   (D)

Figure 5. *NONSECRETING MACROADENOMA. (A, B) Sagittal and coronal T1WI. The chiasm is markedly compressed and displaced upward. The cavernous sinuses are compressed and displaced laterally. (C, D) Sagittal and coronal T1WI following i.v. injection of gadolinium. The tumor becomes markedly hyperintense.*

Rathke's Cleft Cyst

They are a common incidental finding, very rarely symptomatic. They are of two types: serous, with a signal very close to that of CSF, and mucous characterized by T1 hyperintensity.

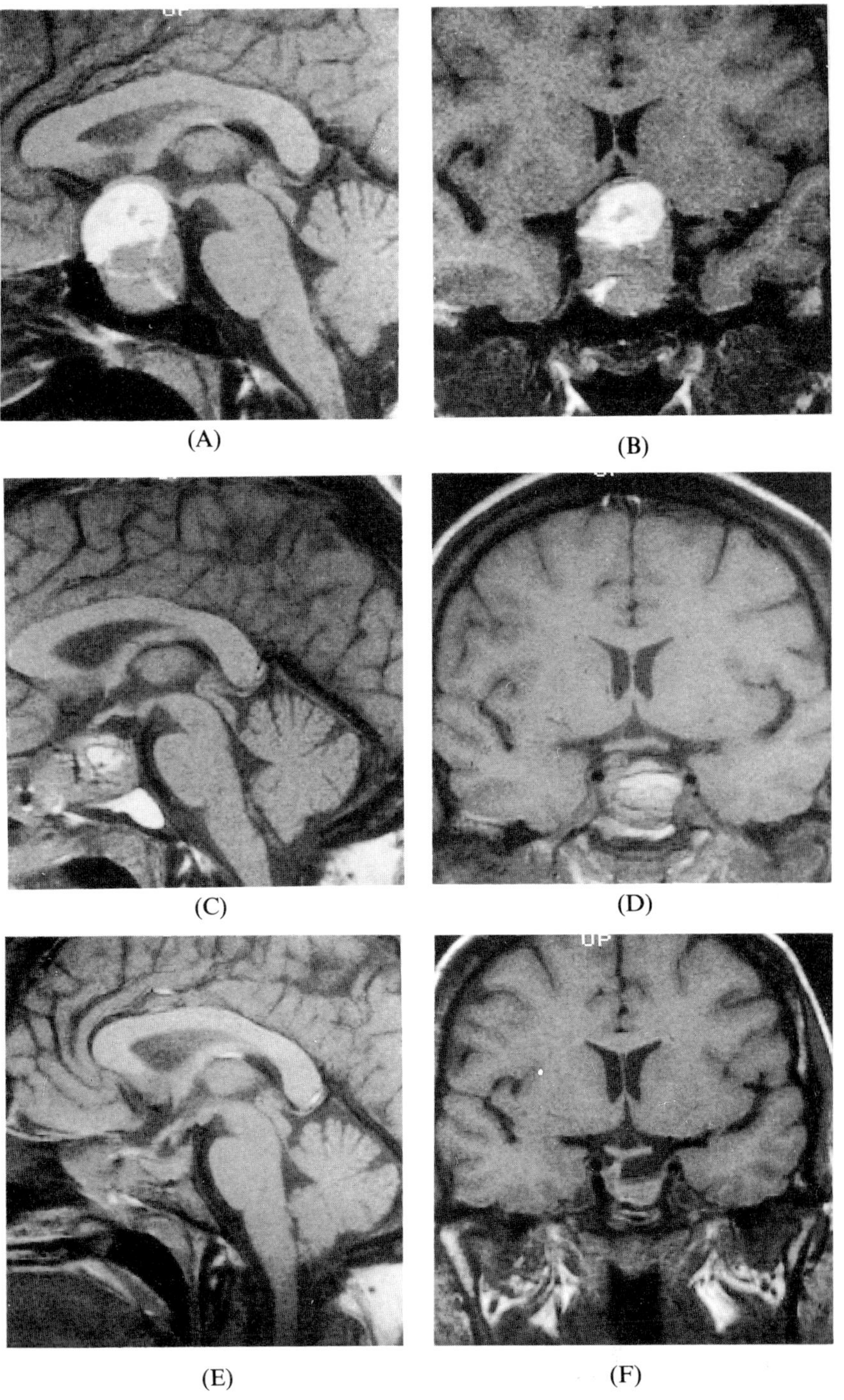

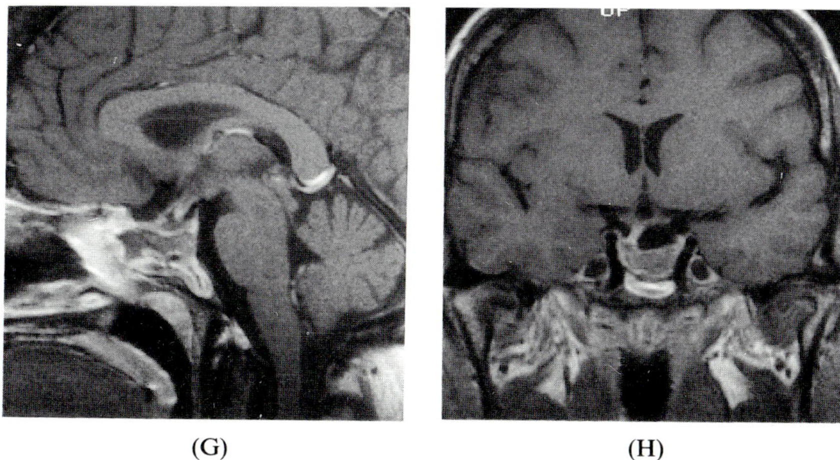

(G)   (H)

Figure 6. *GH SECRETING MACROADENOMA. (A, B) Sagittal and coronal precontrast T1WI. Inhomogeneous very large macroadenoma with superior hyperintense hemorrhagic component. The chiasm is markedly compressed and elevated. (C, D) Early postoperative MR (5 days, transsphenoidal surgery). Marked changes with complete removal of the suprasellar component of the tumor. The chiasm is free; inhomogeneous material with bloody components is present within the sella cavity and sphenoid sinus. (E, F) Late postoperative MR (90 days). The chiasm and the suprasellar cisterns are completely free. There is still some tissue within the sella cavity, isodense and homogeneous. (G, H) After i.v. injection of gadolinium there is marked enhancement within the sphenoid sinus, around the residual tissue and also a minimum enhancement of the intrasellar tissue. This most likely represents residual tumor since the patient still has elevated GH levels.*

Arachnoid Cysts and Epidermoids

Arachnoid cysts are usually differentiated from epidermoids because the latter are usually hyperintense to CSF on proton density images. However, sometimes a definite distinction may be very difficult since both have signals very close to that of CSF, hypointense in T1WI and hyperintense in T1WI.

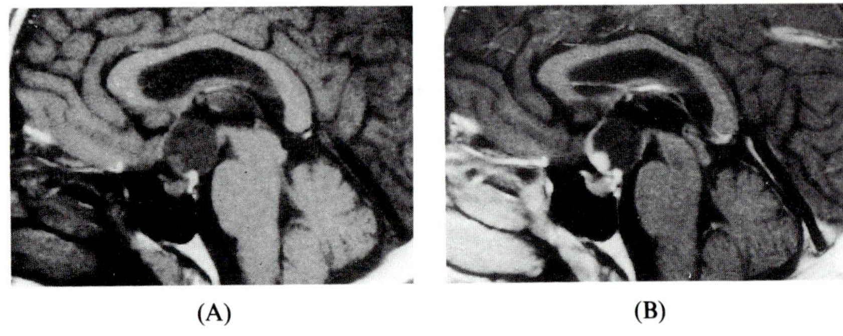

(A)   (B)

Figure 7. *CRANIOPHARYNGIOMA. (A) T1W sagittal precontrast view. The tumor is mainly cystic with a small anteroinferior mural nodule. (B) After Gd-DTPA injection the nodule and the capsule become markedly hyperintense.*

Meningioma

These tumors may be located in different positions with respect to the sella; parasellar, within the cavernous sinus, at the level of the tuberculum, from the diaphragm sellae or from the anterior clinoids. Meningioma from the planum sphenoidal or from the optic nerves may extend within the sella or in the suprasellar region. They are usually slow growing and the most common clinical presentation is either visual field defects or oculomotor disturbance with diplopia.

Meningiomas are most frequently isointense in T1WI and less commonly hypointense. They may be either iso- or hyperintense in T2WI [25] (Fig. 8). Recognition of small isointense tumors may be difficult and the use of Gd-DTPA enhancement is mandatory. These tumors usually enhance markedly. When in the cavernous sinus they may encase the carotid siphon that is usually restricted; this is not the case with cavernous sinus extension of pituitary adenomas.

Chiasmatic and Hypothalamic Glioma

They are mostly tumors of infancy, frequently associated with neurofibromatosis. They may have different growth patterns although not different histologically; optic chiasm, optic nerves,

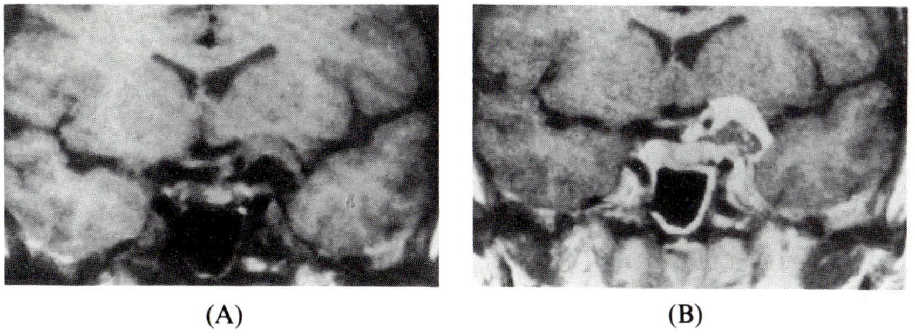

(A)   (B)

Figure 8. *LEFT PARASELLAR MENINGIOMA. (A) Precontrast T1W coronal view. The deepest component has no signal due to heavy calcification within the tumor mass. (B) After gadolinium the isointense soft component becomes markedly hyperintense. The supraclinoid portion of the carotid is encased and elevated.*

hypothalamus and optic radiations may be involved with different degrees of severity and combinations of extension (Fig. 9).

They are usually isointense in T1WI and slightly hyperintense in T2WI. In patients with neurofibromatosis differential diagnosis must be made with benign hamartomas; these usually do not enhance with contrast.

Histiocytosis X

Granulomas of Langerhans cells may be found in the hypothalamus or pituitary stalks both isolated or in the systemic form of histiocytosis X. The most common clinical presentation is diabetes

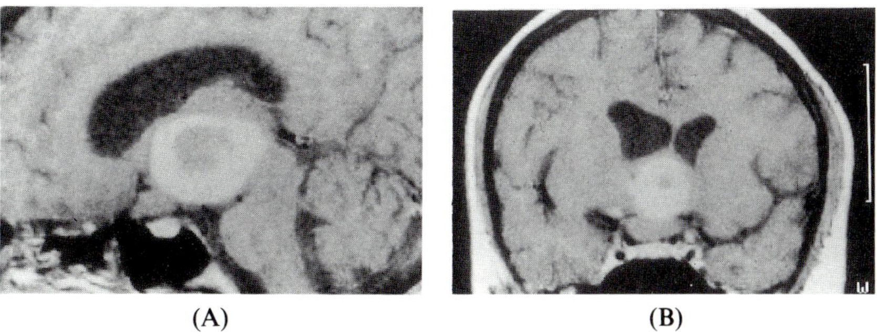

(A)   (B)

Figure 9. *HYPOTHALAMIC GLIOMA. (A, B) Sagittal and coronal T1WI post Gd injection. The hypothalamic-chiasmatic portion of the tumor does not enhance while the main component within the third ventricle enhances.*

insipidus. In these cases the posterior pituitary hyperintensity is lost: the pituitary stalk is thickened and a slight T2 hyperintensity may be found. Sometimes gadolinium enhancement is present. Differential diagnosis with hypothalamic glioma may be difficult and may require biopsy [26].

Hamartomas of the Tuber Cinereum

These are not neoplasms but sessile nodules of neural tissue histologically similar to normal hypothalamus located in the postero-superior part of the tuber cinereum and hanging down in the interpeduncular cistern. They are frequently found in precocious puberty, are usually isointense to brain parenchyma and do not enhance with contrast [27].

Rare Conditions

Abscesses, meningeal infections, sarcoidosis, aneurysms, dural fistulae are rare conditions that must be kept in mind in the differential diagnosis of lesions in the sellar and parasellar region.

References

1. Triulzi F, Scotti G. La RM nella patologia sellare e parasellare. Rivista di Neuroradiologia, 1988;1:75-93.
2. Kucharczyk W, Montanera WJ. The sella and parasellar region. In: Atlas S.W. ed. Magnetic resonance imaging of the brain and spine. Raven Press, 1991:625-667.
3. Colombo N, Berry I, Kucharczyk J, et al. Posterior pituitary gland: appearance in MRI in normal and pathologic states. Radiology 1987;165:481-485.
4. Fujisawa I, Asato R, Nishimura K, et al. Anterior and posterior lobes of the pituitary gland: assessment by 1.5 T MR imaging. J Comput Assist Tomogr 1987;11:214-220.
5. Fujisawa I, Asato R, Kawata M, et al. Hyperintense signal of the posterior pituitary and T1-weighted MRI: an experimental study. I Comput Assist Tomogr 1989;13:371-377.
6. Kucharczyk J, Kucharczyk W, Berry I, et al. Histochemical characterization and functional significance of the hyperintense signal on MR images of the posterior pituitary. AJNR 1988;9:1079-1083.
7. Kucharczyk W, Lenkinski RE, Kucharczyk J, et al. The effect of phospholipid vesicles on the NMR relaxation of water: an explanation for the appearance of the neurophypophysis? AJNR 1990;11:693-700.
8. Triulzi F, Scotti G, Beccaria L, et al. Anterior pituitary hyperintensity on T1-weighted MRI in the newborn. Neuroradiology 1991;33:273-275.
9. Cox TD, Elster AD. Normal pituitary gland: changes in shape, size, and signal intensity during the 1st year of life at MR imaging 1. Radiology 1991;179:721-724.
10. Brismar K. Growth hormone secretion in empty sella syndrome. J Endocrinol Invest 1982;5:417-422.

11. Merle P, Georged AM, Goumy P, et al. Primary empty sella turcica in children. Pediatr Radiol 1979;8:209-213.
12. Stanhope R, Hindmarsh P, Kendall B, et al. High resolution CT scanning of the pituitary gland in growth disorders. Acta Pediatr Scand 1986;75:779-786.
13. di Natale B, Scotti G, Pellini C, et al. Empty sella in children with pituitary dwarfism, does it exist? Paediatrician 1987;14:246-252.
14. Pellini C, di Natale B, De Angelis R, et al. Growth hormone deficiency in children: role of magnetic resonance imaging in assessing aetiopathogenesis and prognosis in idiopathic hypopituitarism. Eur J Pediatr 1990;149:536-541.
15. Fujisawa I, Kikuchi K, Nishimuea K, et al. Transection of the pituitary stalk: development of an ectopic posterior lobe assessed with MR imaging. Radiology 1987;165:487-489.
16. Kelly WM, Kucharczyk W, Kucharczyk J, et al. Posterior pituitary ectopia: and MR feature of pituitary dwarfism. AJNR 1988;9:453-460.
17. Scotti G, Triulzi F, Chiumello G, et al. New imaging techniques in endocrinology: magnetic resonance of the pituitary gland and sella turcica. Acta Paediatr Scand 1989;356:5-14.
18. Triulzi F, Scotti G, Anzalone N, et al. La risonanza magnetica nella diagnosi del diabete insipido. In: Pardatscher K, ed. Neuroradiologica. del Centauro, Udine, 1989.
19. Davis PC, Hoffman JC, Spencer T, et al. MR imaging of pituitary adenoma. CT, clinical and surgical correlation. AJNR 1987;8:107-112.
20. Peck WW, Dillon WP, Normal D, et al. High resolute MR imaging of microadenomas at 1.5 T: experience with Cushing disease. AJNR 1988;9:1085-1091.
21. Pojunas KW, Daniels DL, Williams AL, et al. MR imaging of prolactin-secreting microadenomas. AJNR 1986;7:209-212.
22. Newton DR, Dillon WP, Norman D, et al. Gd-DTPA-enhanced MR imaging of pituitary adenomas. AJNR 1989;10:949-953.
23. Scotti G, Anzalone N, Triulzi F, et al. MR evaluation of post-surgical changes in trasphenoidal surgery for pituitary adenomas. Rivista de Neuroradiologia 1991;4:57-61.
24. Pusey E, Kortman KE, Flannigan BD, et al. MR of craniopharyngiomas: tumor delineation and characterization. AJNR 1987;8:439-444.
25. Bradac GB, Riva A, Schoiner W, et al. Cavernous sinus meningiomas: an MRI study. Neuroradiology 1987;29:578-481.
26. Moore JB, Kulkarn R, Crutcher DC, et al. MRI in multifocal eosinophilic granulamatosis: staging disease and monitoring response to therapy. Am J Pediatr Hemayol Oncol 1989;11:174-177.
27. Burton EM, Ball WS Jr, Crane K, et al. Hamartomas of tuber cinereum: comparison of MR and CT findings in 4 cases. AJNR 1989;10:497-502.

Intracranial Vascular Malformations

Anne G. Osborn

*Department of Radiology, University of Utah, Salt Lake City,
Utah, USA*

Pathologists divide basic vascular malformations into four basic types: 1) arteriovenous malformations; 2) venous vascular malformations; 3) capillary telangiectasias and 4) cavernous angiomas. Each of the four types has specific features of the pathology which forms the foundation for the various imaging findings in this disease spectrum; pertinent clinical and demographic data and finally typical angiographic, CT and MR imaging studies.

Arteriovenous malformations (AVMs)

AVMs can be parenchymal, dural or mixed.

A. Arteriovenous malformation, parenchymal:
    1. Congenital
    2. Most common *symptomatic* vascular malformation
    3. Rarely multiple; no sex predilection
    4. Age at presentation: 20-40 y; 80% symptomatic by age 50
    5. Location: found in all areas (70-93% supratentorial)
    6. Pathology: (Fig. 1)
        - tortuous tightly packed mass of enlarged arteries, dilated draining veins
        - no capillary bed; no normal brain within malformation
        - surrounding brain often atrophic, gliotic; associated hemorrhage frequent
        - calcification common
        - vascular supply: pial or mixed pial-dural

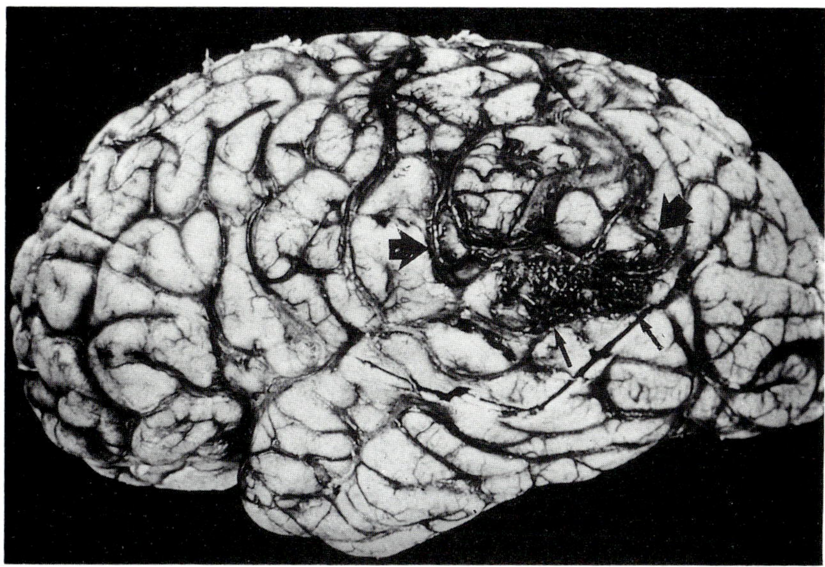

Figure 1. *ARTERIOVENOUS MALFORMATION. Gross pathology specimen from a patient with an unruptured arteriovenous malformation. Note enlarged arteries (large arrows) feeding a tightly packed mass of dilated smaller arteries and draining veins (small arrows). (Case courtesy of Armed Forces Institute of Pathology, Washington, D.C.)*

7. Associated aneurysm in 7-9%
8. Presentation: subarachnoid hemorrhage, headache, seizure, neurological deficit
9. Risk of hemorrhage: 2-3%/year (very recent data indicates risk of hemorrhage may be as high as 4%/year, cumulative). Each hemorrhagic episode carries 10-30% risk of death, 25% long term morbidity. Size of AVM, presence/absence of hypertension no value in predicting rupture. Incidence of hemorrhage is similar in infratentorial and supratentorial locations.
10. Angiography: (Fig. 2)
    - tightly packed mass of enlarged feeding arteries, tortuous draining veins
    - AV shunting ("early draining veins"); "steal" from adjacent vessels common
    - 7-9% associated aneurysm (secondary to high flow states)

- mass effect subtle unless hemorrhage is present
- may be "cryptic" (no detectable angiographic abnormalities); partially thrombosed AVM may have only subtle blush, early draining vein

11. CT: (Fig. 3)
    - hemorrhage, associated atrophy common
    - serpiginous iso-or hyperintense foci with strong enhancement following contrast
    - Ca^{++} frequent

12. MR: (Fig. 4)
    - tightly packed "honeycomb" appearance; mixed signals often seen
      a. serpiginous "flow voids"; absent signal in Ca^{++} foci
      b. foci of increased signal in thrombosed/slowly flowing vessels
      c. associated hemorrhage in different stages of evolution, hemosiderin ring
    - surrounding brain may have
      a. atrophy
      b. gliosis
      c. hemorrhage
      d. edema
    - MR angiography shows nidus well but to date visualization of afferent arteries and venous drainage is better depicted with conventional angiography

13. SPECT or PET scanning can evaluate perfusion status of adjacent brain

B. Arteriovenous malformation, dural:
    1. Etiology: considered acquired, not congenital
       - traumatic
       - atherosclerotic
       - spontaneous
    2. Incidence: 10-15% of all intracranial vascular malformations
    3. Age peak 40-60 y
    4. Common locations:
       - base of skull
       - posterior fossa

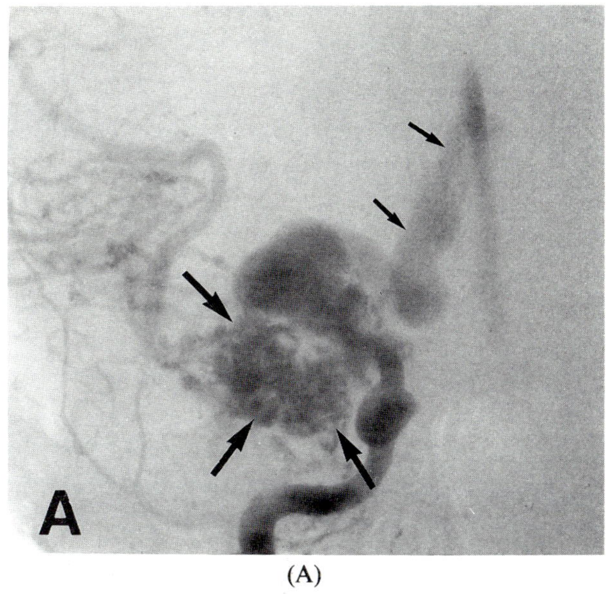

(A)

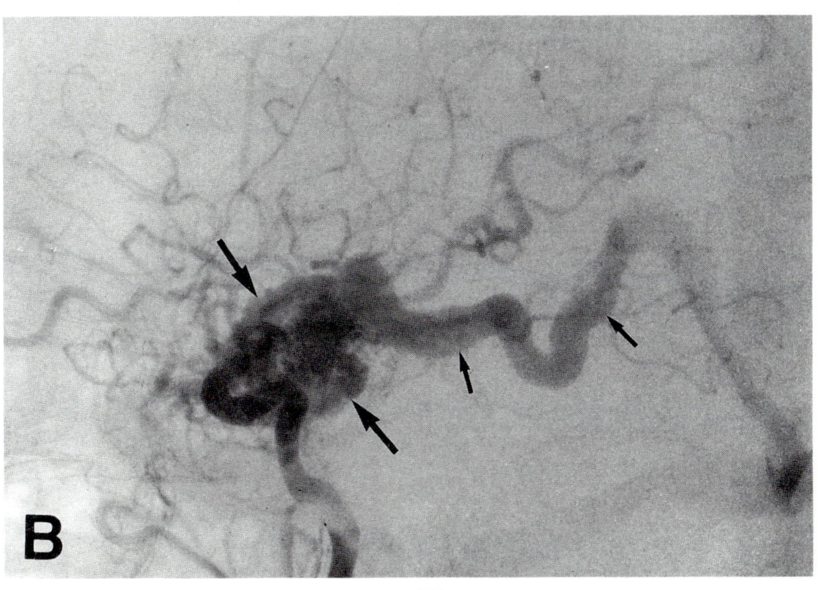

(B)

Figure 2. *ARTERIOVENOUS MALFORMATION. AP (A) and lateral (B) view of carotid angiogram in a patient with a large right temporal AVM shows a tightly packed mass and dilated arteries (large arrows) with early draining veins (small arrows).*

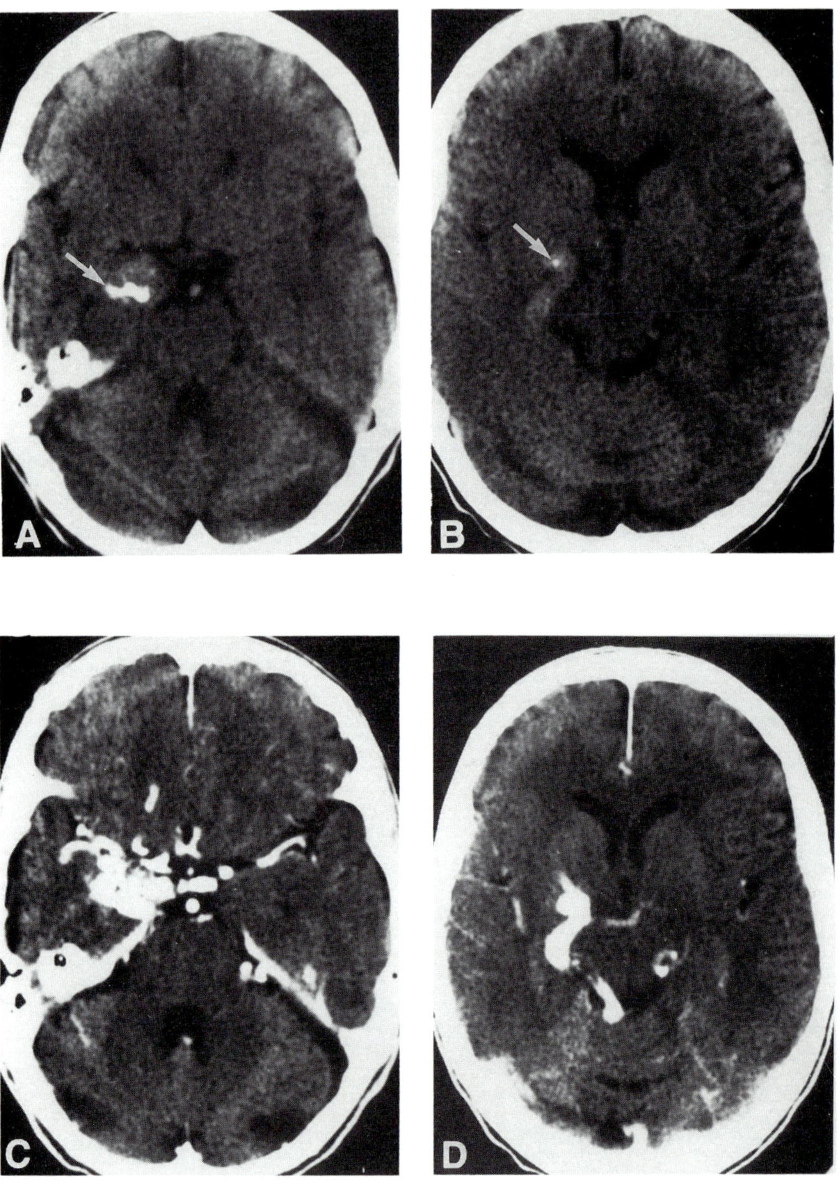

Figure 3. *ARTEREOVENOUS MALFORMATION. Same patient as Figure 2. Plain (A, B) and contrast-enhanced (C, D) CT scans in a patient with a large temporal lobe arteriovenous malformation. The enlarged vessels are seen as slightly hyperdense, serpentine structures on the noncontrast scans; also note dystrophic calcification and phleboliths (A, B, arrows).*

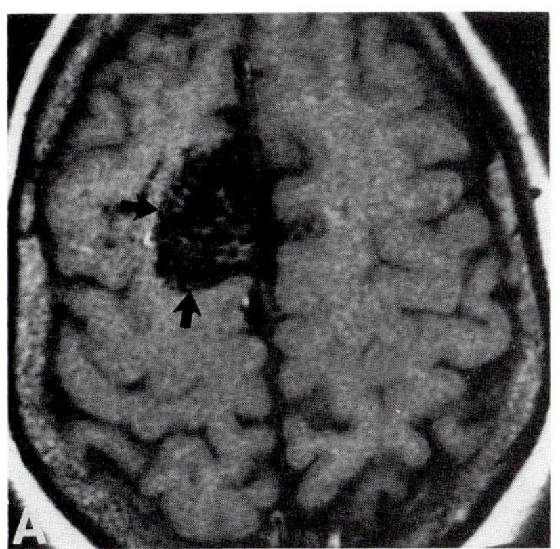
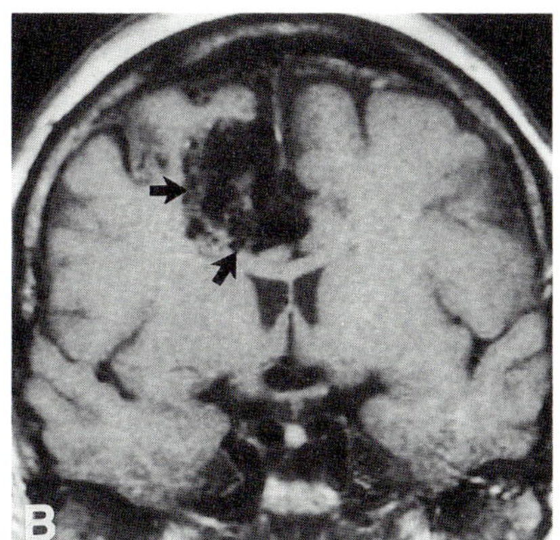
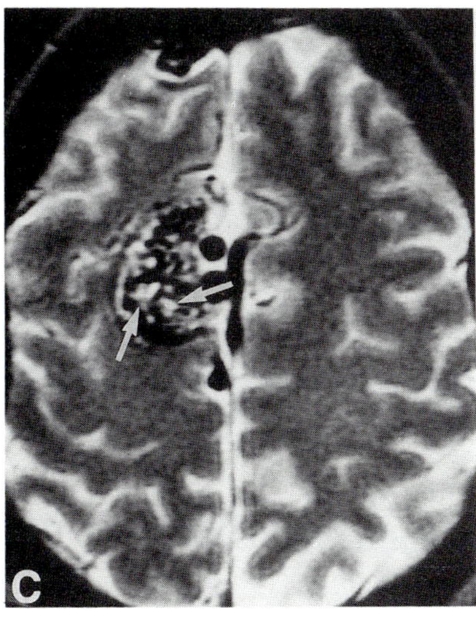

Figure 4. *PARENCHYMAL AVM. Axial (A) and coronal (B) T1-weighted MR scans in a patient with a large unruptured posterior frontal arteriovenous malformation (arrows). Note the tightly packed mass of vessels has little mass effect. T2-weighted scan (C) shows only small foci of gliotic brain (arrows) within the AVM.*

5. Clinical
   - hemorrhage rare
   - pulsatile tinnitus, exophthalmus, etc. (related to location)
6. Pathogenesis, theory of:
   - thrombosis of dural sinus
   - recanalization
   - arterial fistulization
7. Imaging findings (Fig. 5):
   - Site of fistula, AVM best depicted with angiography
   - In absence of veno-occlusive disease or dilated cortical veins, MR may be normal
   - Dilated cortical veins without a parenchymal nidus on MR is suggestive of DAVF with veno-occlusive disease. Complication common and include subdural/parenchymal hemorrhage, venous infarction.

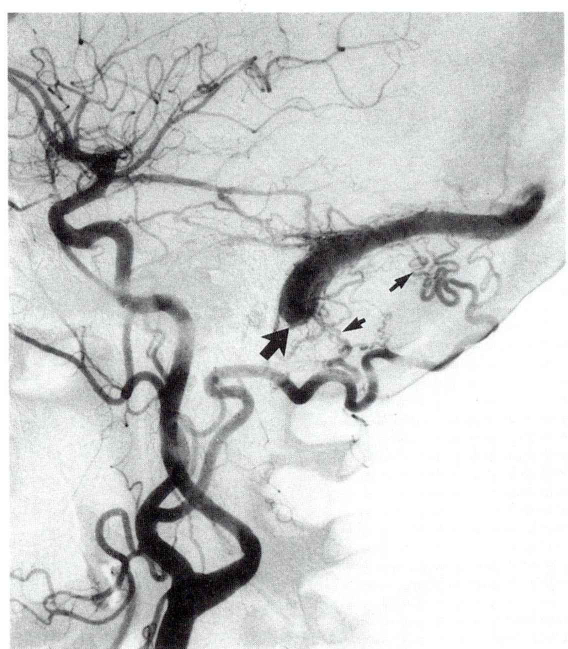

Figure 5. *DURAL AVM. Lateral view of a common carotid angiogram in a patient with a posterior fossa dural AVM. Note multiple enlarged dural perforating branches (small arrows) arising primarily from the occipital artery. The transverse sinus is opacified early but is occluded near the sigmoid sinus (large arrow).*

Venous Malformations

While classically considered a type of intracranial vascular malformation, some investigators have recently theorized that these are not true vascular malformations at all but instead represent extreme anatomic variants of venous drainage ("developmental venous anomalies" or "DVAs").

A. Venous malformation
1. Most common incidental vascular malformation at autopsy (2%)
2. Sites: cerebellar, deep cerebral white matter (most common = frontal, cerebellar)
3. Pathology:
    - arteries normal; dilated medullary veins. No increase in number or size of feeding vessels
    - normal intervening brain parenchyma between vessels
4. Presentation:
    - usually found incidentally on CT or MR
    - seizure, headache; hemorrhage relatively rare
5. Usually solitary
6. Angiography (Fig. 6)
    - arterial phase normal
    - capillary phase normal or faint blush
    - dilated medullary veins ("Medusa head") draining into enlarged transcortical vein. Pathognomonic.
7. CT (Fig. 7)
    - usually normal on NECT
    - stellate tangle of vessels draining into sharply defined transcortical vein that drains superficially into dural sinus or into deep subependymal veins
    - usually frontal or cerebellar near angle of ventricle
8. MR (Fig. 8)
    - linear tubular structure
        a. low signal ("flow void") typical; may show flow-related enhancement on gradient echo studies
        b. may see paradoxical high signal if slow flow present
    - hemorrhage, adjacent gliosis uncommon

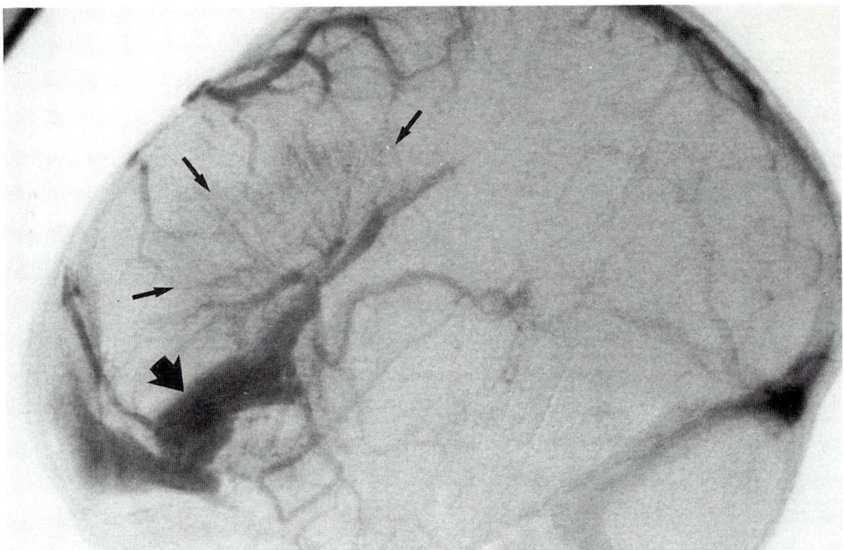

Figure 6. *VENOUS MALFORMATION. Three-month-old infant with subcutaneous soft tissue mass on his forehead that appears when he cries. Venous phase left internal carotid angiogram, lateral view, shows a large frontal venous angioma (small arrows) that empties into a huge transcortical draining vein (large arrow). A sinus pericranii was seen on very late venous phase films (not shown).*

Capillary telangiectasias

While commonly found in the spinal cord and brain at autopsy, these are uncommonly identified on imaging studies. Recent studies indicate that capillary telangiectasia and cavernous angioma may represent a spectrum within a single pathological entity.

A. Capillary telangiectasias
   1. Common; rarely symptomatic; usually found at autopsy (second only to venous angioma)
   2. Sites: pons most common; cerebral cortex; spinal cord
   3. Multiple lesions common
   4. Pathology (Fig. 9): abnormally dilated capillaries separated by normal interstitial neural tissue
   5. CNS involvement in Osler-Weber-Rendu disease is very rare (most head and neck lesions in this disease are in the nasal/oral mucosa or scalp (Fig. 10)

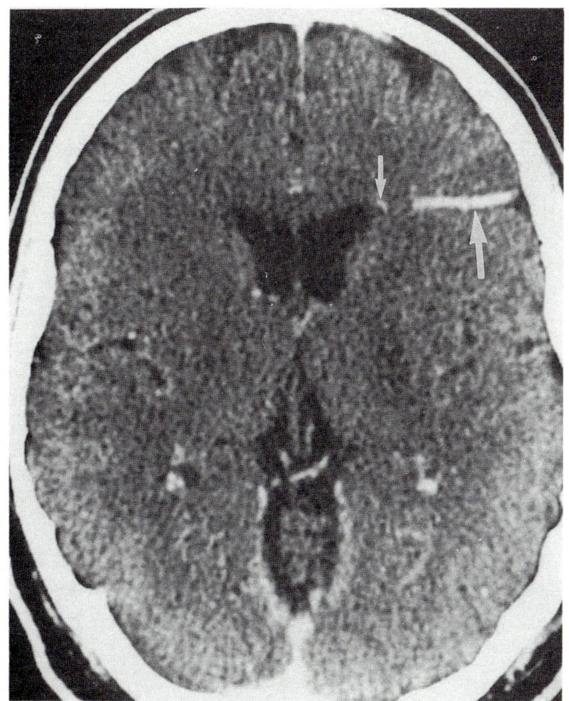

Figure 7. *VENOUS MALFORMATION. Post-contrast axial CT scan in a patient scanned for persistent headaches following trauma. A small tuft of vessels near the frontal horn of the left lateral ventricle (small arrow) drains into a large transcortical vein (large arrow).*

6. Angiography: Intracranial studies usually negative
7. CT: often negative. May have faint ill-defined hyperdensity on enhanced studies
8. MR: multiple foci of hypointense signal on T2W1 (Fig. 11). May have faint enhancement on T1W1 with contrast.

Cavernous angiomas

While uncommonly identified on imaging studies prior to the advent of MRI, these lesions are now easily identified because of their blood degradation products.

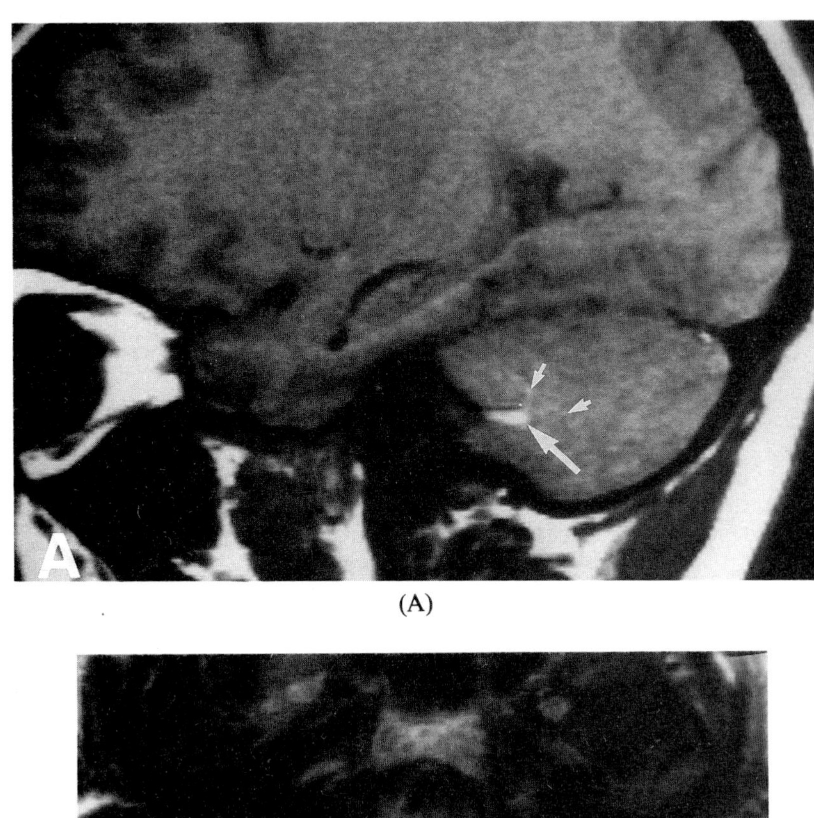

(A)

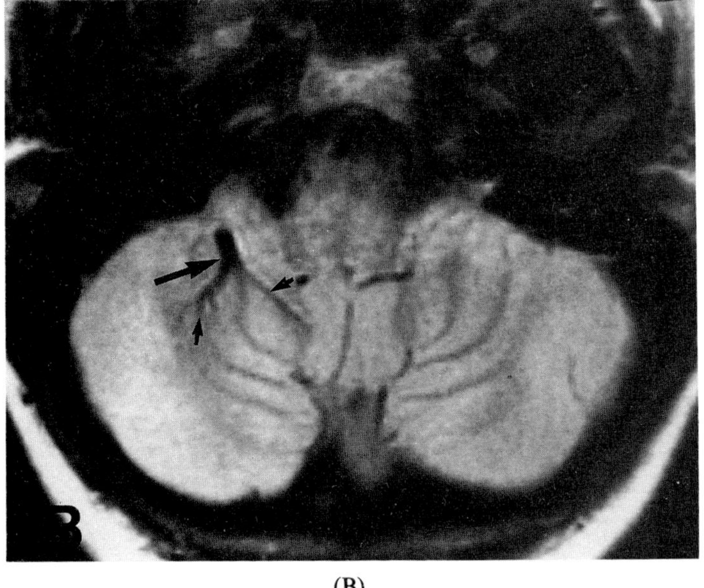

(B)

Figure 8. *VENOUS MALFORMATION. Sagittal T1-weighted* (A) *and axial "proton density" MR scan* (B) *in a 26-year-old man with a cerebellar venous angioma. The dilated transcortical vein is indicated by the large arrows; tributaries are indicated by small arrows.*

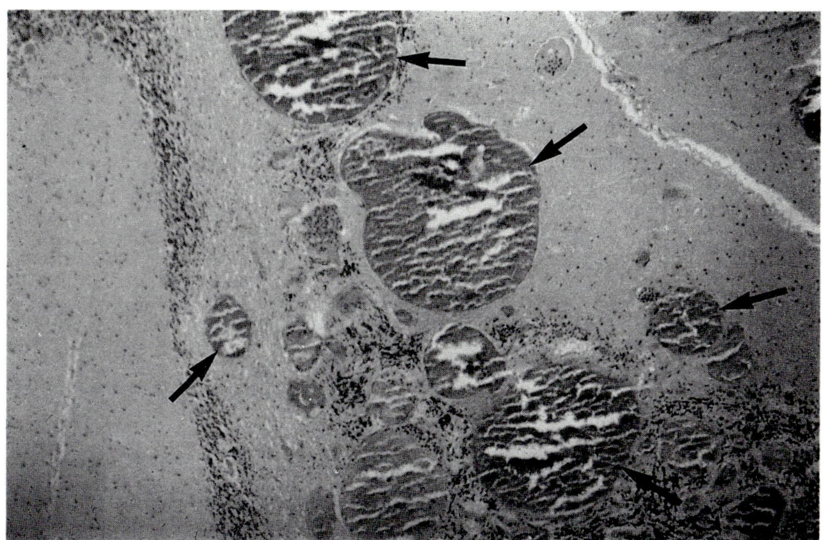

Figure 9. *CAPILLARY TELANGIECTASIAS. Photomicrograph of a capillary telangiectasia in the cerebellum. Note the dilated capillaries (arrows) are separated by normal neural tissue.*

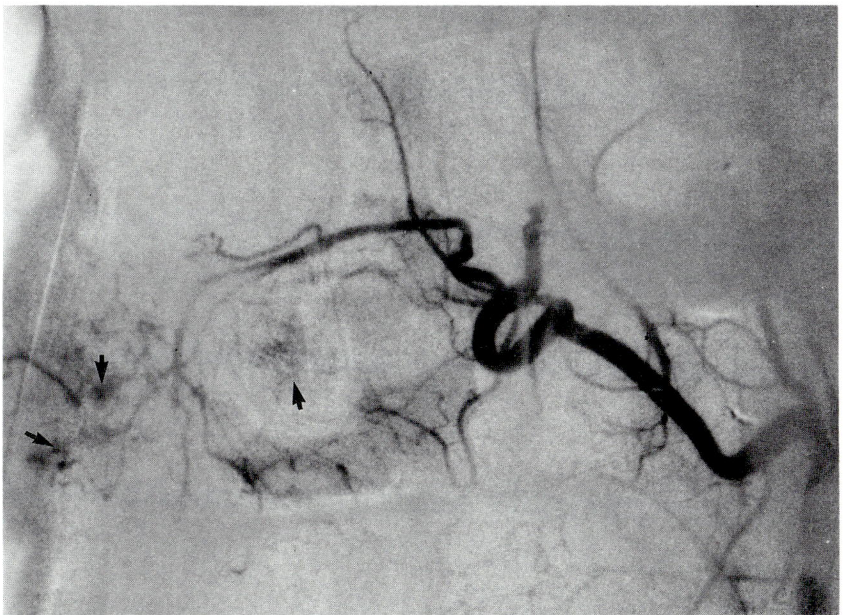

Figure 10. *CAPILLARY TELANGIECTASIAS. Selective maxillary angiogram in a patient with Osler-Weber-Rendu disease and frequent bouts of epistaxis. Note multiple telangiectasias in nasal mucosa (arrows). (Case courtesy Dr T. H. Newton, San Francisco).*

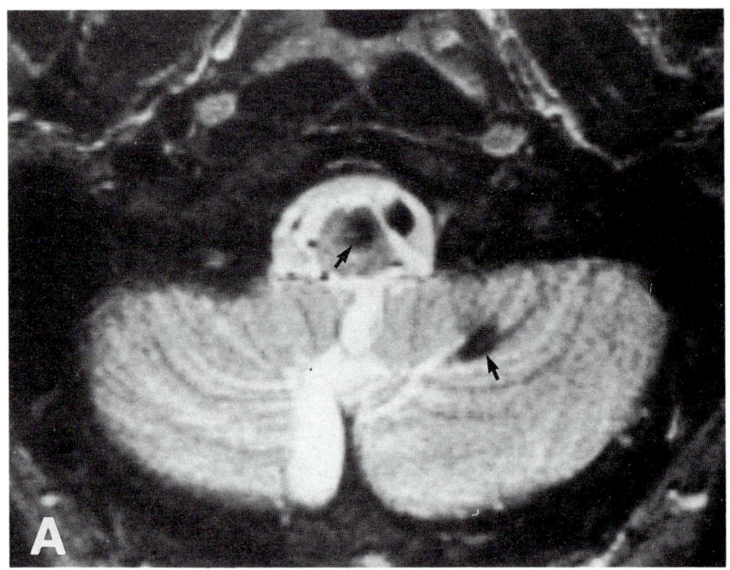

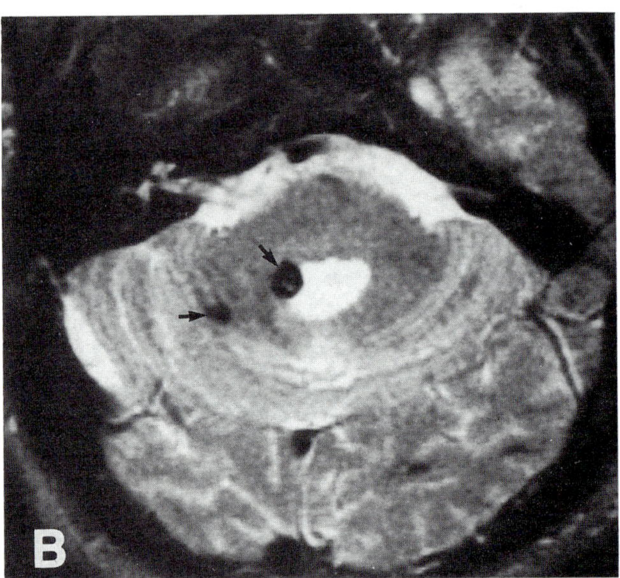

Figure 11. *CAPILLARY TELANGIECTASIAS. Axial T2-weighted scans in a patient with multiple capillary telangiectasias (seen as foci of decreased signal) (A, B arrows).*

A. Cavernous angiomas
   1. Most common vascular malformation seen at MR (especially with gradient echo scans)
   2. Sites: anywhere
   3. 50% multiple; 80% in familial
   4. Age: 20-40 y
   5. Presentation: 60% seizure; 20-30% hemorrhage; 20-25% focal or progressive neurological deficit

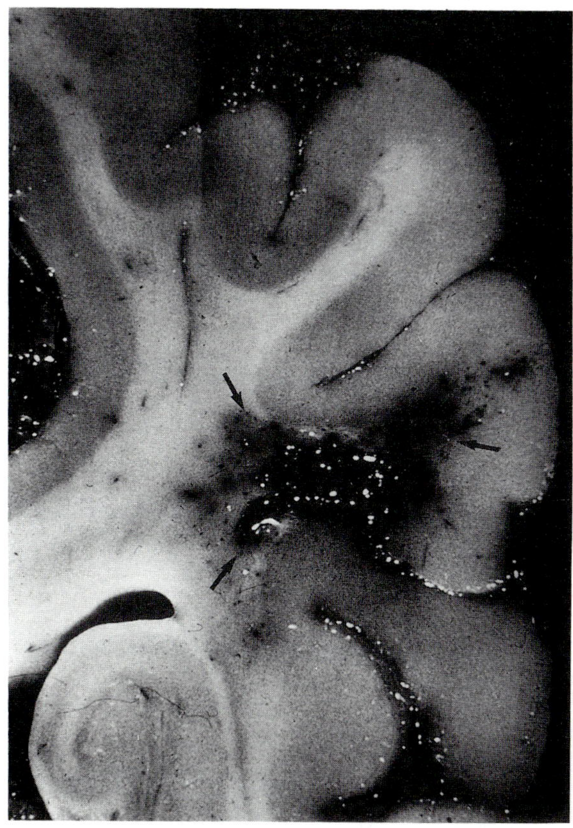

Figure 12. *CAVERNOUS ANGIOMA. Gross specimen of a cavernous angioma (arrows) shows evidence for subacute and chronic hemorrhage central thrombi and peripheral hemosiderin staining, respectively. (Case courtesy of Armed Forces Institute of Pathology, Washington, D.C.)*

6. Pathology (Fig. 12): endothelial-lined sinusoidal spaces without intervening neural tissue (distinguishes these from capillary telangiectasias); hemorrhage in different stages of evolution commonly present. Histological heterogeneity common.

7. Overt annualized bleeding rate recently reported at < .1%/year

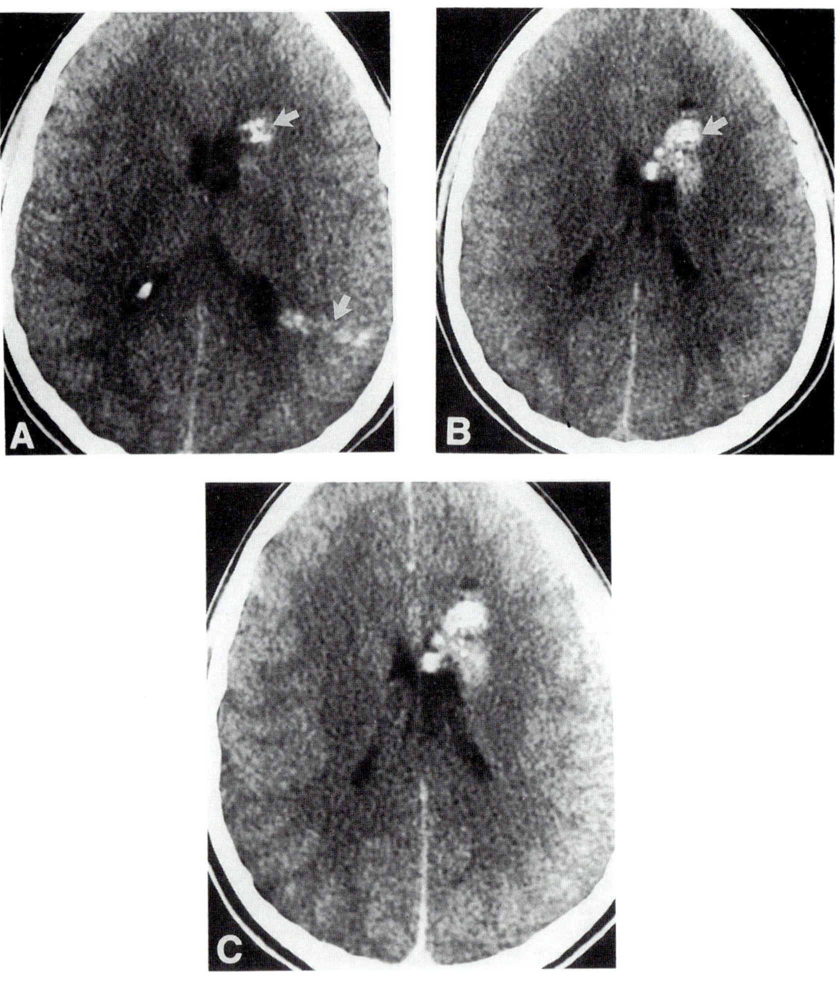

Figure 13. *CAVERNOUS ANGIOMAS. Axial noncontrast CT scans in a 19-year-old male with his first seizure show two calcified lesions in the left hemisphere (A, B, arrows). Little change is noted after contrast administration (C). Cavernous angiomas.*

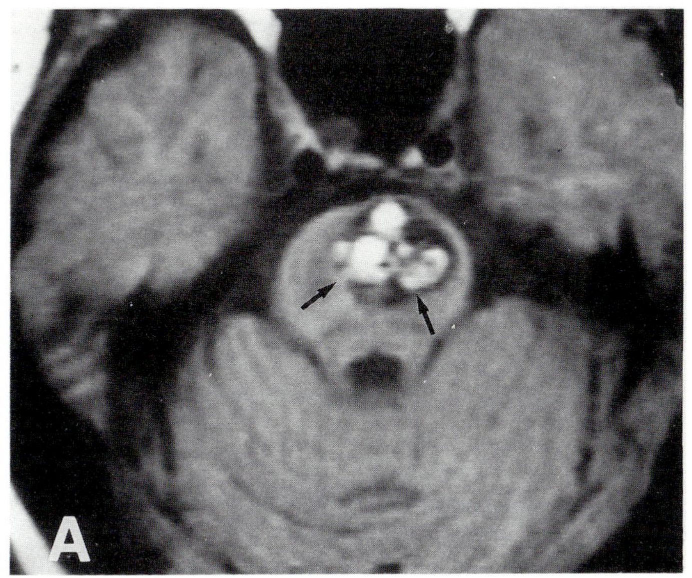

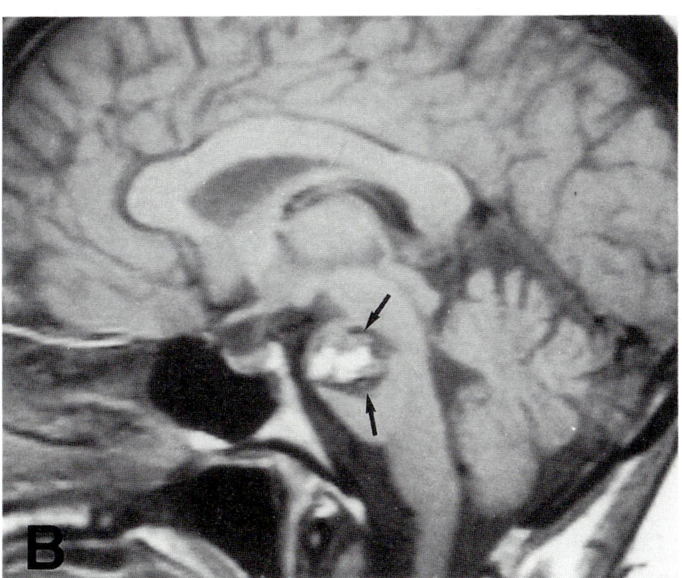

Figure 14. *CAVERNOUS ANGIOMA. Axial* (A) *and sagittal* (B) *T1-weighted MR scans show the classic well-delineated mixed signal lesion (arrows) characteristic of a cavernous angioma that has hemorrhaged on several occasions.*

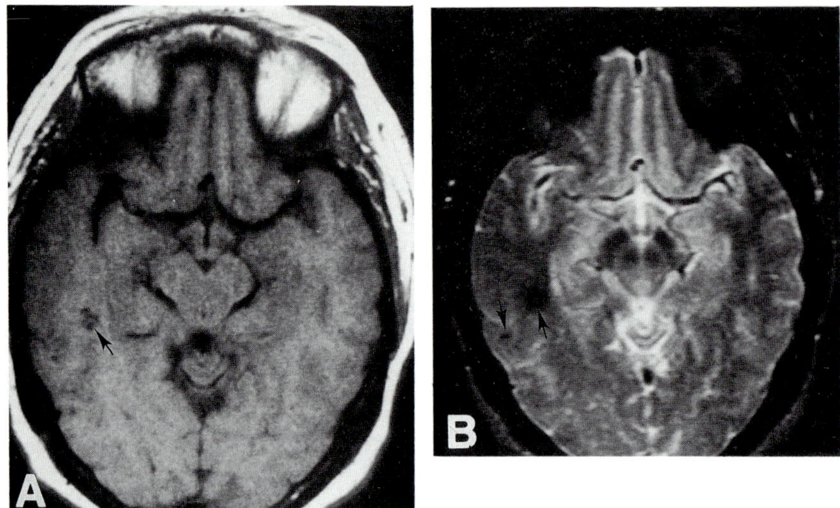

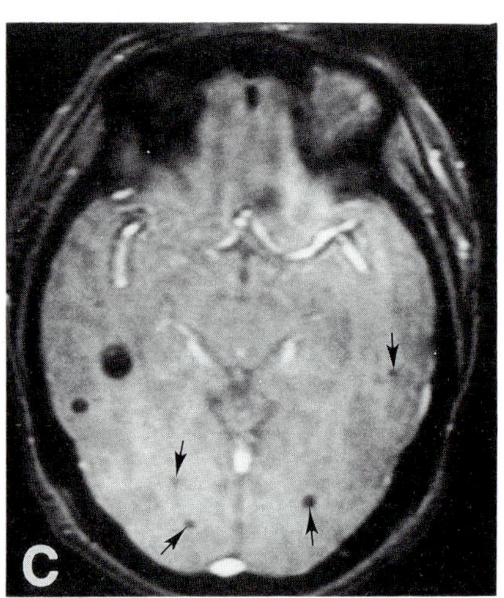

Figure 15. *CAVERNOUS ANGIOMAS. Axial T1-weighted scan in a woman with multiple cavernous angiomas. Only one definite lesion is noted on the T1-weighted study (A, arrow) while two are identified on the T2-weighted image (B, arrows). When a gradient echo scan was performed, multiple additional lesions became apparent (C, arrows). Gradient echo scans are exquisitely sensitive to magnetic susceptibility effects and therefore even relatively small foci of hemosiderin can be detected.*

8. Angiography:
   - usually normal
   - occasionally faint blush on capillary/venous phase
9. CT (Fig. 13)
   - often hyperdense on NECT; occasionally calcified
   - enhancement varies from none/minimal to striking (uncommon)
   - edema usually absent but on occasion is striking
10. MR: complex internal structure with variable appearance. Common:
   - mixed signal mass with reticulated core of low and high - signal foci (Fig. 14)
   - surrounding low signal rim (secondary to hemosiderin deposition)
   - gradient - echo (GRE) scans show "blooming" of low signal due to magnetic susceptibility effect of hemosiderin; may demonstrate flow in residual patent vessels. *GRE scans often demonstrate multiple small lesions not seen on T2W1* (Fig. 15).

References

1. Smith HJ, Strother CM, Kikuchi Y, et al. MR imaging in the managment of supratentorial intracranial AVMs. AJNR 1988;9:225-235.
2. Atlas SW, Mark AS, Fram EK, Grossman RI. Vascular intracranial lesions: applications of gradient-echo MR imaging. Radiology 1988;169:455-461.
3. Toro VE, Geyer CA, Sherman JL, et al. Cerebral venous angiomas: MR findings. J Comp Asst Tomogr 1988;12:935-940.
4. Brown RD, Weibers DO, Forbes G. The natural history of unruptured intracranial arteriovenous malformations. J Neurosurg 1988;68:352-357.
5. Goulao A, Alvarez H, Monaco RG, et al. Venous anomalies and abnormalities of the posterior fossa. Neuroradiol 1990;31:476-482.
6. Rapacki TFX, Brantley MJ, Furlow TW Jr, et al. Heterogeneity of cerebral cavernous hemangiomas diagnosed by MR imaging. J Comput Assist Tomogr 1990;14:18-25.
7. DeMarco JK, Dillon WP, Halbach VV, Tsuruda JS. Dural arteriovenous fistulas: evaluation with MR imaging. Radiology 1990;175:193-199.
8. Marchal G, Bosman H, Van Fraeyenhoven L, et al. Intracranial vascular lesions: optimization and clinical evaluation of three-dimensional time-of-flight MR angiography. Radiology 1990;175:443-448.
9. Graves VB, Duff TA. Intracranial arteriovenous malformations: current imaging and treatment. Invest Radiol 1990;25:952-960.
10. Rigamonti D, Johnson PC, Spetzler RF, et al. Cavernous malformations and capillary telangiectasia: a spectrum within a single pathological entity. Neurosurg 1991;28:60-64.

Clinical Applications of MR Angiography in the Head and Neck

Anton N. Hasso

Loma Linda University Medical Center, Department of Radiation Science, Loma Linda, California, USA

Introduction

In order to acquire MR images which highlight vessels, one must exploit the potentially high contrast of blood. Blood has a high water content, and therefore its "spins" should provide an intense MR signal. However, the usual appearance of blood is either as a signal void or as a smearing artifact across the image in the phase encoding direction. Occasionally the signal of blood is bright, if the spins just enter the imaging slice as they are encoded. These entering spins have not been saturated by the RF pulses. The transposition of longitudinal magnetization from one region into another is referred to as time-of-flight effect [9,13].

When the spins of in-plane flowing blood move between RF excitation and encoding, they will acquire an additional motion induced phase change at the time of the echo. This phenomenon occurs when moving spins flowing along a magnetic field gradient accumulate a phase shift with respect to stationary spins. The additional phase change will have two deleterious consequences which consist of spatial misregistration and spin dephasing within the voxel, leading to smearing or signal loss [8,9].

The flow sensitivity of MRI is based on both the time-of-flight and the phase change effects [1,7,13]. These flow phenomena are the basic tools of MR angiography (MRA) and can be used to differentiate between flowing and stationary spins. Both these effects normally occur simultaneously during MRI which makes it necessary to suppress one effect and enhance the other effect in order to obtain diagnostic MRA studies. For time-of-flight MRA, phase shift effects are reduced by using flow compensated sequences. The phase changes are compensated for by incorporating additional gradient pulses of specific amplitude, a technique known as gradient motion rephasing, velocity compensation, or gradient moment nulling. Additional cancellation of phase dispersion is accomplished by using short TE's and small isotropic voxels [9,12]. Phase change effects are particularly useful for quantification of flow as well as for visualization of slow flow through vessels [2].

Three Dimensional (3-D) Imaging

Spatial localization is achieved in 2-D imaging by the combination of the slice selection, phase encoding and read or frequency encoding gradients. 3-D imaging employs the same three gradients and adds an additional phase encoding step for slice selection after the initial gradient pulse which selects the volume to be imaged. This second phase encoding step increases the imaging time proportionately by the number of phase encoding steps for slice selection, i.e., the number of partitions. An imaging volume with 32 partitions will be 32 times as long as a single slice acquisition. The great advantage of GRE techniques in 3-D imaging is the speed of acquisition because of the short TR's. These short TR's allow volume imaging within a reasonable examination time according to the formula:

3-D imaging time =
        TR × NEX × phase encoding steps × partitions

Because of the improved signal to noise ratio, only one excitation is needed in most MRA applications, resulting in 3-D imaging times which are within reasonable limits. For example, an examination of 32 partitions utilizing a TR of 50 msec takes approximately 6.5 minutes [9,16].

MRA Sequences

The finest resolution and anatomic fidelity to date utilizes MRA sequences that exploit the influx of the unsaturated spins (time-of-flight effects), short echo times, small voxels and velocity compensation in order to maximize contrast between stationary and moving tissues and minimize dephasing of spins across the voxel. In order to obtain diagnostic MRA examinations, it is essential to utilize velocity compensation gradients with a TE of 10 msec or less and choose thin contiguous slices of less than 1.5 mm [9,15,16].

The signal of the unsaturated inflowing spins is usually large enough to differentiate blood vessels from the surrounding stationary tissue. 3-D gradient echo (FLASH or FISP) sequences are utilized with small (15-30°) flip angles and thin contiguous partitions. Flow compensation is utilized in the slice selection and read encoding directions to correct for first order motion (velocity) effects. Both 2-D sequential slice imaging and volume acquisition techniques are used to create high resolution 3-D data sets of the volume of interest. The imaging slab thickness may range from 32 to 64 mm with an effective thickness of 1-1.25 mm for each partition.

The resulting images have flat gray/white matter differentiation, but flow is very bright (Fig. 1A). The individual partitions may be viewed on a monitor or on hard copy X-ray film. In order to further enhance the visualization of the vessels, the data set is run through a post processing routine called maximum intensity projection (MIP). The MIP algorithm creates projections in which flowing vessels show up as the brightest objects in a relatively transparent background of stationary tissue. All the vessels within the slab or block of tissue may be viewed as a single static image (Fig. 1B). When these MIP projections are created at multiple viewing angles and shown in a cine mode, a 3-D view of the vessels may be seen in various projections or rotations [1,4-6,16] (Fig. 2).

The larger the 3-D imaging slab, the more partitions one must use to keep the section thickness within a reasonable range. Optimally, one would like both to maximize spatial resolution and to minimize dephasing effects by decreasing section thickness, yet minimize imaging time by decreasing the number of partitions. These objectives can be met by judicious selection of the plane of the original partitions that make up the 3-D data set. For example, the midline deep venous system of the brain is best depicted on sagittal images while the circle of Willis is best viewed on axial images (Fig. 2). In some applications, it may be necessary to obtain 3-D slabs in two or three planes [10-12].

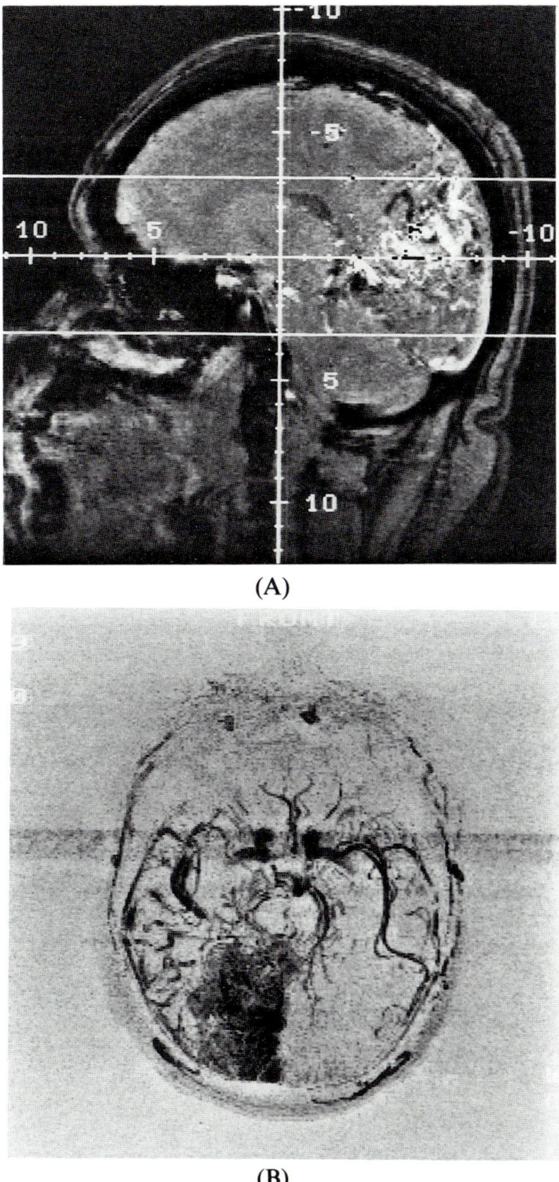

(A)

(B)

Figure 1. *RIGHT PARIETO-OCCIPITAL AVM. (A) Sagittal gradient echo localizer image in an adult. The parallel lines demonstrate the level of the MRA examination. Note that on this two-dimensional gradient echo image, most of the vessels are bright. (B) Axial MRA scan. FLASH 3-D 25°/40/13. The vessels show the same bright signal intensity (reversed to black on white for display). The localization and extent of the AVM is well shown.*

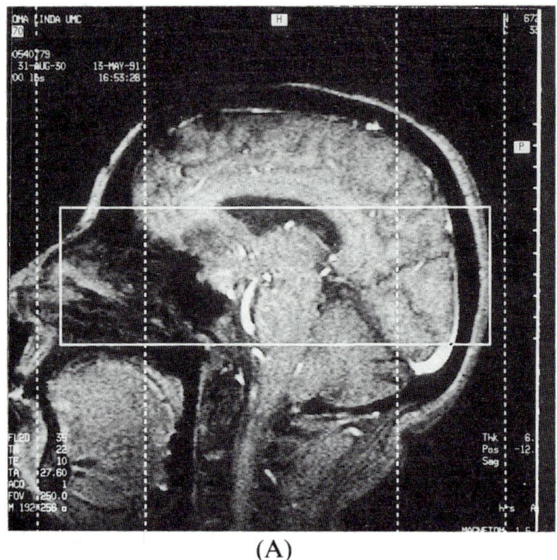

(A)

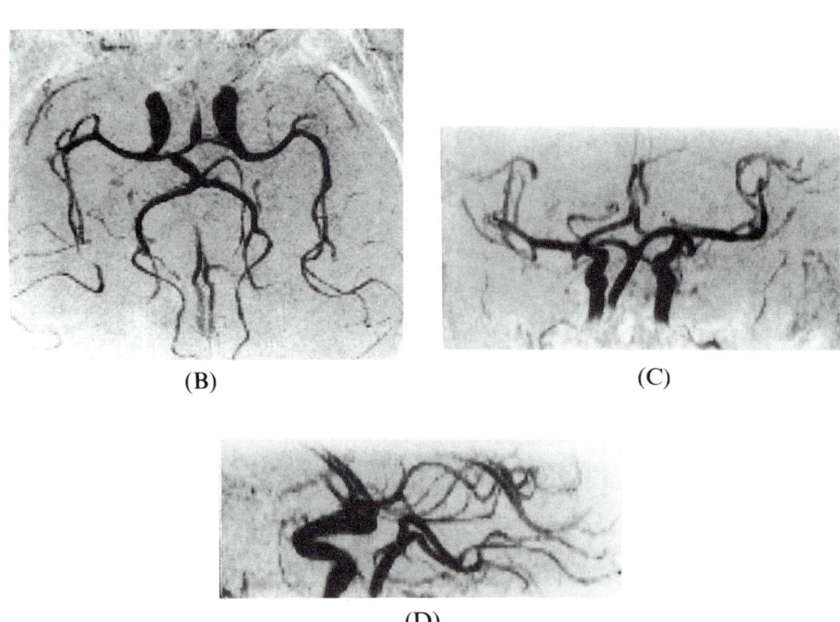

(B)   (C)

(D)

Figure 2. *NORMAL CIRCLE OF WILLIS.* (A) *Sagittal gradient echo localizer image. The "box" outlines the axial slab through the circle of Willis. The dotted vertical lines represent anterior and posterior presaturation pulses used to eliminate breathing motion (anteriorly) or venous and dural sinus flow (posteriorly). (B) Axial view of the circle of Willis. (C) Coronal and (D) Sagittal views of the circle of Willis obtained from the same axial slab. The MRA data sets may be rotated in all directions.*

It is essential to view the individual projection images along with the 3-D projection slab. For example, slowly filling aneurysms may not be seen on the slab images, but may be visible on the individual projection images. Some severe carotid stenoses may not be optimally viewed on the MRA data sets, but will be readily depicted on the individual projection scans.

Enhanced MRA

Visualization of slow flowing vessels is improved after Gd-DTPA enhancement. The addition of gadolinium improves the depiction of the vasculature by shortening the T1 of blood. The existing time-of-flight enhancement of the FISP sequence is even further enhanced by the wash-in of even more fully relaxed flowing spins due to the T1 shortening effect of gadolinium. The increased signal is most apparent in veins and dural sinuses. The increased signal in fast flowing arteries is much less apparent since these structures already have bright signal on MR angiograms [3,14].

An added benefit to the use of gadolinium is lesion conspicuity. If a lesion markedly enhances with Gd-DTPA on planar spin echo images, it is highly visible on the individual projection and 3-D slab images (Fig. 3). Since the MIP algorithm records the maximum intensity along a ray, it will project all brightly enhancing lesions along with the bright blood vessels.

In certain applications of MRA, the use of gadolinium is essential. We have found Gd-DTPA enhancement useful in demonstrating dural sinus invasion by meningiomas and/or skull base tumors. If a particular dural sinus is not seen on the unenhanced scans, one cannot be certain if it is occluded or if it does not have sufficient moving spins. The demonstration of non-filling is of greater diagnostic significance following gadolinium injection. This lack of filling after gadolinium administration indicates obstruction of the dural sinus.

Applications

Extracranial Cervicocranial Vessels

MRA has been shown to be useful in demonstrating occlusive disease of the cervicocranial circulation (Fig. 4). Occasionally, lesser amounts of stenosis are overgraded as severe stenosis (Fig. 5). This

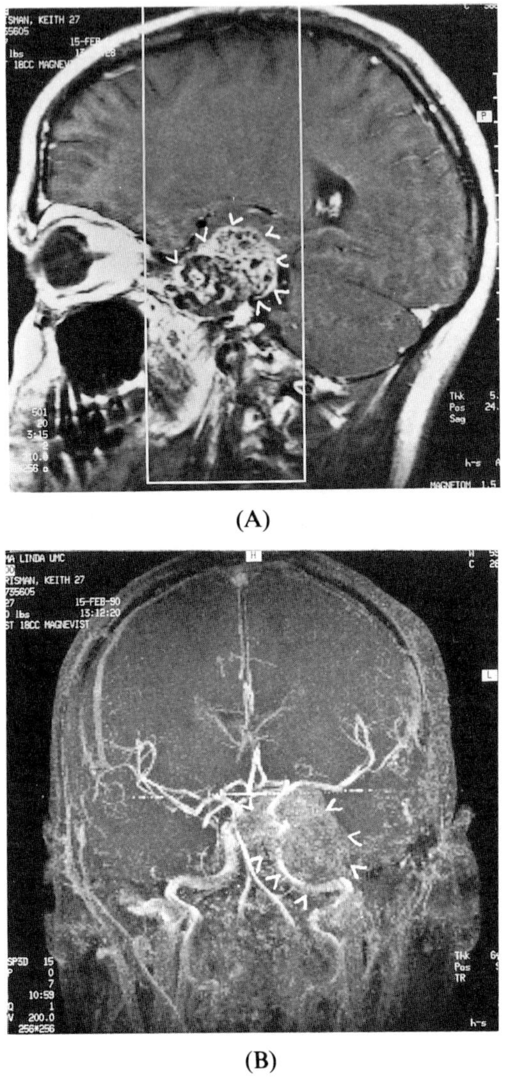

(A)

(B)

Figure 3. *LEFT PETROUS APEX MYXOCHONDROMA. (A) Sagittal spin echo image following gadolinium-DTPA administration in young adult male. The heterogeneously enhancing tumor extends upward from the skull base into the parasellar region (arrowheads). The vertical parallel lines demonstrate the level of the MRA examination. (B) Coronal MRA scan. FISP 3-D 15°/40/7 with gadolinium-DTPA enhancement. The enhancing tumor mass (arrowheads) is well seen along with its relationship to the left cavernous and supraclinoid internal carotid artery segments. The vessel is irregularly narrowed in several sites by the circumferential tumor.*

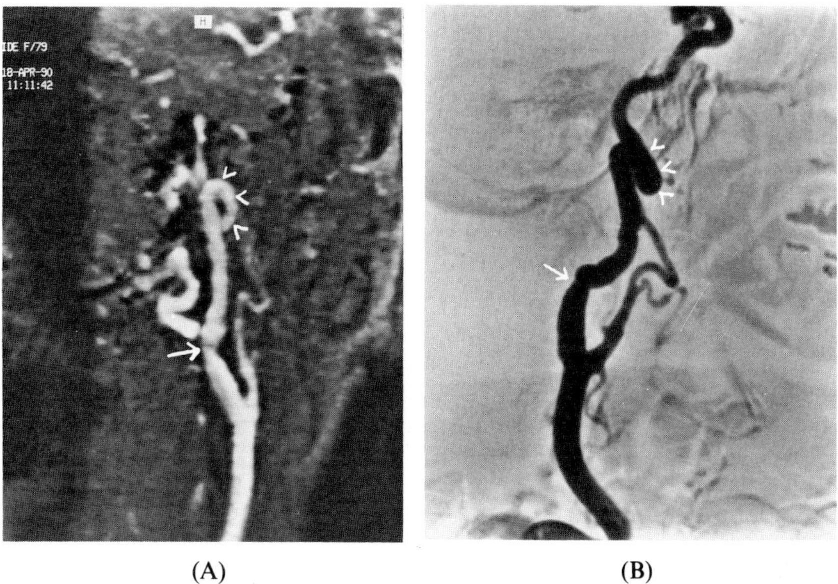

(A)   (B)

Figure 4. *STENOSIS OF THE RIGHT INTERNAL CAROTID ARTERY.
(A) Oblique sagittal MRA scan. The cervicocranial vessels are well seen with
a complete loop in the right distal internal carotid artery (arrowheads). A
kink with an associated stenosis is noted in the right proximal internal
carotid artery (arrow). There is a superimposed vessel beyond the area of
stenosis which represents the right vertebral artery. Note the presaturation
pulse (asterisks) which is utilized to eliminate incoming flow from the venous
structures. (B) Conventional selective right common carotid artery angiogram. This oblique sagittal view shows the loop of the distal internal carotid
artery (arrowheads) and the site of stenosis (arrow). Note that the stenosis
is somewhat more prominent on the MRA than on the conventional
angiogram.*

error is produced by the presence of turbulent flow distal to the
stenosis, which results in signal loss due to phase-contrast effects,
despite the application of flow compensation. Problems with turbulent flow are decreased by the application of very short TE's (7
msec or less) which minimize the phase errors and allow the acquisition of diagnostic quality images without cardiac gating. Some
situations with low flow such as severely stenotic arteries, time-of-
flight effects may be reduced by saturation effects. This problem is
partially resolved by acquiring the 3-D data set in the axial projection and then viewing the projection images in the coronal or sagit-

151

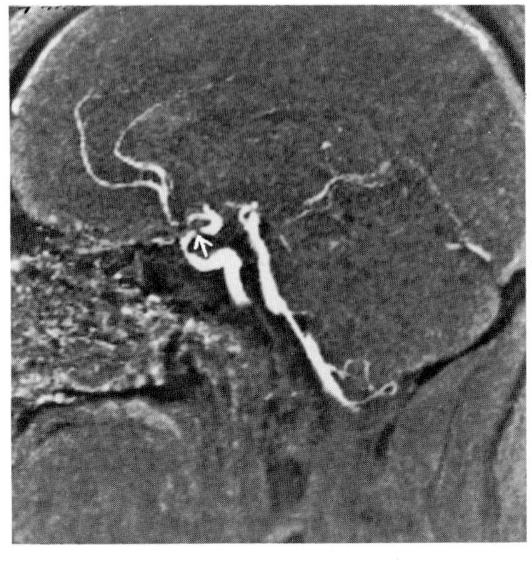

(A)

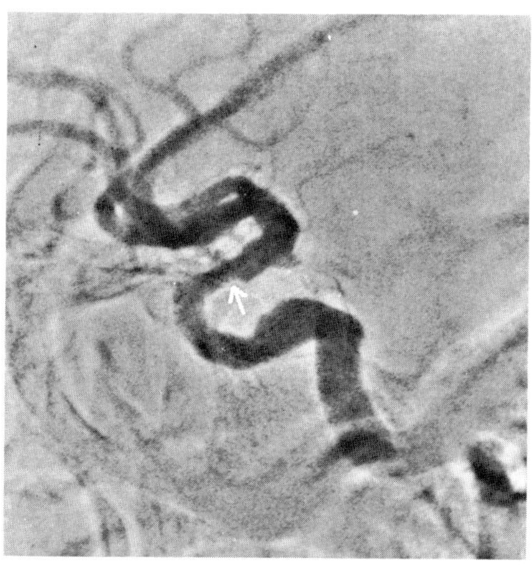

(B)

Figure 5. *CRITICAL STENOSIS, SUPRACLINOID PORTION LEFT INTERNAL CAROTID ARTERY. (A) Sagittal MRA scan. The circle of Willis vessels are well seen. There is a critical stenosis of the supraclinoid portion of the left internal carotid artery (arrow). (B) Conventional selective left internal carotid artery angiogram. The segmental irregularity and site of stenosis are clearly visible (arrow). The degree of stenosis are overestimated on the MRA when compared to the conventional angiogram.*

tal planes. This technique maximizes time-of-flight effects since the flow in the cervicocranial vessels is generally perpendicular to the direction of data acquisition [11].

Carotid ulcerations may not be detected with MRA because the relative stasis of blood within these lesions fails to produce adequate flow contrast [6,11]. In such cases, duplex sonography of the carotid bifurcation may be helpful. On the other hand, MRA is more accurate that sonography in differentiating a severely stenotic vessel from an occluded one. This distinction is important, because a stenotic vessel may be amenable to surgery, while a thrombosed one may not. MRA can demonstrate the whole length of the internal carotid artery from its origin in the neck to its intracranial bifurcation, which sonography is generally unable to accomplish because of the dense skull base (Fig. 4).

Intracranial Vessels

Preliminary studies show that MRA has a role in the evaluation of a variety of intracranial vessels. In a study of aneurysms, MRA detected 17 of 19 the typical congenital berry form. This technique can define the circle of Willis sufficiently to allow detection of intracranial aneurysms as small as 3-4 mm (Figs. 6 and 7). Aneurysms with slow flow or giant aneurysms that are partially thrombosed are difficult to detect on the projection images. However, a review of the conventional spin echo images and/or the injection of gadolinium will help in detecting some of these lesions [15].

The current applications of MRA in intracranial aneurysms is limited to certain clinical situations such as the evaluation of patients with severe pulsating headaches. MRA can also be used as a noninvasive screening examination in patients with a family history of aneurysm or in patients with a phobia about aneurysms. In searching for mycotic aneurysms or elucidating a suspected aneurysm seen on spin echo MR or CT scans, MRA may prove to be useful. MRA is not indicated in patients with subarachnoid hemorrhage or evidence of other intracranial catastrophes.

MRA has proven to be a good means for detecting and characterizing intracranal AVM's (Fig. 1). Techniques of 3-D MRA can delineate the nidus and major feeding vessels of AVM's without invasive angiography. Occasionally, the hyperdynamic afferent

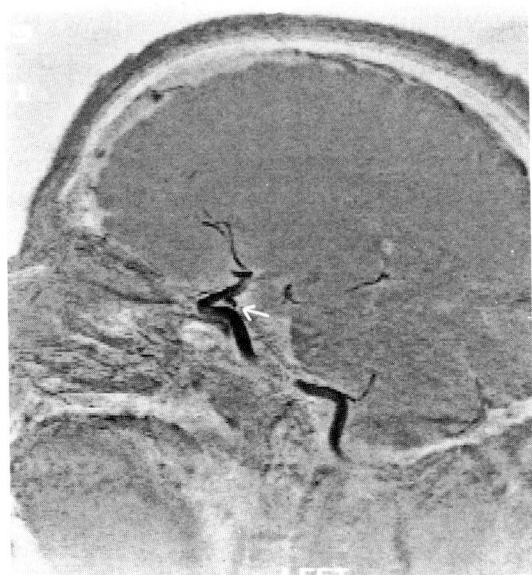

Figure 6. *SMALL ANEURYSM, RIGHT SUPRACLINOID INTERNAL CAROTID ARTERY. The small (3-4 mm diameter) aneurysm is clearly visible on this selective sagittal MIP study (arrow). The MIP study of all the partitions did not show the aneurysm.*

arteries may not be completely seen because of incomplete rephasing of the moving spins. In such instances, presaturation techniques can be utilized to allow the different vascular territories contributing to the AVM to be mapped. For example, if an AVM appears to be fed by multiple arteries, a presaturation pulse may be applied to one feeding vessel without effecting the other major intracranial branches. The presaturation pulse eliminates the signal only within that portion of the AVM supplied by the presaturated vessel, allowing clear depiction of the other feeding vessel(s) [5,6,12].

Depiction of venous angiomas may be accomplished by MRA. In one study, 13 of 14 venous angiomas were detected on detailed thin slab acquisitions. Gadolinium has to be injected in order to see the slowly flowing veins which are generally not seen on time-of-flight angiographic techniques [10].

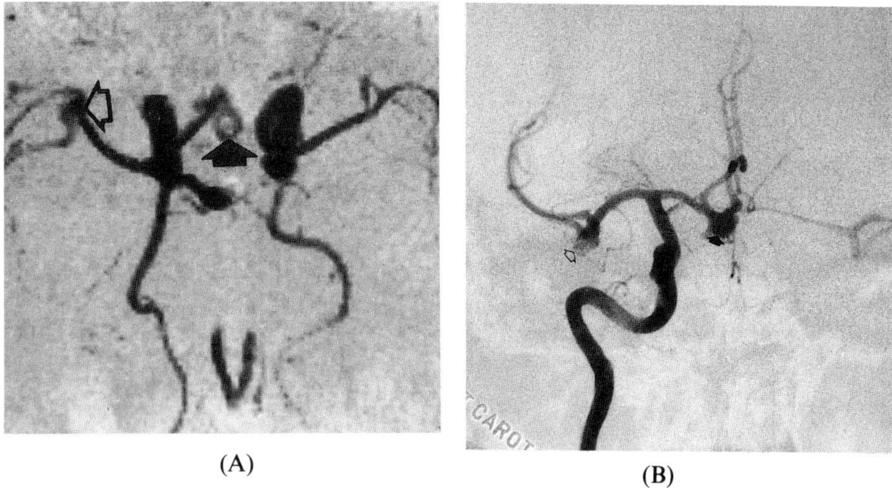

Figure 7. *TWO ANEURYSMS OF THE CAROTID CIRCULATION. (A) Axial MRA image in an elderly female. FLASH 3-D 25°/40/13. The aneurysm of the anterior communicating artery (closed arrowhead) shows slow flow centrally as an area of low signal and high flow peripherally at the site of maximum vortex activity. Another aneurysm in the bifurcation of the right middle cerebral artery is seen (open arrowhead). (B) Conventional selective right internal carotid artery angiogram. The anterior communicating artery aneurysm fills homogeneously (closed arrowhead). The right bifurcation middle cerebral artery aneurysm shows partial filling (open arrowhead).*

Head and Neck Tumors

We have utilized MRA to evaluate a variety of mass lesions of the head and neck. Injections of gadolinium are utilized in most cases, either to improve visualization of the cranial veins (for example, meningiomas invading the dural sinuses) or for improved lesion conspicuity. The MRA studies follow spin echo examinations of the lesions, because there are inherent difficulties in covering large regions of interest with MRA. Once the tumor is localized, however, it is possible to focus on a region of interest. The relationships of these tumors to the vessels are clearly shown on the MRA studies.

Conclusions

We conclude that MRA can play a role in providing useful information about the intra- and extracranial circulation, which when used in conjunction with standard MRI can facilitate the preoperative planning of patients with a variety of vascular lesions. Particular applications include carotid occlusive disease, aneurysms, AVM's or patients with head and neck neoplasms. MRA cannot substitute for conventional angiography in all cases and is not indicated in patients with subarachnoid hemorrhage.

References

1. Afidi RJ, Masaryk TJ, Haacke EM, Lenz GW, Ross JS, Modic MT, Nelson AD, LiPuma JP, Cohen AM. MR angiography of peripheral, carotid, and coronary arteries. AJR 1987;149:1097-1109
2. Bendel P, Buonocore E, Brockisch A, Besozzi MC. Blood flow in the carotid arteries: quantification by using phase-sensitive MR imaging. AJR 1989;152:1307-1310
3. Creasy JL, Price RR, Presbrey T, Goins D, Partain CL, Kessler RB. Gadolinium-enhanced MR angiography. Radiology 1990;175:280-283
4. Edelman RR, Wentz KU, Mattle H, Zhan B, Liu C, Kim D, Laub G. Projection arteriography and venography: initial clinical results with MR. Radiology 1989;172:351-357
5. Edelman RR, Wentz KU, Mattle HP, O'Reilly GV, Candia G, Liu C, Zhao B, Kjellberg RN, Davis KR. Intracerebral arteriovenous malformations: evaluation with selective MR angiography and venography. Radiology 1989;173:831-837
6. Edelman RR, Mattle HP, Atkinson DJ, Hoogewoud HM. MR angiography. AJR 1990;154:937-946
7. Gullberg GT, Wehrli FW, Shimakawa A, Simons MA. MR vascular imaging with a fast gradient refocusing pulse sequence and reformatted images from transaxial sections. Radiology 1987;165:241-246
8. Keller PJ, Drayer BP, Fram EK, Williams KD, Dumoulin CL, Souza SP. MR angiography with two-dimensional acquisition and three-dimensional display. Radiology 1989;173:527-532
9. Laub GA, Kaiser WA. MR angiography with graident motion refocusing. J Comput Assist Tomogr 1988;123:377-382
10. Marchal G, Bosmans H, Van Fraeyenhoven L, Wilms G, Van Hecke P, Plets C, Baert AL. Intracranial vascular lesions: optimization and clinical evaluation of three-dimensional time-of-flight MR angiography. Radiology 1990;175:443-448
11. Masaryk TJ, Ross JS, Modic MT, Lenz GW, Haacke EM. Carotid bifurcation: MR imaging. Radiology 1988;166:461-466
12. Masaryk TJ, Modic MT, Ross JS, Ruggieri PM, Laub GA, Lenz GW, Haacke EM, Selman WR, Wiznitzer M, Harik SI. Intracranial circulation: preliminary clinical results with three-dimensional (volume) MR angiography. Radiology 1989;171:793-799
13. Pernicone JR, Siebert JE, Potchen EJ, Pera A, Dumoulin CL, Souza SP. Three-dimensional phase-contrast MR angiography in the head and neck: preliminary report. AJNR 1990;11:457-466

14. Rippe DJ, Grist TM, Uglietta JP, Fuller GN, Boyko OB. Case Report. Carotid body tumor: flow sensitive pulse sequences and MR angiography. J Comput Assist Tomogr 1989;13:874-877
15. Ross JS, Masaryk TJ, Modic MT, Ruggieri PM, Haacke EM, Selman WR. Intracranial aneurysms: evaluation by MR angiography. AJNR 1990;11:449-455
16. Ruggieri PM, Laub GA, Masaryk TJ, Modic MT. Intracranial circulation: pulse-sequence considerations in three-dimensional (volume) MR angiography. Radiology 1989;171:785-791

Magnetic Resonance of Multiple Sclerosis and White Matter Disease

Giuseppe Scotti

Department of Neuroradiology, Ospedale San Raffaele, Milano, Italy

Introduction

The role of neuroradiology in the diagnosis of Multiple Sclerosis (MS) and other diseases of the white matter begins with the advent of CT. Before 1972, the neuroradiologist was involved only in the differential diagnosis, to rule out by means of angiography or pneumoencephalography tumors either intracranial or spinal, or vascular ischemic lesions.

For years CT has played an important role, although frequently disappointing [1,2,3]. With CT the white matter can be differentiated from gray matter; the white matter has a higher content of myelin, hence lipids containing atoms of carbon that have a low attenuation coefficient. For this reason the white matter is hypodense with respect to the gray matter.

However, foci of demyelination causes an increase in water within the white matter, reflected in a further subtle hypodensity that cannot always be clearly detected or defined.

Magnetic Resonance has proven to be far superior to CT in diagnosis of white matter lesions, due to its sensitivity to white matter changes, higher spatial resolution and multiplanar capabilities [4,5,6,7].

In T1WI the white matter appears slightly hyperintense with

respect to gray matter while in T2WI the white matter becomes hypointense with respect to gray matter. The difference in signal is due to the low content of mobile protons in the phospholipids of myelin that is responsible for relatively long T1 and T2 shortening with respect to the gray matter where a higher concentration of mobile protons is found.

The demyelinating process is characterized by a disruption of the blood brain barrier, inflammatory perivascular reaction, myelin loss and then by a local increase of water concentration. Lately axonal degeneration may be found. The phenomenon that causes recognition of the plaque at MR is then totally nonspecific and reflects merely a focal increase in water content.

Gadolinium injection shows the disruption of the blood-brain barrier when present and has proven to be of a very great help in better diagnosing MS and understanding its clinical evolution [8,9,10,11].

Technique

T2-weighted spin echo (SE) sequences are more sensitive than T1-weighted ones for the demonstration of lesions in MS. A moderately T2-weighted sequence, where the cerebrospinal fluid (CSF) signal is slightly less intense than that of normal white matter, is optimal for demonstrating periventricular lesion. A more heavily T-2 weighted sequence, in which lesions intensity is greater than that of gray matter, but in which CSF intensity is not excessive, is optimal for demonstrating subcortical lesions. It is desirable to obtain the thinnest slice which provides an adequate signal-to-noise ratio in a reasonable period of time; axial 5 mm thick slices are more convenient. Sagittal cuts are very useful to demonstrate plaques in the corpus callosum and brain stem.

Gd-DTPA enhancement is common in MS lesions, where it also indicates the presence of inflammation.

Enhancement occurs in almost all new lesions which appear during serial monthly scans of patients with relapsing-remitting or secondary progressive MS. Scanning should commence at least 5 minutes after injection of Gd-DTPA, as most lesions display maximum enhancement 5-30 minutes post-injection.

Multiple Sclerosis

CT has produced the first relevant improvement in understanding some pathological aspects of the disease. Plaques are not infrequently visible as foci of hypodensity, mainly in the supratentorial periventricular white matter. Small plaques, particularly in the corpus callosum, in the subcortical areas, in the brain stem and posterior fossa in general are not easily recognized. There is no way to distinguish recent from old plaques when, as usual, they coexist in the same patient.

Only iodinated contrast medium differentiates active from silent plaques: disruption of the blood brain barrier in the acute plaques produces enhancement that may become more obvious using a double dose and performing delayed scans.

MR is, however, definitely superior to CT: much smaller plaques can be detected and critical areas such as the corpus callosum [12] and the brain stem are easily investigated employing sagittal or coronal sections.

While CT, with and without contrast is possible in about 50% of patients non selected for type or phase of the disease, MR has a 90% positive yield in the same group while the positivity raises up to 100% in cases of definite MS. MR is more sensitive than laboratory tests like evoked potentials or CSF oligoclonal bands in patients with definite MS.

As with CT, it is not possible to differentiate new from old plaques. Retrospectively old plaques may be recognized because they decrease in size due to the reduction of edema.

Plaques tend to be periventricular, frequently have an oval shape with a radial distribution along medullary veins and the major axis oriented perpendicular to the lateral wall of the ventricle (Fig. 1).

The most common locations are in the deep white matter of the hemispheres: cerebellar peduncles (Fig. 2) brain stem (Fig. 3) medial longitudinal fasciculus located immediately in front of the aqueduct (Fig. 4) and corpus callosum (Fig. 5) are also frequently involved.

Particularly useful is MR in patients that present with a first episode of optic neuritis: not infrequently asymptomatic plaques may be seen in the brain parenchyma (Fig. 6). They may eithcr be contemporary to the episode of optic neuritis or indicate previous episodes. The same is true for other clinical presentations: many

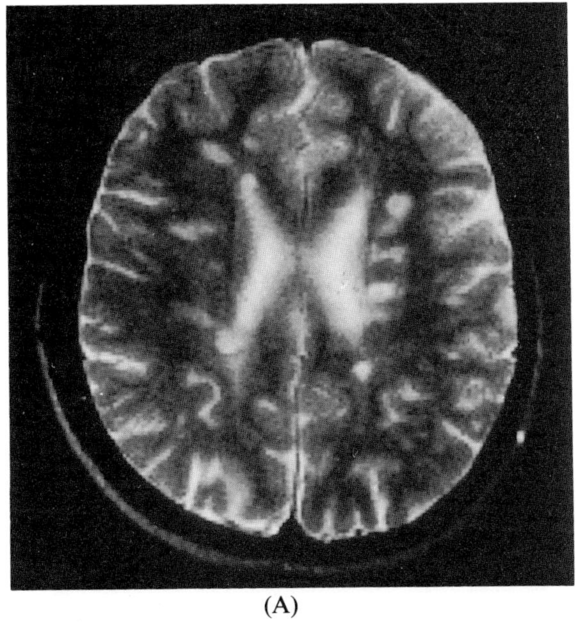

(A)

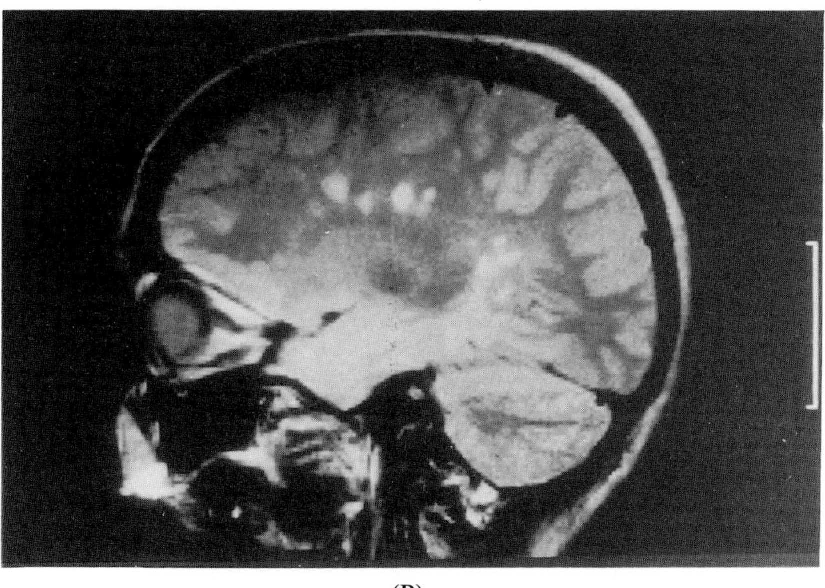

(B)

Figure 1. *CLASSICAL MS. (A and B) Axial and sagittal T2WI. Plaques are hyperintense with respect to normal parenchyma. They are mainly periventricular and have oval shape with a major transverse axis.*

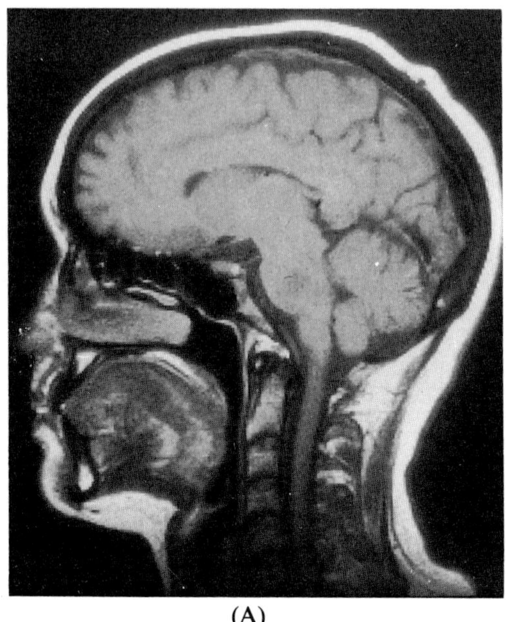

(A)

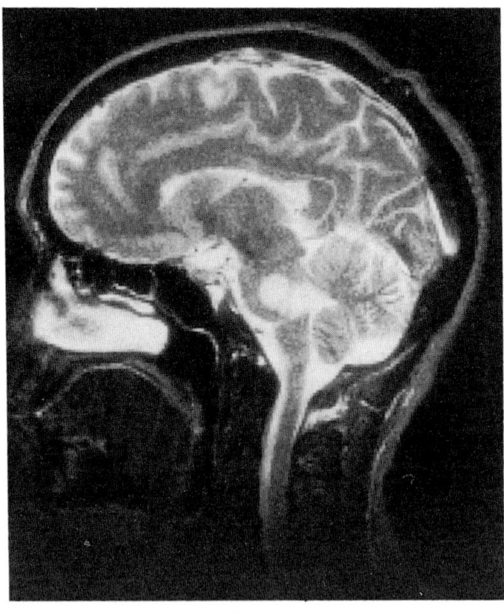

(B)

Figure 2. *BRAIN STEM MS. Large plaque in the brain stem and middle cerebellar peduncle. (A) The lesion is slightly hypointense and is barely seen. (B) T2WI. The plaque is hyperintense and is clearly seen.*

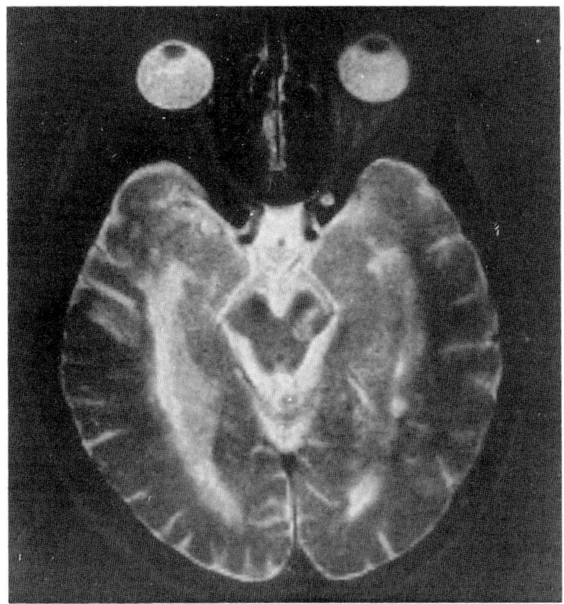

Figure 3. *PEDUNCULAR MS. T2WI, axial plane. Plaque is in the left cerebral peduncle.*

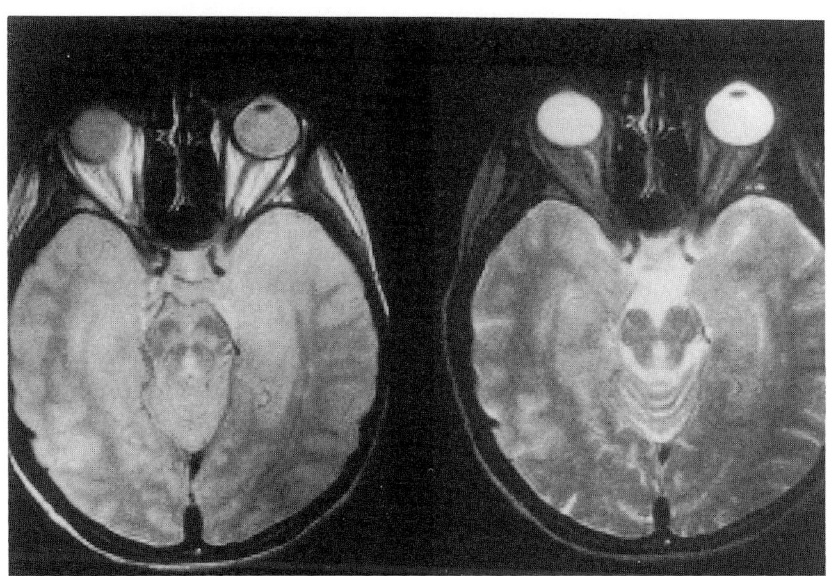

Figure 4. *MEDIAL, LONGITUDINAL FASCICULUS IN MS. Proton density (left) and T2WI. Hyperintensity due to demyelination is seen in the medial longitudinal fasciculus, in front of the aqueduct.*

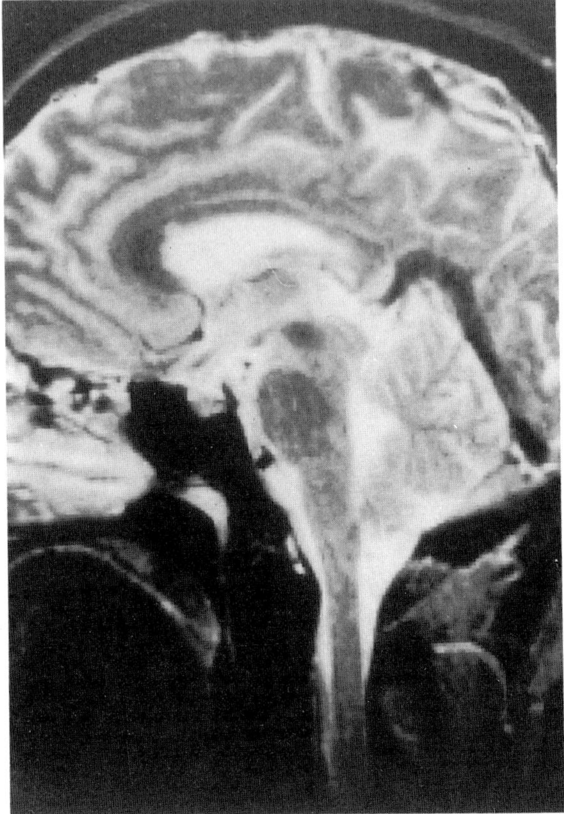

Figure 5. *CORPUS CALLOSUM MS. Midline sagittal T2WI. Small plaque in the anterior third of the Corpus Callosum.*

more plaques, frequently inactive are found in patients at the first clinically recognized episode of MS (Fig. 7).

Gd-DTPA provides the only way to differentiate recent from old plaques: recent plaques show a focal hyperintensity in T1WI. Sometimes Gd allows identification of hyperacute plaques that have not yet produced a signal change in T1 or T2WI: Gd is in fact able to demonstrate the disruption of the blood brain barrier before the formation of the inflammatory infiltrate and subsequent formation of edema (Fig. 8).

Gd enhancement may have different shapes: ring enhancement probably reflects reactivation of an old plaque while a nodular homogeneous enhancement indicates a recent plaque.

The demonstration in the same patient at the first clinical poussée of acute enhancing plaques together with chronic non-enhancing plaques confirms that MS is not a monophasic disease and provides

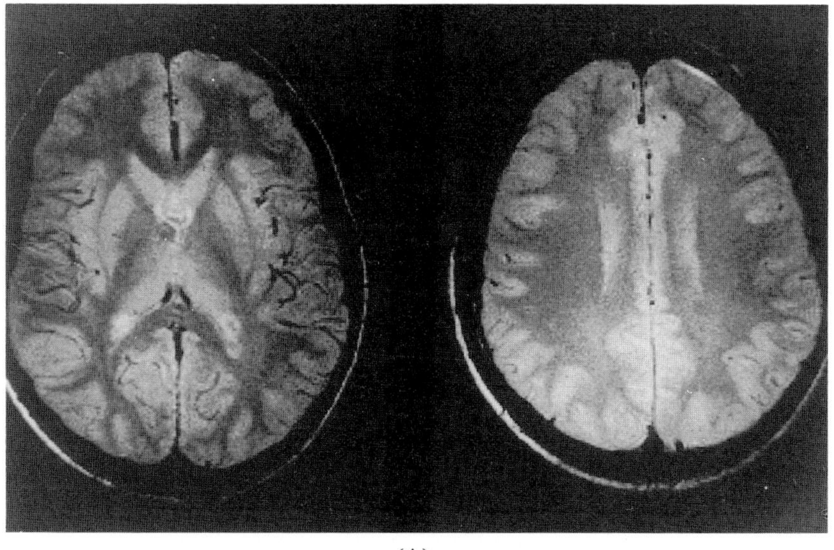

(A)

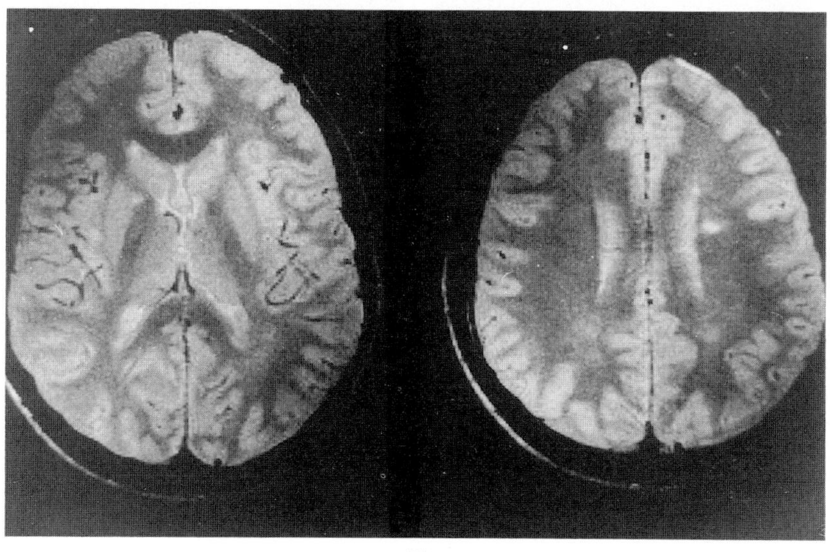

(B)

Figure 6. *OPTIC NERVE MS. (A) Proton density axial slices in a patient with the first episode of optic neuritis. No clinical CNS signs. No white matter abnormalities are seen in the brain. (B) Same patient two months later, when a second episode of optic neuritis occur. Proton density axial slices at the same level as (A). Two foci of demyelination are now seen, one in the anterior limb of the right internal capsule and the second in the deep frontal white matter on the left side.*

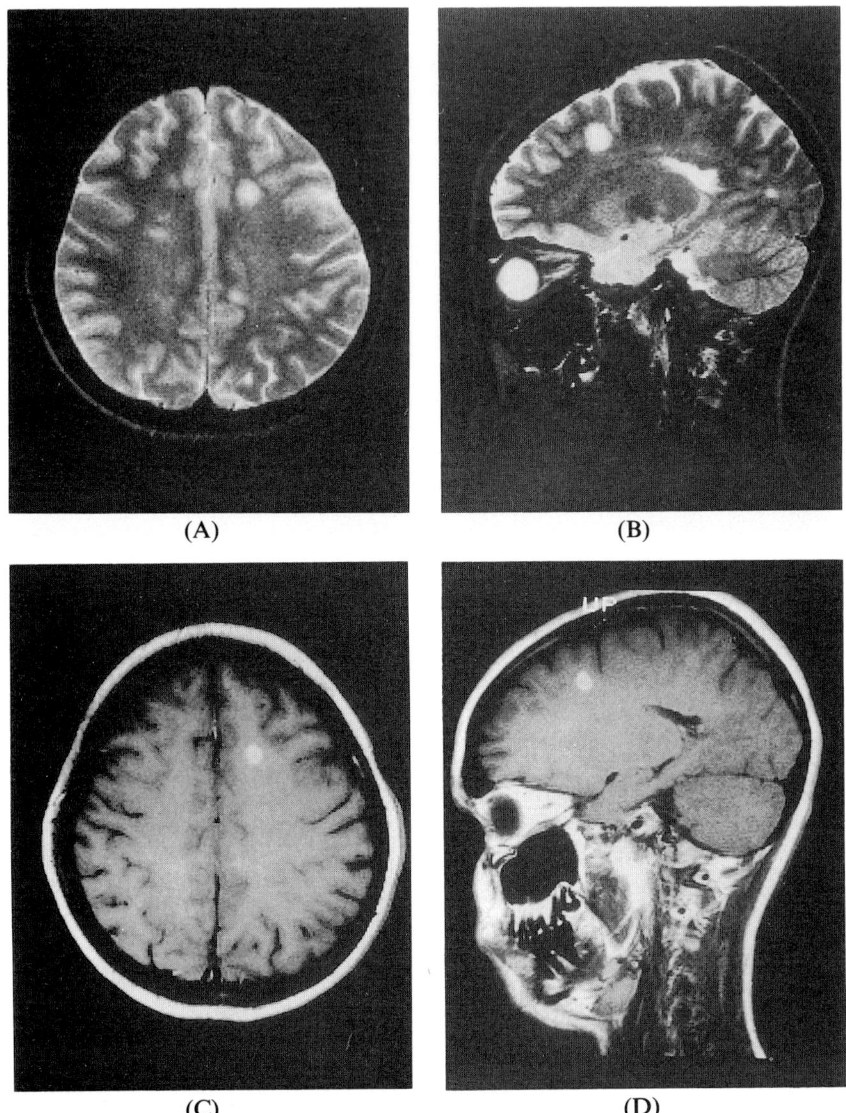

(A)   (B)

(C)   (D)

Figure 7. *ACTIVE PLAQUE AND CONTRAST. First episode of MS in a 24-year-old woman. (A, B) T2WI, axial and sagittal. At least five foci of hyperintensity are seen in the white matter of both hemispheres. The left frontal plaque is larger and brighter than the others. (C, D) T1WI, axial and sagittal, following i.v. injection of Gd-DTPA. Only the left frontal plaque enhances. This is probably the only active plaque. The others correspond to previous lesions, clinically silent.*

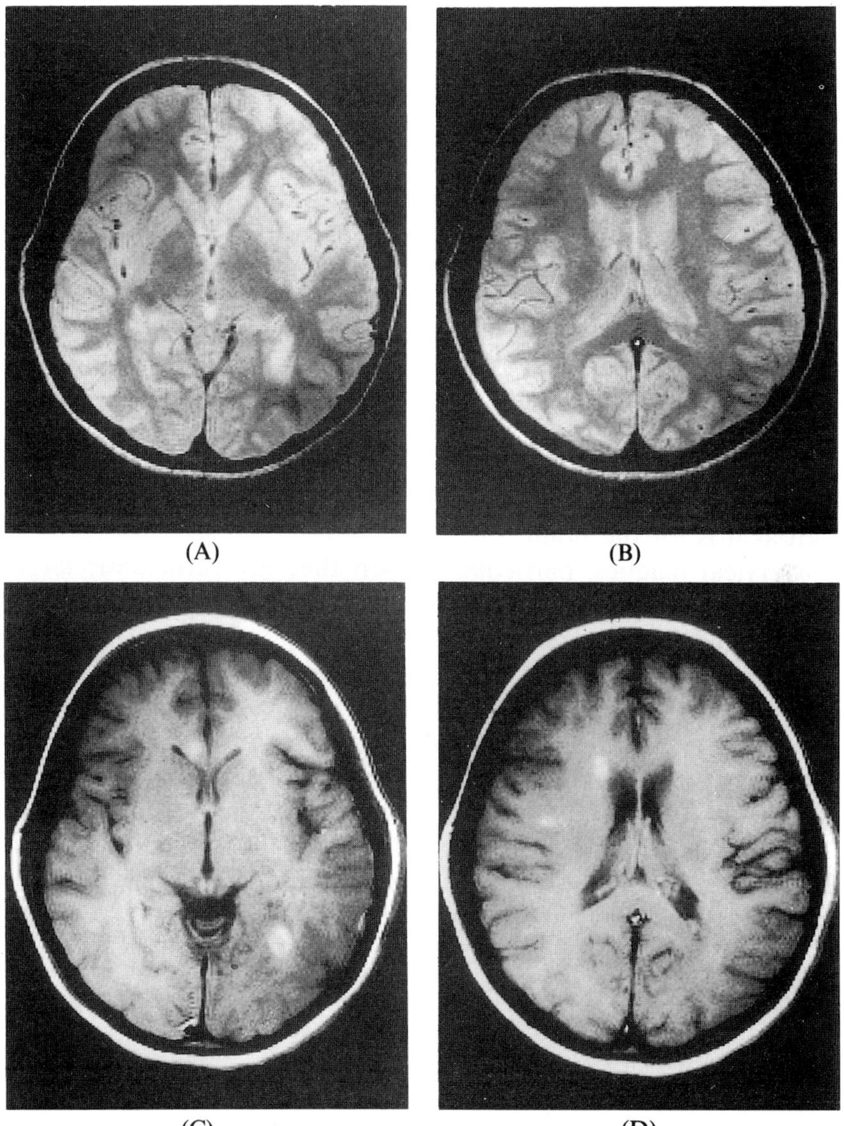

(A)

(B)

(C)

(D)

Figure 8. *RELAPSING MS.* (A, B) *Axial T2WI. Only one area of abnormal signal is clearly seen posterolaterally to the left trigone.* (C, D) *Following Gd injection the left peritrigonal plaque enhances. Three more foci become evident in the right hemisphere corpus callosum, subcortical frontal operculum and lateral to the frontal horn. These represent hyperacute plaques with blood-brain barrier disruption but without parenchymal changes detectable in proton density sequences.*

useful criteria for differential diagnosis with other diseases affecting the white matter like Acute Disseminated Encephalomyelitis (ADEM):

Some authors have performed Gd enhanced scans every two weeks and have demonstrated a high subclinical activity in the formation of plaques [13,14,15,16,17]. The knowledge of this phenomenon has provided a useful indication for clinical models in therapeutic trials [18].

Spinal Cord Multiple Sclerosis

Plaques in the spinal cord are less easily seen than in the brain since MRI is less sensitive in demonstrating small lesions in the cord as it is for the brain.

Cervical plaques, particularly when they are sufficiently large, involve about one level and produce some swelling of the cord, may be detected (Fig. 9).

The positive yield is much lower for the thoracic cord. A commonly used criterium in a patient suspected of having cord localization of MS, is to scan the brain in search of asymptomatic plaques. If this test is positive the diagnosis is easily made; a negative brain MRI, however does not rule out a diagnosis of MS.

The higher frequency of detection of spinal cord MS plaques in the cervical region probably reflects a better resolution of MR for this topographical region more than a much higher frequency of occurrence of plaques in the vertical cord.

Differential Diagnosis

Diagnosis of MS is a clinical diagnosis that must be supported by clinical history, age of the patient, other laboratory data such as evoked potentials and CSF oligoclonal bands.

The MR appearance of a plaque is, in fact per se, nonspecific.

In front of multiple, diffuse white matter focal lesions, other disease entities such as vasculitis, radiation damage [19,20] and subcortical atherosclerotic encephalopathy (Binswanger's disease)

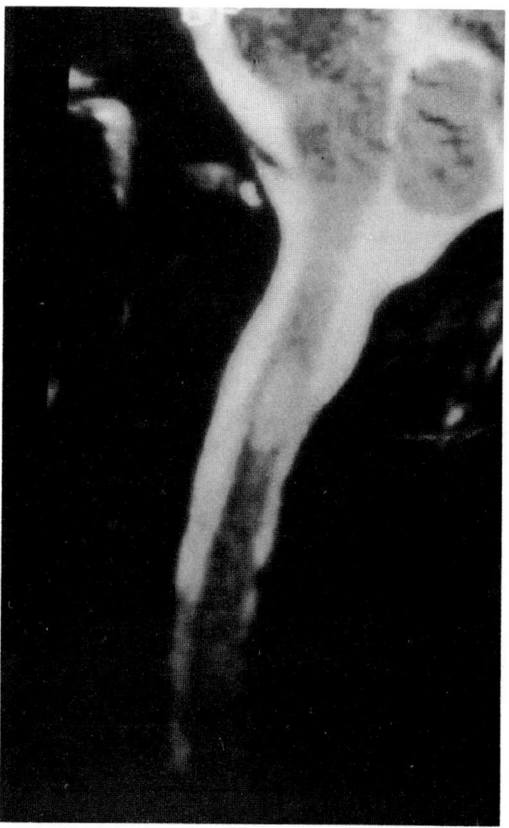

Figure 9. *SPINAL CORD MS. Spinal cord plaque. T2W sagittal image. Large focus of increased signal at C2-C3, with mild cord widening.*

[21] must be taken into consideration (Fig. 10). Acute disseminated encephalomyelitis (ADEM) [22] has a very similar appearance but knowledge of a previous viral infectious episode or vaccination and the monophasic aspect of the demyelinating foci will lead to the diagnosis.

In some rare cases plaques may be very large and simulate the diagnosis of a tumor both clinically and morphologically. Short term follow-up and close clinical observation will lead to the diagnosis.

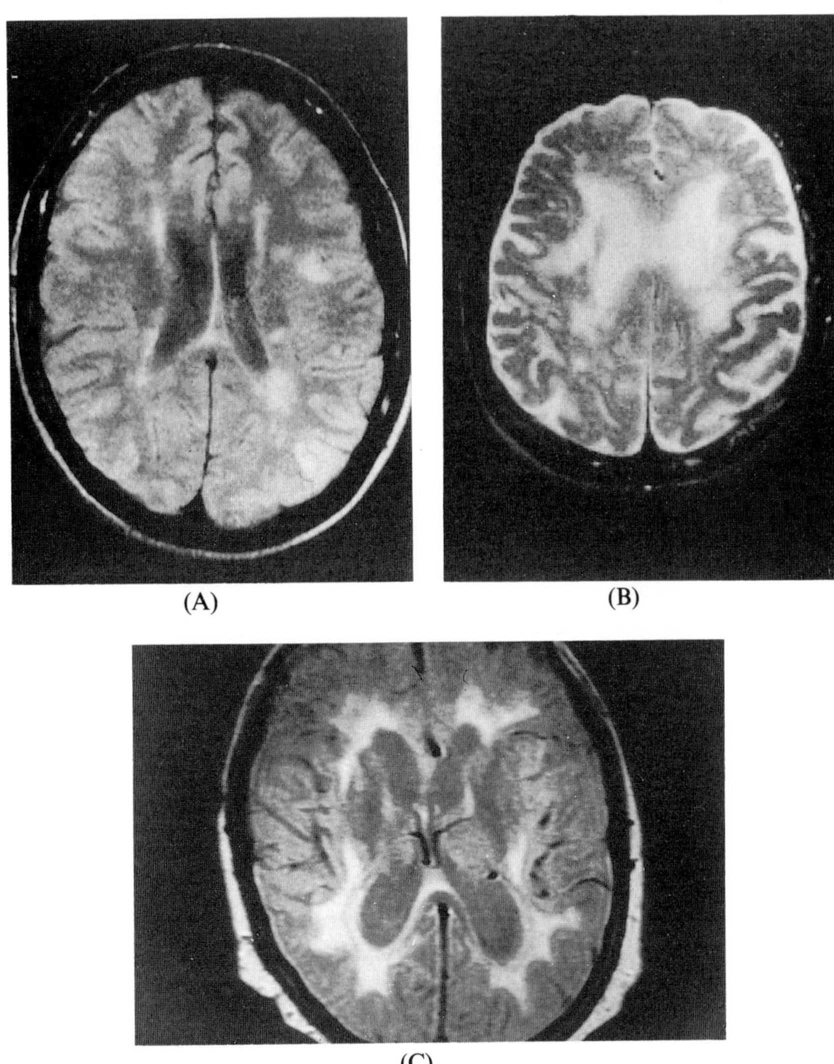

Figure 10. *DIFFERENTIAL DIAGNOSIS OF MS.* (A) *Lupus vasculitis.* (B) *Binswanger's disease.* (C) *Radiation injury.*

References

1. Barret L, Drayer B, Shin C. High-resolution computed tomography in multiple sclerosis. Ann Neurol 1985;17:33-38.

2. Ebers GC, Vinuela FV, Feasby T, Bass B. Multifocal CT enhancement in MS Neurology 1984;34:341-346.

3. Heinz ER, Drayer BP, Haenggeli CA, Painter MJ, Crumrine P. Computed tomography in white-matter disease. Radiology 1987;130:371-378.

4. Kirshner HS, Tsai SI, Runge VM, Price AC. Magnetic resonance imaging and other techniques in the diagnosis of multiple sclerosis. Arch Neurol 1985;42:859-863.

5. Scotti G, Scialfa G, Biondi A, et al. Magnetic resonance in multiple sclerosis. Neuroradiology 1986;28:319-323.

6. Young IR, Hall AS, Pallis CA, et al. Nuclear magnetic resonance imaging of the brain in multiple sclerosis. Lancet 1981;II:1063-1066.

7. Lukes SA, Crooks LE, Aminoff MJ, et al. Nuclear magnetic resonance imaging in multiple sclerosis. Annals of Neurology 1983;13:567-572.

8. Grossman RI, Gonzales-Scarano F, Atlas SW, Galetta S, Silberberg DH. Multiple sclerosis: gadolinium enhancement in MR imaging. Radiology 1986;161:721-725.

9. Grossman RI, Braffman BH, Brorson JR, Goldberg HI, Silberberg DH, Gonzales-Scarano F. Multiple sclerosis: serial study of gadolinium-enhanced MR imaging. Radiology 1988;169:117-122.

10. Miller DH, Rudge P, Johnson G, Kendall BR, et al. Serial gadolinium enhanced magnetic resonance imaging in multiple sclerosis. Brain 1988;111:927-939.

11. Kappos L, Staedt D, Rohrbach E, Keil W. Gadolinium-DTPA-enhanced magnetic resonance imaging in the evaluation of different disease courses and disease activity in multiple sclerosis. Neurology 1988;38 (suppl 1):255.

12. Simon JH, Holtas SL, Schiffer RB, Rudick RA, et al. Corpus callosum and subcallosal-periventricular lesions in multiple sclerosis: detection with MR. Radiology 1986;160:363-367.

13. Thompson AJ, Kermode AG, Wicks D, et al. Major differences in the dynamics of primary and secondary progressive multiple sclerosis. Ann Neurol 1992;29:53-62.

14. Koopmans RA, Li DKB, Oger JJF, et al. Chronic progressive multiple sclerosis: serial magnetic resonance brain imaging over six months. Annals of Neurology 1989;26:248-256.

15. Miller DH, Rudge P, Johnson G, et al. Serial gadolinium enhanced magnetic resonance imaging in multiple sclerosis. Brain 1988;111:927-939.

16. Grossman RI, Braffman BH, Brorson JR, et al. Multiple sclerosis: serial study of gadolinium-enhanced MR imaging. Radiology 1988;169:117-122.

17. Bastianello S, Pozzilli C, Bernadi S, et al. Serial study of gadolinium-DTPA MRI enhancement in multiple sclerosis. Neurology 1990;40:591-595.

18. Miller DH, Barkhof F, Berry I, Kappos L, Scotti G, Thompson AJ. Magnetic resonance imaging in monitoring the treatment of multiple sclerosis: cec guidelines. J Neurol Neuros Psych 1991:in press.

19. Curnes JT, Laster DW, Ball MR, Moody DM, Witcofski RL. Magnetic resonance imaging of radiation injury to the brain. AJNR 1986;7:389-394.

20. Dooms GC, Hecht S, Brant-Zawadzki M, Berthiaume Y, et al. Brain radiation lesions: MR imaging. Radiology 1986;158:149-155.

21. Kinkel WR, Jacobs L, Polachini I, Bates V, Heffner RR. Subcortical arteriosclerotic encephalopathy (Binswanger's disease). Computed tomographic, nuclear magnetic resonance and clinical correlations. Arch Neurol 1985;42:951-959.

22. Atlas SW, Grossman RI, Goldberg HI, Hackney DB, Bilaniuk LT, Zimmerman RA. MR diagnosis of the acute disseminated encephalomyelitis. JCAT 1986;10:798-801.

Imaging of Cerebral Ischemia and Stroke

Anton N. Hasso
Loma Linda University Medical Center, Department of Radiation Science, Loma Linda, California, USA

Introduction

Cerebral ischemia may be global or focal. Global ischemia is usually caused by hypoxia from lack of oxygenation or hypoperfusion from decreased cardiac output. Focal ischemia has a variety of causes and presents in a variety of ways. This presentation is primarily a discussion of focal ischemia and its appearance on MRI of the central nervous system. The sensitivity and/or specificity of corresponding CT data (conventional and contrast enhanced) will also be reviewed.

Categories of Ischemia

The categories of cerebral ischemia are primarily based on their pathophysiological cause or location within the brain. In some categories, the MR signal intensities are sufficiently distinctive to allow for specific characterization of the lesions during varying pulse sequences [1]. In all cases, the diagnosis of ischemia or stroke is aided by clinical history and neurological examination.

Pale Infarction

Acute

MRI offers greater sensitivity and possibly better specificity in the detection of acute stroke than other traditional methods. The MR findings in early infarction are loss of gray matter-white matter contrast and mass effect (in some cases). These changes are evident on T1-weighted images by T1 lengthening and on proton density weighted images by increase in proton density. Acute infarcts show up as sharply marginated areas of increased intensity on T2-weighted images due to the early cytotoxic edema (Figs. 1A and 2A and B). This latter finding is particularly useful since CT scans may be normal or equivocal in early acute infarction. The mass effect in acute strokes is better appreciated by MR than by CT due to significant increased tissue contrast. MR scans and/or MR angiograms may be used to document occlusion of the internal carotid artery or its branches [2,3](Figs. 1 and 2).

Subacute

Subacute infarcts are characterized by the same sharply marginated areas without mass effect. The T2 prolongation in ischemic lesions corresponds to the CT appearance of areas of decreased attenuation and abnormal contrast enhancement. MRI following gadolinium-DTPA administration offers similar enhancement patterns which may be helpful in differential diagnosis (Fig. 3). Mild focal enhancement may be seen in areas of luxury perfusion. Gyriform enhancement is seen in areas of endothelial proliferation.

Chronic (mature)

MR scans of some chronic infarcts show two distinct zones of alteration in signal intensities. The zone of more severe tissue damage (usually further from the nutrient vessel) demonstrates decreased CSF-like intensity. The zone of less severe tissue damage (usually closer to the nutrient vessel) appears intense on T2-weighted images and represents a zone of gliosis. This is apparently due to a varied host response or may be a reflection of the severity of the ischemic episode.

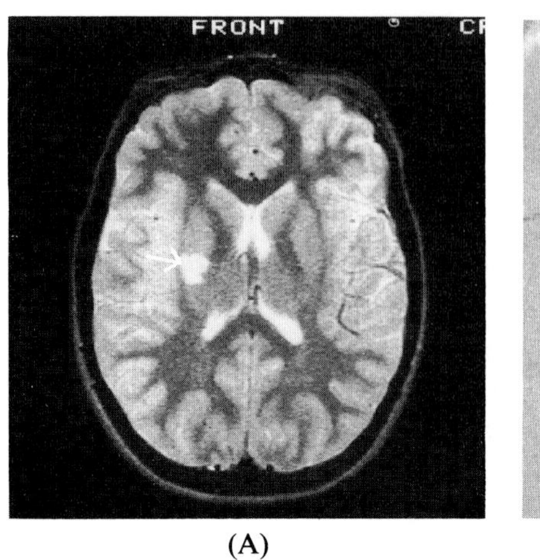
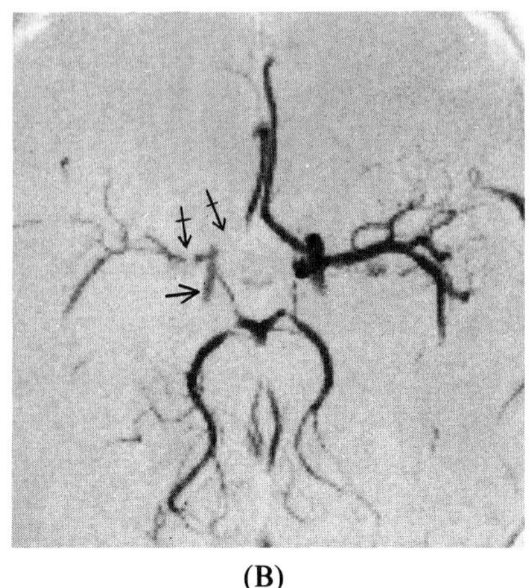

(A)   (B)

Figure 1. *RIGHT INTERNAL CAROTID OCCLUSION AND INFARC-
TION. (A) Axial T2-weighted MR scan in a young girl. There is a focal
sharply marginated area of high signal involving the posterior portion of the
right lenticular nucleus and adjacent posterior internal capsule (arrow). (B)
Axial MR angiogram through the circle of Willis. There is significant narrowing of the right internal carotid artery in its supraclinoid portion (arrow).
There are stenoses and/or occlusions of the proximal portions of the right
anterior and middle cerebral arteries (crossed arrows). There is poor flow
into the right middle cerebral artery branches. This most likely represents an
idiopathic arteriopathy or vasculitis.*

MR scans of most cases of chronic infarction show significant T1
prolongation with an area of CSF-like intensity and adjacent cortical atrophy or ipsilateral ventricular enlargement (encephalomalacia). The MR appearance corresponds to the CT findings of decreased attenuation, focal enlargement of the cisternal spaces or
cortical sulci, and encephalomalacia. In all chronic infarcts, both CT
and MR scans show no mass effect.

Lacunar

Lacunar infarcts are usually found in hypertensive patients due to
the development of lipohylanosis in the deep perforating vessels
(lenticulostriate, thalamic or pontine). The MR features include
circular or elliptical areas of decreased intensity signal on T1-
weighted images and increased intensity signal on T2-weighted
images (Fig. 4). These lesions are often multiple and deep seated

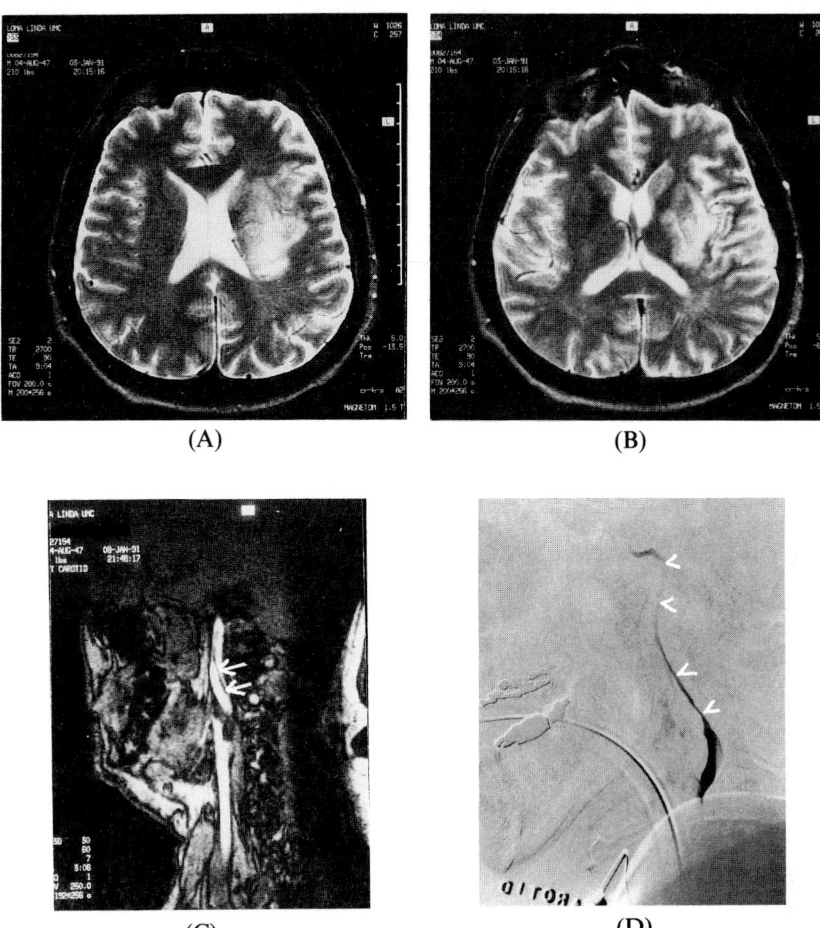

(A)   (B)

(C)   (D)

Figure 2. *LEFT CAROTID DISSECTION AND LARGE LEFT MIDDLE CEREBRAL ARTERY INFARCTION. (A, B) Axial T2-weighted MR scans of the brain in an adult male. There is an extensive area of high signal involving the deep portions of the left hemisphere, including the internal capsule, lateral basal ganglia, external capsule, corona radiata and corticobulbar tracts. (C) Single partition image from a sagittal MR angiogram (30° flip angle, TR 60/TE 7). There is a dissection of the cervical portion of the left internal carotid artery (arrows). (D) Conventional selective left internal carotid artery angiogram. There is a long segment dissection of the cervical portion of the left internal carotid artery extending up into the cavernous sinus (arrowheads).*

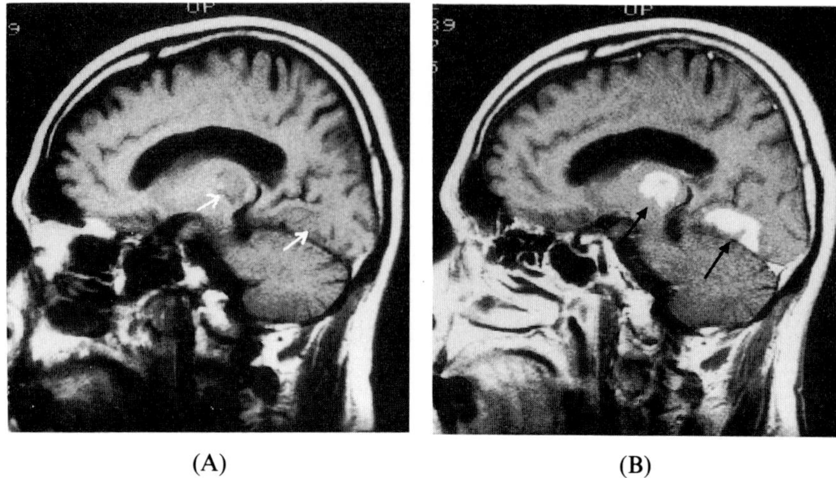

(A)   (B)

Figure 3. *SUBACUTE INFARCTION INVOLVING TERRITORIES SUPP-LIED BY THE DISTAL BASILAR ARTERY. (A) Sagittal T1-weighted MR scan in an elderly male. There are areas of T1 lengthening involving the pulvinar of the left thalamus and inferior portion of the left occipital lobe (arrows). (B) Sagittal MR scan following gadolinium-DTPA administration. There is profound enhancement in the areas of infarction corresponding to sites of subacute infarction with endothelial proliferation (arrows). The areas involved are both supplied by the distal basilar artery through the thalamoperforator vessels and the occipital branch of the left posterior cerebral artery.*

within different portions of the brainstem [4]. Lacunar infarcts in the thalami, basal ganglia, internal capsules, pons or medulla are all well seen with MR scans. Enlargement of the Virchow-Robin spaces may mimic the appearance of chronic lacunes [5,6].

White matter (borderzone)

Ischemic lesions which are located between adjacent vascular terri-tories are termed borderzone infarcts. A similar "watershed" zone is present within the periventricular and central white matter representing the region between the cortical and deep medullary vessels. White matter borderzone infarcts may have the same histologic characteristics as lacunar infarcts and may occur in patients with hypertension or chronic hypoperfusion [7] (Fig. 4).

MR scans show patchy and confluent areas of increased intensity signal on proton density weighted and T2-weighted images. These

176

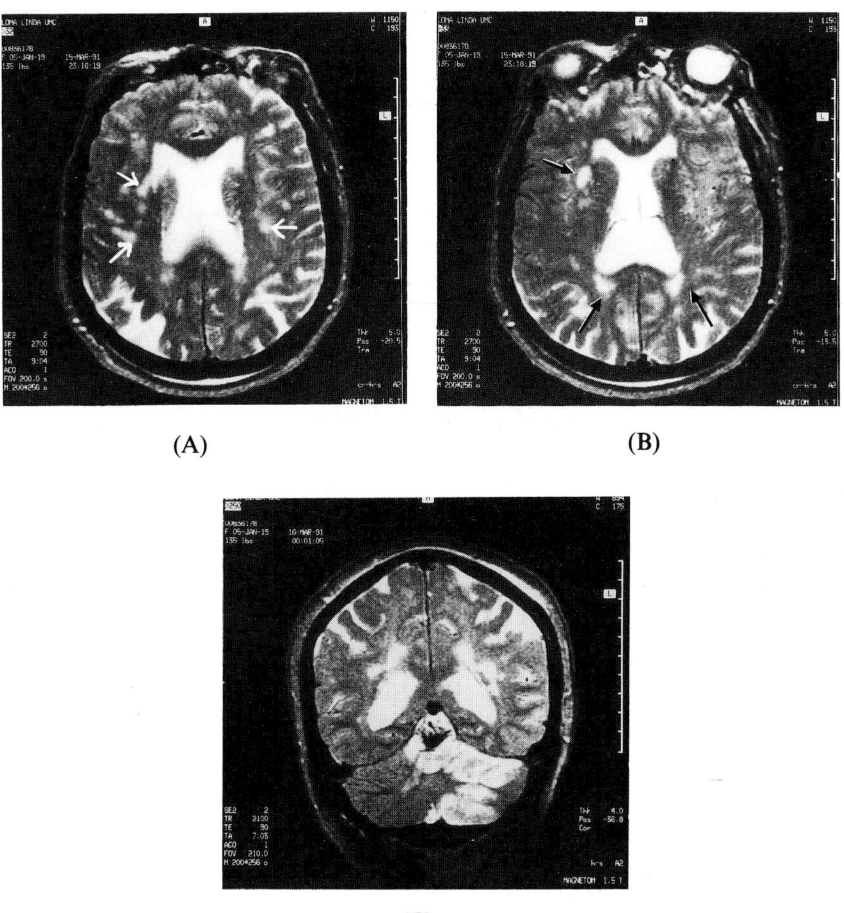

(A)

(B)

(C)

Figure 4. *MULTIPLE INFARCTIONS OF VARYING ETIOLOGIES. (A, B) Axial T2-weighted MR scans of the brain in an elderly hypertensive female. There are multiple lacunar-like infarctions involving the deep white matter of both cerebral hemispheres (arrows). There are multiple patchy areas of T2 lengthening adjacent to the atria of the lateral ventricles which may represent deep white matter infarction due to chronic hypoperfusion or other microangiopathy (arrows, B). (C) Coronal MR scan through the cerebrum and cerebellum. The multiple patchy periventricular areas of high signal are again noted. These changes are most compatible with a microangiopathy, either related to chronic hypoperfusion (cardiac disease) or hypertension. In addition, there is focal infarction in the cerebellum and vermis involving the territories of both the left superior cerebellar and posterior inferior cerebellar arteries.*

areas of bright signal are more readily apparent on MR scans than on CT scans which demonstrate areas of decreased attenuation.

Hemorrhage and Hemorrhagic Infarction

A discussion of intracranial hemorrhage and hemorrhagic infarction needs to distinguish between hyperacute and non-hyperacute lesions. Early (within the first 12 hours following an ictus) hemorrhagic lesions are accurately identified with CT. CT is still the examination of choice in evaluating patients with hyperacute neurological deficits, since the demonstration of hemorrhage and hemorrhagic infarction is extremely important to their clinical management.

Lesions greater than several hours old may be identified with gradient echo images and/or by the oxyhemoglobin effects on standard spin echo images. Over the course of approximately five or less days, there is significant T1 shortening. This apparently occurs with the formation of methemoglobin, which is paramagnetic. There is parallel T2 shortening which increases over a period of a few days. The T2 shortening may be obscured by the very intense T1 shortening, even on the T2-weighted images. Subacute hemorrhagic lesions are more readily diagnosed on MR since these lesions remain bright on MR scans beyond the time when the clots become isodense or hypodense on CT images [8,9,10].

The diagnosis of hemorrhagic infarction is similarly more specific with MR than with CT. A rim zone of T1 lengthening (infarct) surrounds an area of T1 shortening (blood). The dual zone appearance is accentuated as the hemorrhagic infarct gets older.

Conclusion

MR scans are ideal for the evaluation of cerebral ischemia and stroke. They provide a high degree of gray matter-white matter differentiation allowing for the identification of edema in early infarction. Depiction of minute alterations in contrast and subtle mass effect is improved over X-ray CT. There is excellent visualization of superficial cortical and posterior fossa ischemic lesions due to the lack of bone artifacts. The precise localization of brainstem and peritentorial infarcts is improved by the ability to view complex structures in two or more othogonal planes. Vascular structures are readily identified. Slow or obstructed flow in both arterial and venous channels may be recognized.

The use of MRI in hemorrhage and hemorrhagic infarction is limited in the hyperacute stage. Early on, hemorrhage may be occult on MR scans and should be investigated by CT scanning.

References

1. Baker LL, Kucharczyk J, Sevick RJ, et al. Recent advances in MR imaging/spectroscopy of cerebral ischemia. AJR 1991;156:1133-1143

2. Katz BH, Quencer RM, Kaplan JO, et al. MR imaging of intracranial carotid occlusion. AJNR 1989;10:345-350

3. Brant-Zawadzki M. Routine MR imaging of the internal carotid artery siphon: angiographic correlation with cervical carotid lesions. AJNR 1990;11:467-471 and AJR 1990;155:359-363

4. Brown JJ, Hesselink JR, Rothrock JR. MR and CT of lacunar infarcts. AJR 1988;151:357-372

5. Braffman BH, Zimmerman RA, Trojanowski JQ, et al. Brain MR. Pathologic correlation with gross and histopathology. 1. Lacunar infarction and Virchow-Robin spaces. AJR 1988;151:551-558

6. Jungreis CA, Kanal E, Hirsch WL, et al. Normal perivascular spaces mimicking lacunar infarction: MR imaging. Radiology 1988;169:101-104

7. Marshall VG, Bradley WG Jr, Marshall CE, et al. Deep white matter infarction: correlation of MR imaging and histopathologic findings. Radiology 1988;167:517-522

8. Gomori JM, Grossman RI, Goldberg HI, et al. Intracranial hematomas: imaging by high-field MR. Radiology 1985;157:87-93

9. Grossman RI, Gomori JM, Goldberg HI, et al. MR imaging of hemorrhagic conditions of the head and neck. RadioGraphics 1988;8:441-454

10. Edelman RR, Johnson K, Buxton, et al. MR of hemorrhage: a new approach. AJNR 1986;7:751-756

Imaging of Central Nervous System Infections

Anton N. Hasso

*Loma Linda University Medical Center, Department of
Radiation Science, Loma Linda, California, USA*

Pyogenic Infections

Predisposing factors in cerebritis and brain abscess

- Septicemia or endocarditis
- Sinus or mastoid infections
- Immune compromised patient
- Diabetes
- Congenital heart disease
- Trauma or surgery

Pyogenic Cerebral Infections

Following initial infection, progressive changes occur over a 2-3
week period. Initially, a focal or multifocal cerebritis occurs which
consists of vascular congestion with petechial hemorrhages and
tissue edema. Later on in the intermediate stage, there is cerebral
softening with necrosis. These areas of necrosis will appear as low
attenuation on CT and hypointense on short TR MR images. Over
a period of time, there is liquefaction and cavitation with
subsequent capsule formation. These central areas of necrosis and
liquefaction are surrounded by a capsule consisting of an inner layer
of granulation tissue, a middle collagenous layer and an outer
astroglial layer. Edema is typically seen outside the abscess capsule

This gives the characteristic imaging appearance of a well circumscribed, ring enhancing mass with central necrosis and surrounding edema. Ring enhancement in pyogenic abscesses typically show a smooth, thin ring of enhancement with wall thickness ranging between 1-3 mm (Fig. 1). Small lesions, less than 0.5 cm in diameter, may show homogeneous rather than ring-like enhancement [1,2]. Complications of brain abscesses include rupture into the ventricular system or subarachnoid space, producing ventriculitis and/or meningitis. A wide variety of microorganisms cause brain abscesses. In a majority of cases, a single organism such as staphylococcus streptococcus, tuberculosis, or parasites are identified. In approximately 20% cases, multiple organisms may be found. A variety of opportunistic infections may be seen in immunocompromised and/or AIDS patients. In about 25% of the cases, the abscesses are sterile. The abscess capsule formation tends to be weaker on the inner or white matter side which may be related to fewer blood vessels. The medial thinning of the capsule of the abscess may account for the tendency of the abscess to rupture into the ventricular system and for the formation of donor abscesses (Fig. 1). Bleeding within an abscess is uncommon and is usually due to hemorrhagic venous infarction.

Leptomeningitis and Leptomeningoencephalitis

Purulent leptomeningitis is usually a diffuse process. Hemophilus influenza is the most common cause of purulent meningitis in the first year of life and may result in subdural effusions. Subdural empyemas result when such effusions become infected.

A variety of other organisms such as diplococcus pneumonia, Escherichia coli, staphylococcus aureus, Neisseria meningitidis, and beta streptococcus may produce meningitis at any age in high risk patients. The exudate may produce CSF loculations and pathway obstruction resulting in communicating hydrocephalus. Ependymitis, ventriculitis, and choroid plexitis may result in blockage of the ventricular system, producing obstructive hydrocephalus. Intraventricular septation will lead to the development of ventricular compartmentalization. Ventriculitis or ependymitis can be readily recognized by CT or MRI due to the enhancement of the lining of the ventricular system [3]. Whenever the inflammatory

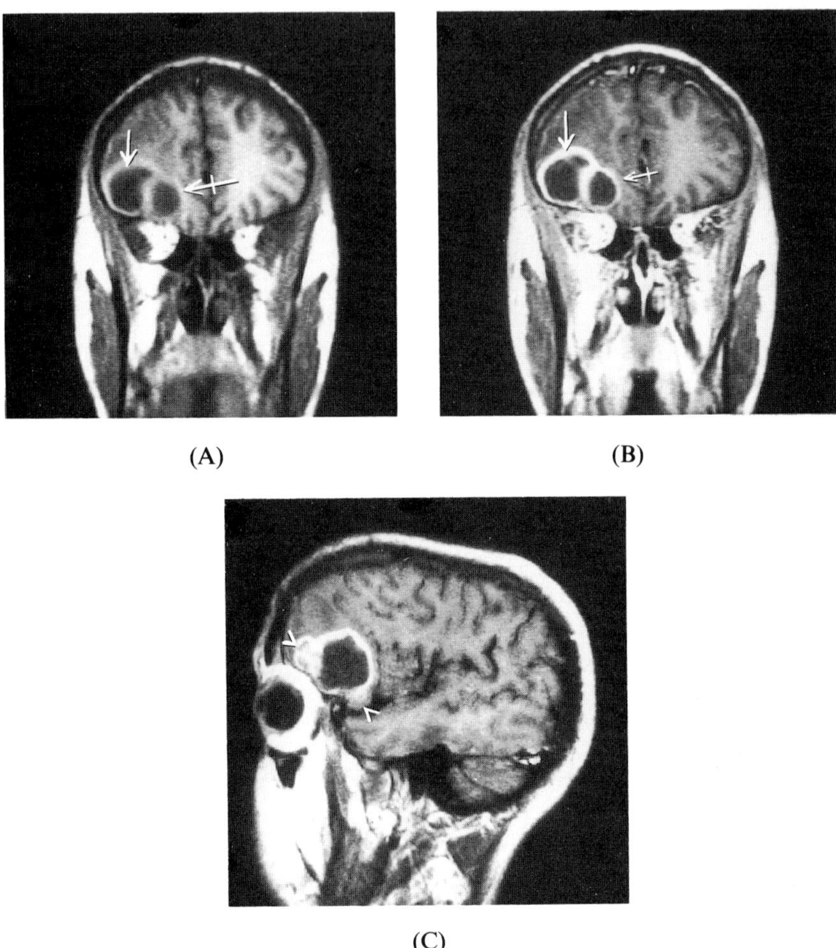

(A)   (B)

(C)

Figure 1. *SBE and right frontal abscesses. (A). Coronal MR scan in a young adult male. There is a large abscess in the right frontal pole (arrow) and a smaller daughter abscess located medially (crossed arrow). (B). Coronal, and (C). Sagittal MR scans following gadolinium-DTPA administration. There is prominent enhancement of the rims of both abscesses (parent abscess, arrow, and daughter abscess, crossed-arrow). The sagittal view (C) documents small budding abscesses which are being formed anteriorly and inferoposteriorly (arrowheads).*

process is localized to the base of the brain, cranial nerve dysfunction may occur. Arteritis and venous thrombosis may result from leptomeningitis leading to cerebral ischemic processes [1,2].

Subdural and Epidural Empyemas

Intracranial extraaxial empyemas are uncommon, but may occur as a result of an extension of a cranial or extracranial infectious process. Epidural empyema usually relates to infections of the paranasal sinuses or mastoid air cells and tympanic cavity. Subdural empyemas may occur as a complication of surgery or of ventricular shunt placement. The capsule of the empyema usually enhances on CT or MRI because of granulation tissue, inflammation of the cerebral surface and/or cortical venous thrombosis (Fig. 2). Prompt diagnosis and treatment of these subdural or epidural effusions is essential. Since there is a poor blood supply in the subdural or epidural spaces, there is no response to antibiotics. Surgical drainage is extremely important [1,2].

Nonpyogenic Infections

Tuberculosis

Tuberculosis meningitis which is encountered in infants and small children is usually part of a generalized miliary tuberculosis, but may appear as a primary tuberculous infection. The leptomeninges at the base of the brain are mainly involved. The complications are similar to those of purulent meningitis and include communicating and noncommunicating hydrocephalus, abscesses and empyemas [1,2]. Multiple cranial nerve involvement and progressive vasculitis leading to cerebral infarctions are common complications. Tuberculomas may be found in the brain parenchyma. These lesions are multiple in the majority of cases. Postcontrast imaging will show homogeneous or ring-like patterns of enhancement. The basal cisterns will also enhance in cases of tuberculous meningitis [4]. Communicating hydrocephalus and cerebral infarction can also be demonstrated.

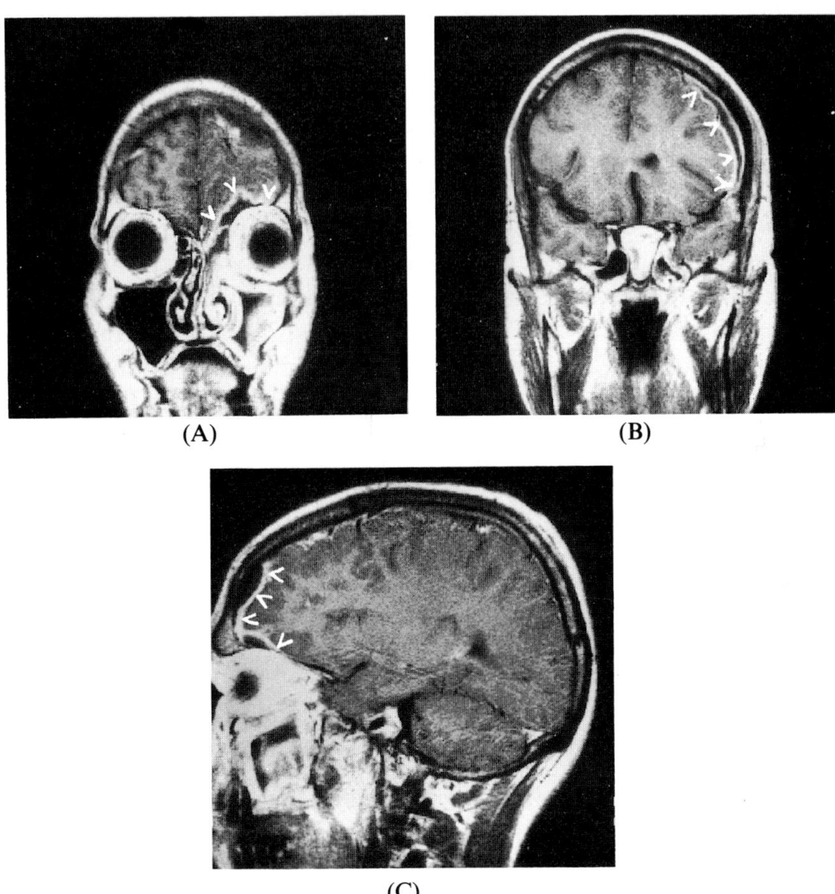

(A) (B)

(C)

Figure 2. *Sinusitis and subdural empyemas. MR scan of the head following gadolinium-DTPA administration in adult male. (A). Coronal view. There is prominent enhancement of the thickened mucosa of the left nasal cavity and left maxillary and ethmoid sinuses. There is a low attenuation lesion in the left frontal pole which is marginated by a dense enhancing reactive membrane (arrowheads). (B). Coronal view obtained more posteriorly from A. There is mucosal enhancement in the left sphenoid sinus. A left frontal subdural empyema with enhancing inner and outer membranes is evident (arrowheads). (C). Sagittal view. The enhancement of the maxillary sinus is well noted. There are subdural empyemas in the left frontal pole with enhancing inner membranes (arrowheads).*

Fungal Infections

The CNS is a common site of involvement of disseminated systemic fungal infections. Opportunistic fungal infections such as candidiasis, cryptococcosis, mucormycosis, nocardiosis, and actinomycosis are often seen. Coccidioidomycosis is more commonly seen in endemic areas and may present as a basilar meningitis with or without cocci granulomas.

The transmission of coccidioidomycosis is by inhalation of the fungus in dust. Coccidioidomycoses involving the CNS manifests itself in a similar manner as other fungal and granulomatous processes. Abnormalities of the subarachnoid spaces can be shown with both CT and MRI following contrast infusions. Cocci may also involve the calvarium and base of the skull as it does in other portions of the skeleton.

Many fungi behave as opportunistic infections attacking the immunocompromised patient. Aspergillus tends to cause parenchymal infection and is most commonly seen in patients receiving chronic corticosteroid therapy (Fig. 3). Mucormycosis is most often seen in diabetic patients and involves the CNS secondary to direct spread from infection in the nasal cavity or paranasal sinuses (Fig. 4). Both of these fungi have a propensity to invade the walls of blood vessels leading to infarction and occasionally hemorrhage [1,2].

Cryptococcus (torulosis) is typically transmitted by inhalation and the primary lesions are most often in the lungs and skin. Lesions in the CNS are disseminated by the hematogenous root. Cryptococcal meningoencephalitis may be fatal within a period of a month. A chronic brain parenchymal inflammatory process may occur with multiple lesions of 1-2 mm in diameter. Cryptococcus can also present as a basal meningitis, if the immune system is functioning. Whenever the immune system is compromised, there is no granulomatous response to a cryptococcal infection [5,6].

Viral Infections

Encephalitis

Encephalitis, in contrast to cerebritis, is a diffuse parenchymal infection that can spread throughout the brain. There are a broad

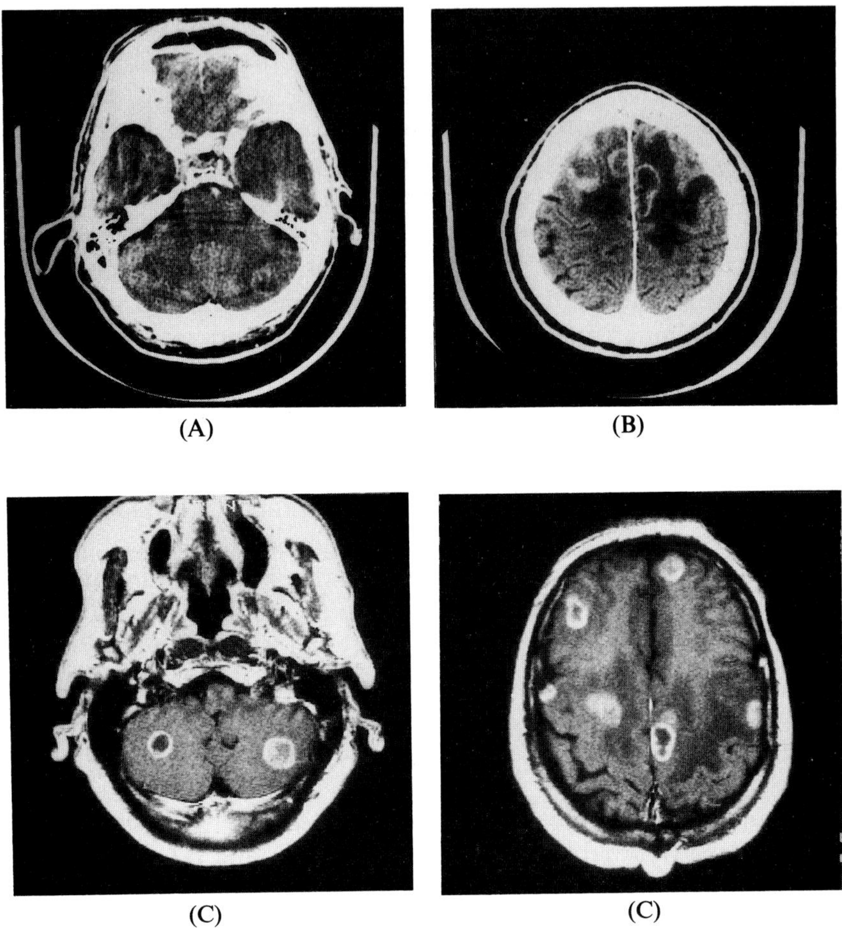

Figure 3. *MULTIPLE CEREBRAL AND CEREBELLAR ASPERGILLOMAS. (A, B). Axial CT scans following intravenous contrast administration in an elderly male. The lesions in the posterior fossa are ill-defined and difficult to identify. The cerebral lesions are seen more distinctly, along with the surrounding vasogenic edema. Some of the lesions show ring enhancement while some smaller lesions show more solid enhancement. (C, D). Axial MR images following gadolinium-DTPA administration. The multiple lesions in both the cerebellar and cerebral hemispheres are readily identified. Lesions close to the surface of the brain are as equally well seen as the lesions that extend deep into the parenchyma. Biopsy of the most superficial right frontal lesion documented an aspergilloma.*

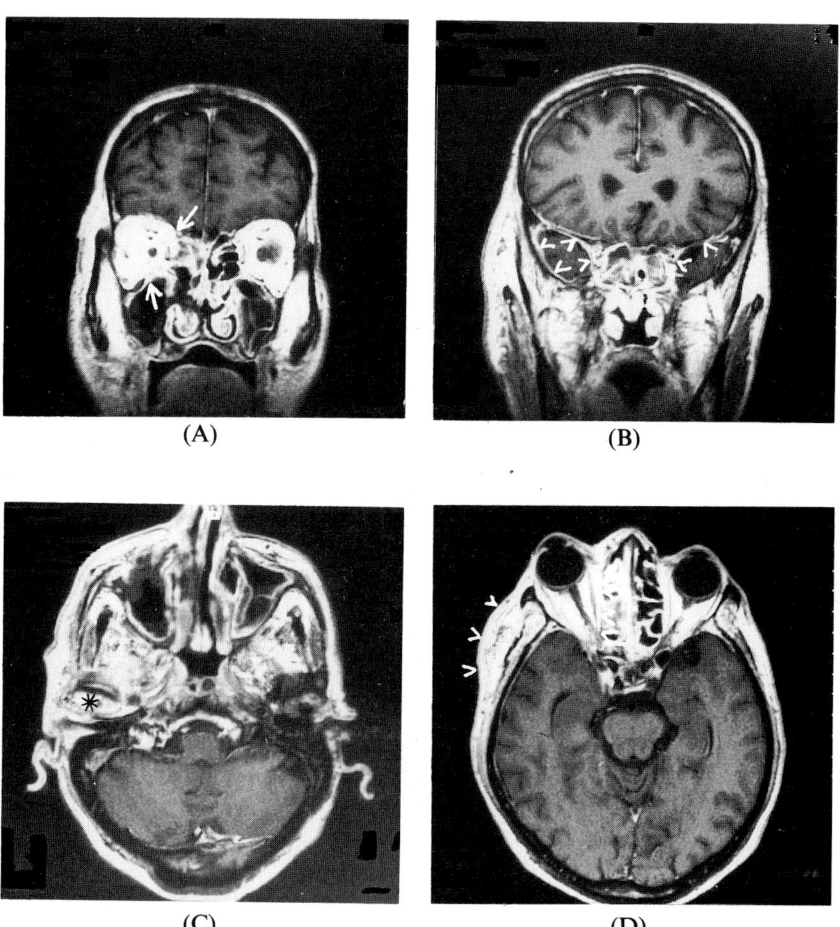

Figure 4. *WIDESPREAD MUCORMYCOSIS OF THE FACE, SINONA-SAL CAVITIES, ORBIT, INFRATEMPORAL FOSSA, TEMPORO-MANDIBULAR JOINT AND MENINGES. MR scans following gado-linium-DTPA administration. (A, B). Coronal views showing extension of the enhanced inflammatory process from the right nasal cavity and ethmoid air cells into the adjacent orbit (arrows, A). There is enhancement of all the walls of the sphenoid sinuses with similar enhancement along the dural margins in the middle cranial fossae (arrowheads, B). (C, D) Axial views. There is septic arthritis surrounding the right temporomandibular joint (asterisk, C). There is dramatic enhancement within the right temporal fossa involving the muscles of mastication and overlying soft tissues. The soft tissue enhancement involves the right temporalis muscle region and the medial portion of the right orbit (arrowheads, B).*

group of organisms that may cause encephalitis including protozoa, Rickettsia, fungi, and bacteria. In most cases, viruses are responsible for the infection.

Herpes simplex virus (HSV) produces an acute and frequently fatal encephalitis in more than 50% of the cases. Although the process may be bilateral, it is predominantly unilateral. HSV involves the neurons and olfactory tract, temporal lobes, cingulate gyrus, and insular cortex. Herpes simplex may also involve the gray matter resulting in necrotic temporal lobes. Herpes encephalitis may be multifocal or diffuse. Treatment with the appropriate antimicrobial agent, if begun early in the course of the disease, can dramatically alter the natural history of the illness. Other common viral encephalitides are caused by members of the arbovirus family including California encephalitis, Eastern equine encephalitis, St. Louis encephalitis and Western equine encephalitis [1,2].

Imaging demonstrates poorly marginated areas of abnormal density or abnormal signal. There may be petechial hemorrhages interspersed with areas of necrosis.

Post infectious encephalitis (PIE)

Encephalitis may occur following viral illnesses or vaccinations. In some cases, no specific virus can be recovered from the CNS. PIE or acute disseminated encephalomyelitis (ADEM) has been described to occur following measles, varicella or rubella infection or vaccination. It is clearly an autoimmune disorder and consists of areas of demyelination showing increased signal on T2-weighted MR images. CT may be normal or show areas of decreased attenuation within the white matter. Treatment with corticosteroids often results in dramatic improvement in the outcome. Unlike multiple sclerosis, there rarely are recurrent episodes of ADEM.

Parasitic Infections

Cysticercosis

Cysticercosis [1,2,7] has a predilection for the CNS. Imaging plays a key role in its diagnosis and treatment. The clinical manifestations vary greatly and depend on the number, size, location and stage of the process. There are four distinct clinicopathologic and radiographic types:

1. The most common type is manifested by brain parenchymal cystic lesions, which may be solitary or multiple, ranging in size from a few millimeters to 6 cm. Many of these lesions terminate as calcified granulomatous processes. An encephalitic form of intraparenchymal cysticercosis may be seen in children. Parenchymal cysticercus not uncommonly may result in calcifications with minimal or no surrounding reaction. These lesions may be solitary or multiple.

2. Meningeal-type of cysticercosis is manifested mainly by ventricular dilatation, indicating diffuse meningeal inflammatory processes. The cysticerci may be seen as lucent cystic lesions in the basal cisterns (racemose cysts).

3. The intraventricular type of cysticercosis is manifested by obstructive hydrocephalus caused by blockage within the various portions of the ventricular system. The cysts may be solitary or multiple. These racemose cysts do not contain a scolex.

4. A mixed type of cysticercosis is often present.

CNS Complications of AIDS

Approximately 1% of the population in the United States is currently human immunodeficiency virus (HIV) sero-positive. There is a 5-9 year incubation period for the virus to be manifested clinically.

AIDS is formed by a DNA retrovirus leading to deficient cell mediated immunity. The virus infects the monocytes and macrophages which in its pure neurologic form leads to the development of microglial nodules which may be visible pathologically in 75-80% of autopsied brains. Clinically, up to 39% of patients will develop neurological symptoms [8,9].

The complications of AIDS includes toxoplasmosis which is caused by toxoplasmas gondii, an obligate intracellular parasite. The clinical manifestations are variable, manifested by meningoencephalitic symptoms, seizures, and pseudotumor cerebri syndrome.

Toxoplasmic granulomas are the result of glial mesenchymal reaction. The granulomas, which may be cystic, are surrounded by edema with microinfarcts due to vasculitis (Fig. 5). Basal ganglia involvement is common, and is seen in 75% of cases. However, lesions may be multiple and may be scattered throughout the brain parenchyma. The inflammatory foci of toxoplasmosis may be difficult to distinguish from CNS lymphoma in AIDS patients. Response to antitoxotherapy or biopsy may be necessary for definitive diagnosis. The lesions of toxoplasmosis typically show a ring or nodular enhancement with surrounding white matter edema. MR is more sensitive than CT in the detection of these lesions [10,11].

Cryptococcosis is another complication of AIDS leading to the development of meningitis. As discussed above, 80% of AIDS patients have no granulomatous reactions since they lack the capability to form an immune response leading to the development of granulomas [5,6]. Imaging will show only the development of hydrocephalus and cortical or central atrophy. If there is a sufficient immune response, an appearance of granulomatous meningitis with enhancement may be evident. Cryptococcosis can extend along the

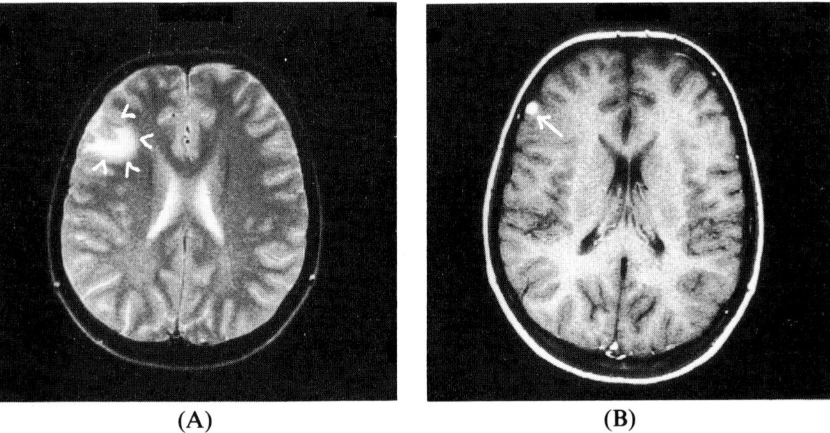

(A)   (B)

Figure 5. *AIDS AND A SOLITARY TOXOPLASMOSIS GRANULOMA. (A) Axial T2-weighted MR scan in an adult. There is a focus of edema in the right frontal lobe (arrowheads). (B) Axial MR scan following gadolinium-DTPA administration. A single nodule of enhancement is noted near the vertex of the right frontal lobe (arrow). Surgical biopsy revealed a toxoplasmosis granuloma.*

Virchow-Robin (V-R)spaces into the brain, but not into the brain parenchyma so there is typically no enhancement. These represent cryptococcomas, along the V-R spaces, but not yet in the brain parenchyma.

Cytomegalovirus (CMV) infections always occur with HIV infections affecting the monocytes and macrophages of the brain. These also cause clumps of microglia. It may lead to the development of subacute white matter encephalitis which start as patchy white matter lesions. It is not known if the CMV or HIV virus causes this response [10,11].

Another complication of AIDS is caused by the latent papovaviruses which leads to the development of progressive multifocal leukoencephalopathy. These lesions are typically multicentric white matter lesions with scalloped borders. Pathologically, there are decreased areas of demyelination and edema secondary to the virus destruction of oligodendrogliocytes. Asymmetric parietooccipital involvement is most characteristic, however, any white matter tracts may be involved including those in the posterior fossa. Gray matter involvement has been demonstrated pathologically and may be detected by MR with greater sensitivity than CT [10,12].

Finally, primary central nervous lymphoma may occur in AIDS patients. Unlike lymphomas in other patients, necrosis typically evident. This again reflects the lack of an immune response which, of course, is typical of AIDS patients [9].

References

1. Rodriguez-Carbajal J, Palacios E. Infectious and parasitic supratentorial disorders. Taveras JM, Ferrucci JT, Eds. In: Radiology, Diagnosis-Imaging-Intervention, Vol. III, Ch. 38, 1988.

2. Rodriguez-Carbajal J, Palacios E. Infectious and parasitic disorders of the posterior fossa. Taveras JM, Ferrucci JT, Eds. In: Radiology, Diagnosis-Imaging-Intervention, Vol. III, Ch. 69, 1988.

3. Chang KH, Han MH, Roh JK, Kim IO, Han MC, Kim CW: Gd-DTPA-enhanced MR imaging of the brain in patients with meningitis: Comparison with CT. AJNR 1990;11:69-76.

4. Chang KH, Han MH, Roh JK, Kim IO, Han MC, Choi KS, Kim CW: Gd-DTPA enhanced MR imaging in intracranial tuberculosis. Neuroradiology 1990;32:19-25.

5. Popovich MJ, Arthur RH, Helmer E: CT of intracranial cryptococcosis. AJNR 1990;11:139-142.

6. Wehn SM, Heinz ER, Burger PC, Boyko OB: Dilated Virchow-Robin spaces in cryptoccol meningitis associated with AIDS: CT and MR findings. J Comput Assist Tomogr 1989;13:756-762.

7. Alarcon, Escalante L, Duenas, Montalvo M, Roman: Neurocysticercosis. Arch Neurol 1989;46:1231-1236.

8. Chrysikopoulos HS, Press GA, Grafe MR, Hesselink JR, Wiley CA: Encephalitis caused by human immunodeficiency virus: CT and MR imaging manifestations with clinical and pathologic correlation. Radiology 1990;176:185-191.

9. Grafe MR, Press GA, Berthoty DP, Hesselink JR, Wiley CA: Abnormalities of the brain in AIDS patients: Correlation of postmortem MR findings with neuropathology. AJNR 1990;11:905-911.

10. Balakrishnan J, Becker PS, Kumar AJ, Zinreich SJ, McArthur JC, Bryan RN: Acquired immunodeficiency syndrome: Correlation of radiologic and pathologic findings in the brain. RadioGraphics 1990;10:201-215.

11. Kupfer MC, Zee CS, Colletti PM, Boswell WD, Rhodes R: MRI evaluation of AIDS-related encephalopathy: Toxoplasmosis vs. lymphoma. Magnetic Resonance Imaging 1990;8:51-57.

12. Chiasson RE, Griffin DE: Progressive multifocal leukoencephalopathy in AIDS. JAMA 1990;264:79-82.

Neuroradiological Diagnosis of Spinal Cord Tumors

Giuseppe Scotti

Department of Neuroradiology, Ospedale San Raffaele, University of Milano, Italy

Introduction

The diagnostic protocol of spinal cord tumors has rapidly changed over the 5 last years.

For many decades, myelography was the gold standard since its first introduction in 1923 by Sicard and Forestier. Despite significant improvements in chemistry and pharmacology of contrast media however, and despite the combined use of myelography and CT (CT myelography), diagnosis of spinal cord tumors remained an invasive and frequently inconclusive procedure prior to the advent of MR.

Precise definition of location and extent of the tumor, particularly intramedullary, identification of solid from cystic components and recognition of previous hemorrhages etc. are information that now can consistently be obtained by MR imaging in a completely safe and noninvasive way.

The knowledge of the extensive semeiology of bony changes retrievable from plain films or CT represents a solid basis for the experienced neuroradiologist but this semeiology will probably remain an ancillary methodology for teaching more than for diagnosis.

The fine observation of modifications of the subarachnoid spaces providing clues to differentiate intradural from extradural, intramedullary from extramedullary mass lesions remains the basis for analysis of MR pictures.

The superiority of MRI over myelography and post myelography CT in the assessment of intramedullary tumors but also of spinal tumors in general is well established [1,2,3,4].

There is no doubt that neuroradiology of spinal cord tumors is now synonymous with MR.

MR imaging of special cord tumors; intradural tumors, intra- or extramedullary, are the basic important abnormalities; extradural tumors, bone tumors or metastases, will be omitted herein.

Technique

The technique of the examination of spinal cord tumors requires slices obtained at least in the sagittal orientation and two types of sequences; T1 and T2 weighted.

The sagittal plane is the most informative since it provides demonstration of a long segment of spine and cord, allowing a good caudo-cranial localization and excellent demonstration of the relationship of spinal cord with bony spinal canal. Axial and coronal views are however, sometimes necessary to better locate lesions particularly in the axial plane and to define their relationships with the extradural space and neural foramina.

The use of paramagnetic contrast agent (Gadolinium) has become mandatory for more precise delineation of lesions and for their characterization [5,6,7].

The suggested protocol should then include sagittal T1 and T2WI followed by Gd injection and sagittal T1WI.

Slice thickness should not exceed 4 mm. Coronal views after Gd may be useful for a better localization of intradural extramedullary tumors.

Clinical Presentation

The clinical suspicion of spinal cord tumor is frequently delayed since the symptoms and signs may be very subtle, nonspecific and misleading.

Pain, mainly radicular, in the upper or lower limbs, gait disturbances with leg stiffness, parhestesias, bladder disturbances may be the presenting signs. Symptoms may be relapsing and remitting. Particularly in children and young patients, scoliosis may be the only symptom for a very long period. Neurologic examination often reveals only minor motor or sensory changes.

Intramedullary Tumors

The most frequent intramedullary tumors are gliomas: of these astrocytomas and ependymomas represent more than 90%; hemangioblastomas are about 5% while other glial tumors fill the rest. Precise prevalence is lacking because any statistic is biased by the criteria of selection (surgical, radiological, pathological). Astrocytomas and ependymomas however are almost equally frequent, except in children, where astrocytomas are more common and in the lumbar region and cauda equina where the most common tumor is the ependymoma.

Astrocytoma

Approximately 36 to 54% of all intramedullary tumors are astrocytomas with a peak incidence in childhood and around the third decade [8,9]. There is no sex predilection.

Astrocytomas may be found at any level in the spinal cord and can extend for one or more segments; the entire cord may sometimes be involved (holocord astrocytomas). The prevalence of astrocytomas decreases in the caudal direction while that of ependymomas increase.

Our personal experience is based on 17 cases diagnosed by MRI and surgically proven [10]. Our findings are in complete agreement with those of the literature and other reported series.

Fusiform expansion of the spinal cord, sometimes with eccentric development due to exophytic growth is usually found. The signal changes are not specific and are characterized by iso-hypointensity in T1WI, slight hyperintensity in PD and hyperintensity in T2WI (Fig. 1). Some tumor nodules however, may remain isointense also in T1WI. Gd injection usually produces a marked enhancement, homogenous more than inhomogeneous. A demarcation relatively clear from the surrounding cord parenchyma may be found. The

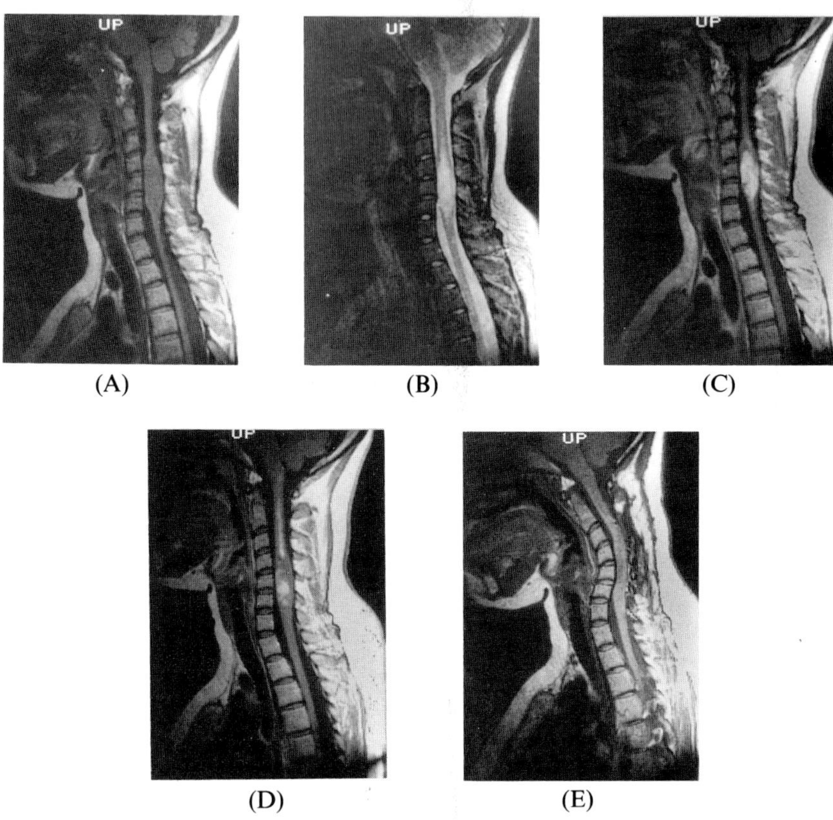

(A)   (B)   (C)

(D)   (E)

Figure 1. *INTRAMEDULLARY ASTROCYTOMA, CERVICAL CORD. (A) T1WI. The cord is enlarged from C4 to C6 by a slightly hypointense space occupying lesion. (B) T2WI. The tumor becomes hyperintense. (C, D) Post gadolinium injection. Marked inhomogeneous enhancement extending cranially along the central canal, that could suggest a wrong diagnosis of ependymoma. (E) One year postoperative follow up. The extensive laminectomy has produced instability of the cervical spine. No recurrent tumor is seen within the spinal cord.*

most interesting and useful finding is however the presence of associated cystic "degeneration" or "transformation" of the cord above or below the tumor nodule [11,12,13,14,15]. Cyst formation is found up to 40% of cases; there is no definite explanation yet as to the precise nature of the cells in the walls of the cyst and the mechanism of formation. Tumor cysts are different than dilated central canal in syringomyelia. They do not need to be surgically removed since they permanently collapse following tumor removal (Fig. 2). The wall of the cyst do not usually enhance. The signal of the cyst is decreased in T1WI and increased in T2WI. Sometimes however due to the high content of proteins the signal of the cyst may be indistinguishable from that of the cord. Paramagnetic substances from the previous hemorrhages may be present both in the tumor nodule and cystic cavities and be recognised mainly because of areas of T2 shortening.

Ependymoma

Ependymoma is the most common primary tumor of the lower spinal cord, conus medullaris and cauda equina but it may occur at any level. They usually are cylindrical elongated masses that cause fusiform expansion of the spinal cord, not dissimilar than astrocytomas. However, they are usually better demarcated, since they frequently have a thin capsule to separate them from the spinal cord. Not dissimilar from astrocytomas cyst formation is very common. Calcification are extremely uncommon while paramagnetic T2 shortening due to the presence of residual hemosiderin from previous hemorrhages is more common than in astrocytomas (Fig. 3).

In our series of 15 surgically proven ependymomas [10] diagnosed by MRI, the signal characteristics do not differ very much from those of astrocytomas to allow a definite preoperative histological diagnosis. The main finding is more inhomogeneity within the tumor nodule with more frequent isointense signal in T1WI and also sometimes in T2WI. Usually however, the tumor nodules are hyperintense in T2WI. Cysts are usually hyperintense in T2 and hypointense in T1. The hemosiderin T2 shortening is more frequently found at the upper and lower poles of the tumor. The associated intramedullary tumor cysts, as for astrocytomas, may extend for many levels above or below the tumor nodule. The cranial extension frequently reaches the medulla, elevating the floor of the lowermost part of the fourth ventricle. To us, this is a pathognomonic sign of tumor cyst versus syringomyelic cavity. In our experience, based on the observation of more than 100 true hydrosyringomyelias, when the dilated central canal extends into the medulla, it does not produce this expansion of the medulla.

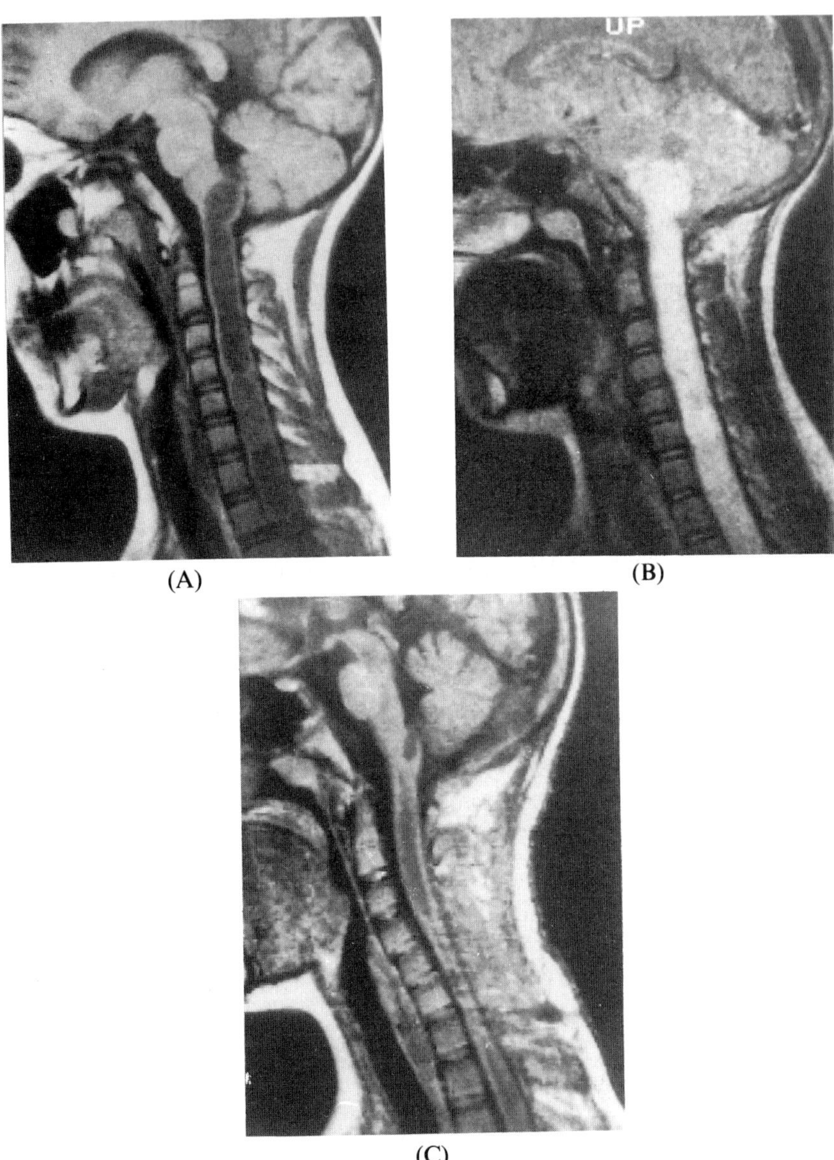

(A) (B) (C)

Figure 2. *INTRAMEDULLARY ASTROCYTOMA. Intramedullary astrocytoma with large cycts extending cranially and caudally. (A) T1WI. The tumor nodule is isointense and may be localized from C4 to C6. An extensive cystic cavity expands the cord cranially and caudally. The cranial end of the cystic cavity deforms and elevates the inferior part of the floor of the fourth ventricle at the level of the medulla. (B) T2WI. The tumor nodule is not well detected due to increased signal intensity similar to that of the cystic component. (C) 15 days after removal of the tumor nodule, the cysts have markedly collapsed.*

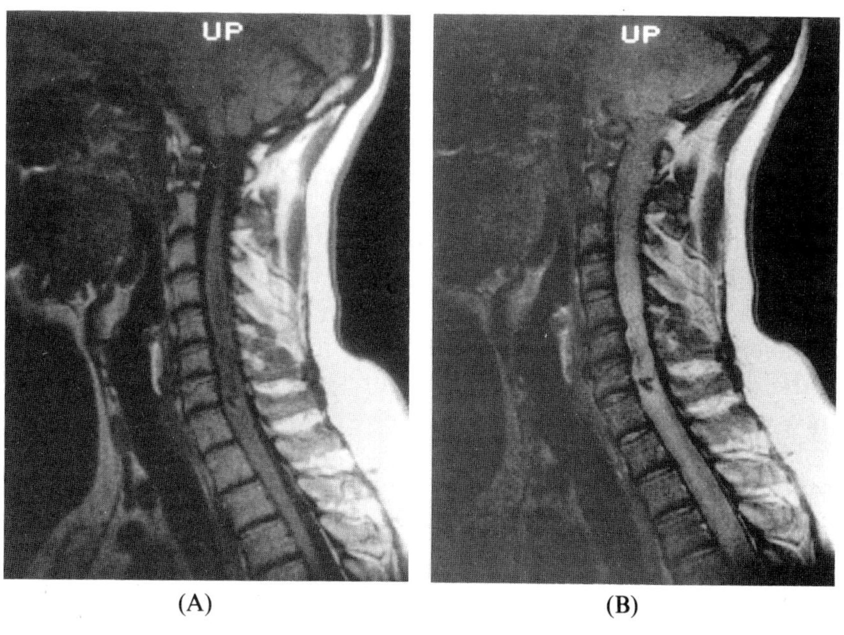

(A)

(B)

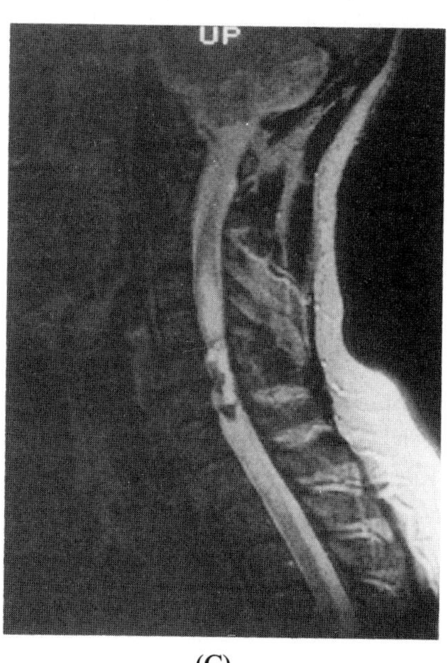

(C)

Figure 3. *INTRAMEDULLARY EPENDYMOMA. (A, B) T1 and T2WI; The tumor has some hemorrhagic components that are seen as paramagnetic effects with T2 shortening. Hyperintensity due to oedema is seen in the spinal cord above and below the tumor nodule.*

Hemangioblastoma

Hemangioblastoma represent about 3-4% of all intramedullary tumors. There is no sex predilection. Their MR appearance consists of tumor nodules slightly and focally expanding the cord, very frequently however associated with the extensive and large cyst [15,16]. Cyst formation is found in more than 70% of cases. The signal characteristics of both nodule and cysts are not very different from those of astrocytomas and ependymomas. Not infrequently, however, a vascular nature of the tumor may be suspected because of the presence of serpiginous structures without signal, representing vessels with flowing blood.

In our series of 6 cases, 5 were associated with intramedullary cysts. Gadolinium injection usually produces a marked enhancement of the nodule.

Other glial intramedullary tumors are very rare, as well as secondary lesions, usually metastatic. No specific morphological or signal aspects allow a differential diagnosis.

Intradural Extramedullary Tumors

These may be divided into primary and secondary. Primary intradural extramedullary tumors are mainly meningiomas and neurofibromas. They are usually recognised particularly in T2WI both because of the distortion of anatomy with compression and dislocation of spinal cord and in particular the T2WI myelographic effect beautifully outlines the contours of the tumor.

Signal intensity varies slightly between the two largest groups, meningiomas and neurinomas. Both tumors follow the general rule of T1 iso or hypointensity and T2 hyperintensity. Meningiomas however, with regard to their intracranial location and due to their histological characteristic, are isointense both in T1 and T2 in one third of the cases. Cystic components within the tumor nodule, though rare, may be encountered in neurofibromas. Calcification is rarely seen almost exclusively in meningiomas. Recognition of extramedullary intradural tumors is easy; only rarely will precise intra- or extramedullary localization be a diagnostic challenge.

Very small tumors, particularly neurofibromas located on the nerve roots may be overlooked. Gd DTPA, however, almost always produces a marked and homogeneous enhancement with clear delineation of tumor and separation from normal cord [18,19].

Neurinoma

Neurinomas, schwannomas and neurilemmomas are synonyms. Neurofibroma is a different entity. Schwannomas do not envelope the adjacent nerve root, which is usually the dorsal sensory root, generally are solitary, and clinically are not typical of neurofibromatosis.

Neurofibromas envelope the dorsal sensory root, frequently are multiple, are usually associated with neurofibromatosis even when single.

Nerve sheath tumors are more commonly intradural extramedullary in location (58%). The remainder are purely extradural (27%), dumbbell shaped, with both an extradural and intradural component (15%) and rarely intramedullary (less than 1%).

In children the most common location is cervical, followed by lumbar and dorsal.

Signal may be heterogeneous with isointense areas mainly due to the fibrous component of the tumor (Fig. 4).

The dumbbell shape is not synonymous of neurinomas; other tumors as ganglioneuromas may develop in a similar fashion (Fig. 5).

Meningioma

Spinal meningiomas are more common in females (60-80%); the average age of presentation is in the fifth and sixth decades.

Meningiomas are primarily intradural extramedullary but can be both intra- and extradural and more rarely purely extradural. The most common location is thoracic in females; in males they are equally found in different locations.

Meningiomas tend to be hypo or isointense to the spinal cord; they are well circumscribed, frequently posteriorly or posterolaterally located with respect to the cord. On T2WI they are more frequently hyperintense (Fig. 6); sometimes areas of signal void due to calcification are seen.

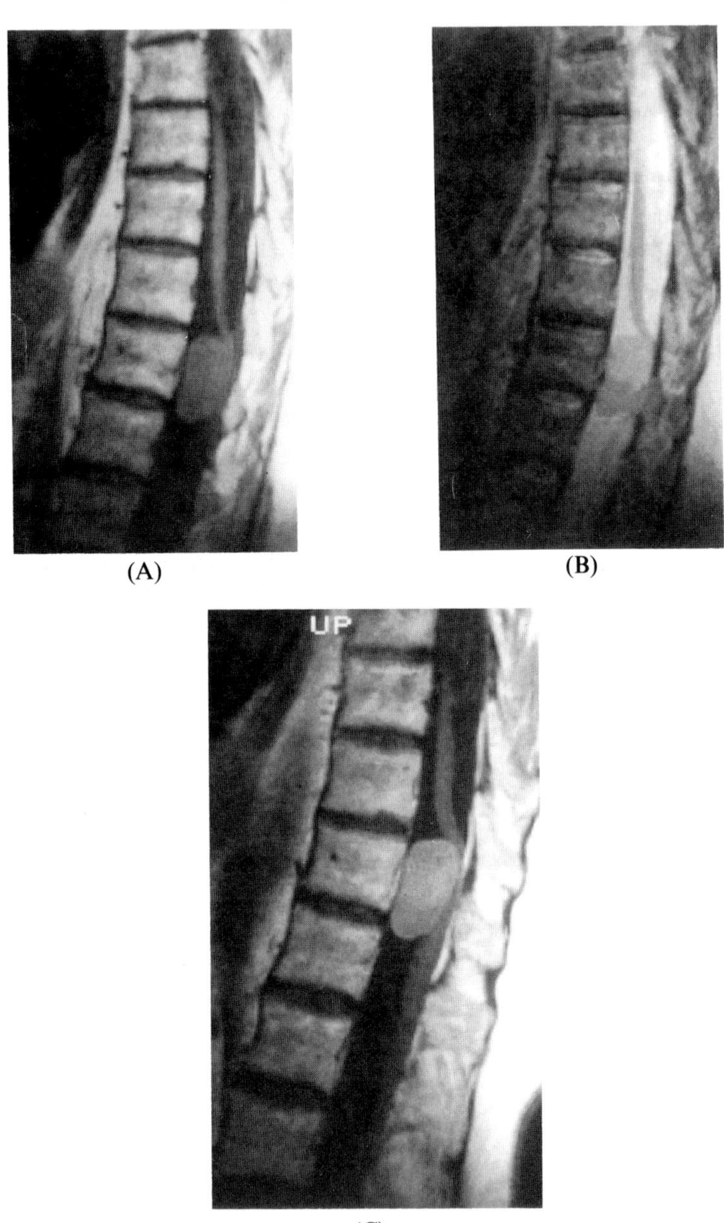

(A)

(B)

(C)

Figure 4. *NEURINOMA.* (A) *T1WI. Heterogeneous signal due to the presence of intratumoral cystic components. The tumor is located posteriorly to the cord from C5 to T1.* (B) *T2WI. The tumor becomes hyperintense.* (C) *Following Gd injection, enhancement of the parenchymatous component is seen while the cystic components are hypointense.*

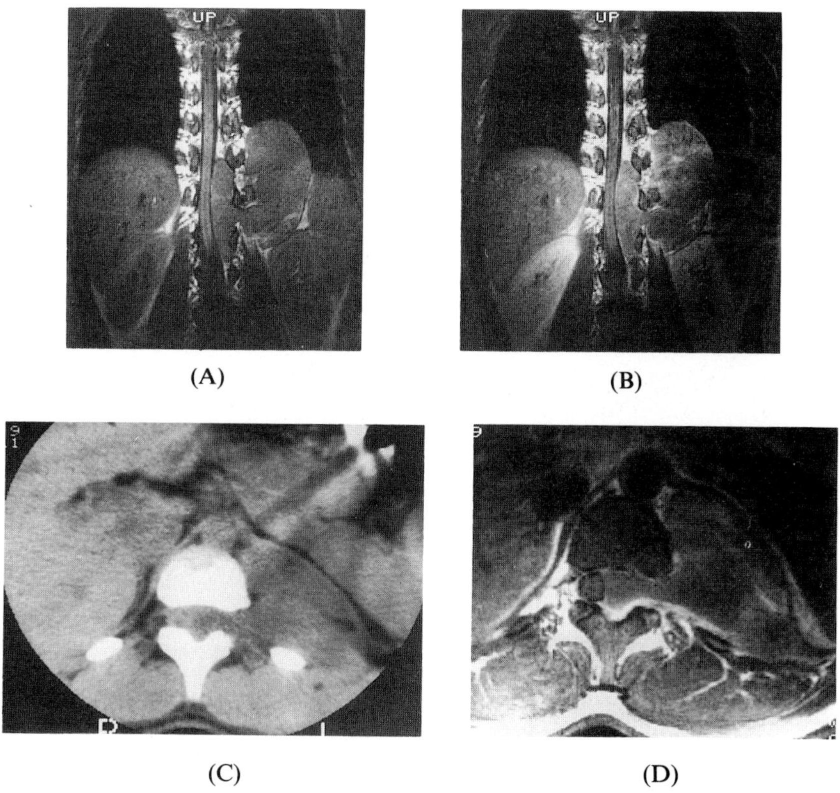

Figure 5. *GANGLIONEUROMA. (A) T1WI. (B) Following Gd injection. Very large dumbbell shaped tumor with intradural extramedullary and paraspinal intrathoracic component. Minimal enhancement is seen following Gd injection. The cord is compressed and displaced contralaterally. (C) Axial CT scan. (D) Axial T1WI at the same level.*

Metastases

Tumor spread within the subarachnoid spaces may occur both with primary intracranial neoplasms and tumors of the other body organs. Meningeal carcinomatosis is better seen by contrast enhanced MRI. Tumor nodules enhance markedly and may be easily recognized while detection with SE T1 or T2WI may sometimes be difficult.

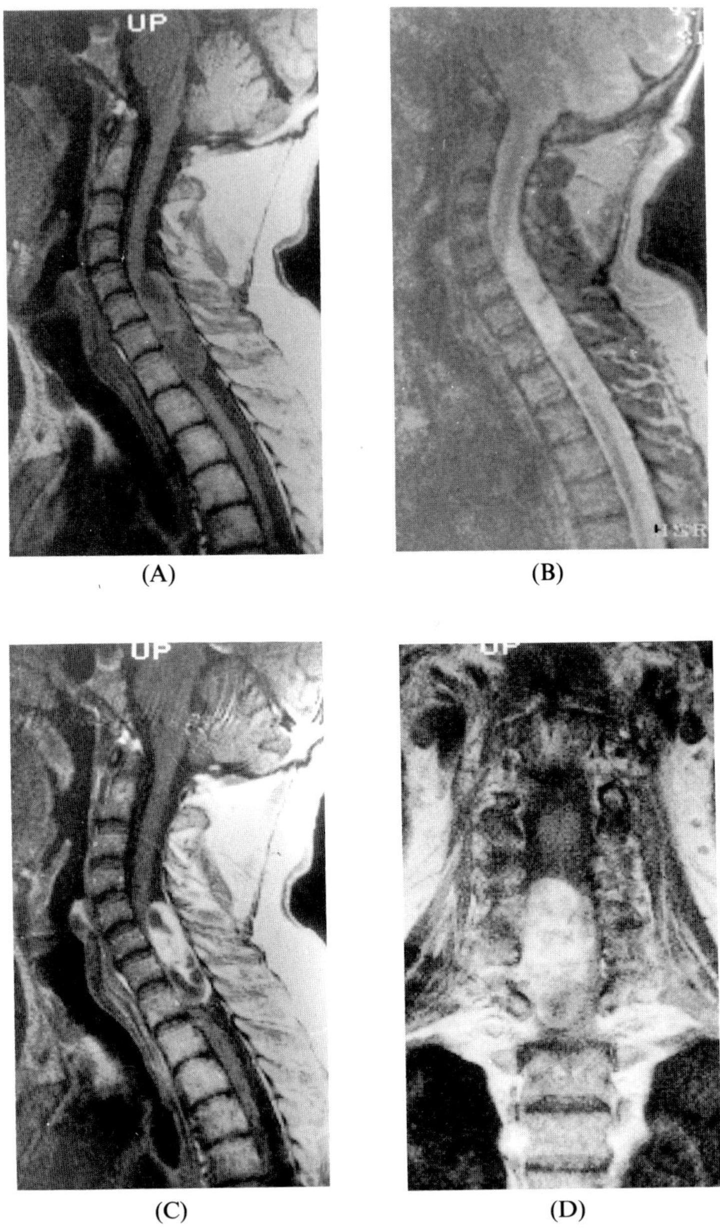

(A) (B)

(C) (D)

Figure 6. *MENINGIOMA. Dorso-lumbar meningioma compressing the lower part of the conus and the origin of the roots of the cauda equina. (A) T1WI. The tumor is isointense. (B) T2WI the tumor is hyperintense with some inhomogeneities; the superior two thirds are more hyperintense. (C, D) Marked enhancement following intravenous injection of Gd-DTPA.*

Conclusions

MRI has proven to be the single most informative and complete modality for the diagnosis of spinal cord tumors.

False negatives exist in the early phases of tumor growth as may happen in gliomas in the brain.

Differential diagnostic problems may arise with inflammatory and vascular lesions. Particularly are dural arteriovenous fistulas of the adult prone to mimic clinically an intramedullary tumor [20]. MRI shows extensive mild cord widening but mainly decreased T1 and increased T2 over many segments, within the spinal cord. Enlargement of dorsal draining veins may only rarely be seen. In these cases it is mandatory to perform a myelogram in search for images of dilated vessels, usually located in the posterior subarachnoid spaces. The definitive diagnosis is made with spinal cord angiography. Embolization or surgery, with occlusion of the fistula, may produce complete return to normal.

Differential diagnosis with syringomyelia is usually not a problem in cases of extensive intramedullary cysts. When a cyst reaches the medulla, the morphology of its cranial aspects is very different from that of syringomyelic cavity since it is tense, rounded and elevating the floor of the lower part of the fourth ventricle.

The tremendous advantage of MR is the capability to directly recognise the tumor nodule, within an extensive enlargement of the cord. This information is crucial in planning the surgical strategy since only the nodule must be removed and not the cysts. Unfortunately, despite this very high sensitivity, the specificity is low. Clear cut differences between astrocytomas and ependymomas are not present.

References

1. Hans JS, Kaufman B et al. NMR imaging of the spine. AJNR 1983;4:1151-1159.
2. Norman D, Mill C et al. Magnetic resonance imaging of spinal cord and canal: potentials and limitations. AJNR 1984;5:9-14.
3. Scotti G, Scialfa G et al. MR imaging of intradural extramedullary tumors of the cervical spine. J Comput Assist Tomogr. 1985;9:1037-1041.
4. Scotti G, Scialfa G. et al. Magnetic resonance diagnosis of intramedullary tumors of the spinal cord. Neuroradiology 1987;29:130-137.
5. Sze G, Krol G. et al. Intramedullary disease of the spine: diagnostic using gadolinium-DTPA enhanced MR imaging. AJR 1988;151:1193-1204.

6. Parizel PM, Beleriaux D et al. Gd-DTPA enhanced MR imaging of spinal tumors. AJR 1989;152:1087-1096.

7. Sze G, Stimac GK et al. Multicenter study of gadopentetate dimeglumine as an MR contrast agent: evaluation in patients with spinal tumors. AJNR 1990;11:967-974.

8. Farwell JR, Dohrman GJ. Intraspinal neoplasms in children. Paraplegia 1977;15:262-273.

9. Shenkin HA, Alpers BJ. Clinical and pathologic features of gliomas of the spinal cord. Arch Neurol Psychiatr 1944;52:87-105.

10. Scotti G, Parazzini C et al. I tumori midollari: diagnostica RM. In: Rosa ML. ed. Neuroradiologia. Centauro, Udine, 1991.

11. Levy WJ, Bay J et al. Spinal cord meningioma. J Neurosurg 1982;57:804-812.

12. Zimmerman RA, Bilaniuk LT. Imaging of the tumors of the spinal canal and cord. Radiol Clin North Am 1988;26:965-1007.

13. Goy AM, Pinto RS et al. Intramedullary spinal cord tumors: MR imaging with emphasis on associated cysts. Radiology 1986;161:381-386.

14. Slaski BS, Bydder GM et al. MR imaging with gadolinium-DTPA in the differentiation of tumor, syninx, and cyst of the spinal cord. J Comput Assists Tomogr 1987;11:845-850.

15. Williams AL, Haughton VM et al. Differentiation by intramedullary neoplasms and cysts by MR. AJNR 1987;8:527-532.

16. Rebner M, Gebarski SS. Magnetic resonance imaging of spinal cord hemangioblastoma AJNR 1985;6:287-289.

17. Silbergeld J, Cohen WA et al. Supratentorial and spinal cord hemangioblastomas: gadolinium enhanced MR appearance with pathologic correlation. J Comput Assist Tomogr. 1989;13:1048-1051.

18. Levine E, Huntrakoon M et al. Malignant nerve-sheath neoplasms in fibromatosis neuro: distinction from benign tumors by using imaging techniques. AJR 1987;149:1059-1064.

19. Scotti G, Scialfa G et al. MR imaging of intradural extramedullary tumors of the cervical spine. J Comput Assist Tomogr 1985;9:1037-1041.

20. Larsson E-M, Desai P et al. Venous infarction of the spinal cord resulting from dural arteriovenous fistula: MR imaging findings. AJNR 1991;12:739-743.

Spinal Dysraphism

Olof Flodmark
Department of Neuroradiology, Karolinska Institutet, Stockholm, Sweden

Introduction

Malformations of the spine may involve mesodermal as well as neuroectodermal structures. Although it is not necessary to find musculo-skeletal and nervous tissue abnormalities in each case the combination is common and variable. The investigation of patients suspected of having a spinal malformation should focus first on evaluation of the neurogenic tissues in order to confirm or exclude a malformation of these structures. When a malformation is found, further radiology must concentrate on a full and detailed mapping of the entire malformation in order to facilitate surgical planning and to avoid complications due to incomplete understanding of the malformation. Plain films of the spine, with or without tomography, may be very important from an orthopedic point of view but is of little or no help in detecting associated malformations of the spinal cord and its coverings. Only direct imaging of the subarachnoid space and its content is of value in this evaluation. Myelography, followed by high resolution CT scanning remains the best method, the "gold standard" in this evaluation. Magnetic resonance imaging (MRI) is a strong contender as it is non-invasive but lacks the same spatial resolution as CT and is time consuming if properly applied. Most obvious is this limitation when the neuroradiologist is requested to rule out a malformation of the spinal cord and meninges. Spinal ultrasonography is of value only during the neonatal period when it may provide useful information for the neuroradiologist.

Neuroradiological Investigation of Spinal Dysraphism

Many factors must be considered in choosing the most appropriate mode of investigating a patient suspected of having a congenital malformation of the spine. Investigation of the bony spine requires different methods than investigation of the spinal canal and its contents. The specificity and sensitivity are different in each imaging modality and vary with pathology. The plane of imaging is important and should influence the choice depending on indication. The amount of radiation involved in a spinal examination is particularly important when investigating infants and children, but also young fertile women.

The use of *neurosonography* in evaluating the spinal canal is limited to the neonatal period. However, the method is harmless and is capable of giving a general idea of the position of the conus and extent of intraspinal lipomas or cysts [1]. The procedure is very operator-dependent and may therefore have a low sensitivity as well as specificity. Spinal sonography has a definite role in the preliminary evaluation of a suspected spinal malformation but can never replace more detailed neuroradiological investigations. The investigation of a neonatal spine may be limited to spinal sonography only if the sonologist is very experienced and if there is in reality no clinical suspicion of a malformation. Even with the slightest clinical suspicion of a malformation, the work-up must include other imaging methods in order to exclude the presence of closed spinal dysraphism.

The best way to investigate the skeletal anomalies is by *plain films,* possibly combined with *conventional tomography.* The transaxial plane of imaging, used in CT, is less useful and it can be very difficult to understand the complex anatomy of segmentation anomalies, particularly in the presence of severe deformation and curvatures of the spine. Plain films, as well as CT of the lower spine carries a very high dose of radiation to the gonads, particularly in females. Thus, the indications for this study must be restricted and carefully evaluated in each individual case. *Skeletal scintigraphy* or bone scan has a high sensitivity but very low specificity. This procedure is very useful as the first investigation of back pain of unknown origin in children. Minor vertebral anomalies may cause abnormal stress and reactive changes may be detected as increased activity on bone scan. Further radiological evaluation can be limited and the radiation restricted when the abnormality is localized.

Neuroradiological investigation of the spinal canal and its contents is best done using *myelography followed by CT scanning,* when spinal malformations are suspected [2-5]. The study should include the entire spinal canal but the following CT scan, which must not be omitted, should be limited to areas with abnormalities or include conus and cauda equina if the myelographic study appears normal. MRI has evolved during the last few years and it has been claimed that MRI will replace all myelography when the equipment becomes more readily available. However, MRI does not have sufficient spatial resolution necessary in the evaluation of spinal malformations and therefore not the same high specificity and sensitivity as myelography with CT. Spinal curvatures can make the interpretation very difficult. It has been shown that diagnoses like hydromyelia are better seen on MR while diastematomyelia and intraspinal dermoids or arachnoid cysts are easily missed on MR imaging, particularly if limited to imaging in the sagittal plane [6,7]. Hence, full evaluation of spinal anatomy using MR requires imaging in all the orthogonal planes using multiple imaging sequences. Such an extensive procedure that takes long time is difficult for the patient to endure and requires general anaesthesia or heavy sedation in children. MR imaging cannot be considered non-invasive under these circumstances.

The neuroradiological investigation has to show all components of the malformation in detail, as it must be possible for the neurosurgeon to plan the reconstructive surgery with all facts available. It is therefore a major advantage if the neuroradiology is performed in the same institution as surgery. This will prevent unnecessary repeat examinations.

Segmentation Anomalies

Many segmentation anomalies with hemi-vertebrae and block-vertebrae will cause spinal deformities requiring orthopedic correction. These obvious malformations may be associated with less obvious malformations in the spinal canal. It is extremely important to exclude tethering of the cord prior to corrective surgery. Congenital scoliosis with early symptoms or painful scoliosis may be caused by diastematomyelia or other forms of closed spinal dysraphism and are situations usually recognised as requiring preoperative investigation of the spinal cord.

Spinal Dysraphism

Spinal dysraphism is divided into two different types. Open and closed (occult) spinal dysraphism represent two different pathological entities thought to have entirely different pathogenesis. Although similarities exist, the two syndromes show some fundamental differences. There is a constant association between cerebral dysgenesis in the form of Arnold-Chiari II malformation and open spinal dysraphism, of which meningo-myelocele is the most important form. Such an association does not exist in closed spinal dysraphism in which Arnold-Chiari II malformation is as rare as in the general population [8].

Open Spinal Dysraphism

The most common form of open spinal dysraphism is *meningo-myelocele (MMC)*. A less common but fatal form is iniencephaly. The incidence of MMC varies within different ethnic groups but is usually quoted to be 1.2 per 1000 live born. MMC is most common in the lumbo-sacral region (80-90%) and is associated with increased interpeduncular distance, wide spinal canal and incomplete closure or absence of the vertebral arches. The neural tube has failed to form properly and the nervous elements remain in a placode ventrally facing the subarachnoid space and dorsally freely exposed. Leaking of cerebro-spinal fluid (CSF) is common as the delicate subarachnoid membranes have ruptured. Associated abnormalities of the spinal cord include hydromyelia in not quite 50% of the cases and a split cord, with or without diastematomyelia, in a little more than a third of the cases. Each case of MMC has an associated Arnold-Chiari II malformation of the brain which may be of varying degree and in a majority of cases (90%) associated with secondary hydrocephalus [8].

There is little need for neuroradiology in the primary diagnosis of MMC. However, prenatal diagnosis of MMC is possible and has become important. Modern ultrasound equipment is capable of demonstrating fetal anatomy so well that increased interpeduncular distance and the meningocele can be reliably identified at 18-20 weeks of gestation. The associated Arnold-Chiari II malformation can also be identified and confirms the diagnosis of MMC. The shape of the skull may be unusual with the "lemon sign." The fetal ventricles are large but completely filled by the choroid plexus. The choroid plexus can be seen to move within the ventricle, "dangling choroid," as the ventricles dilate further due to hydrocephalus. The posterior fossa is small in Arnold-Chiari II malformation and the cerebellum is seen to be compressed along the posterior skull vault. The cisterna magna can no longer be seen and cerebellum has a posteriorly convex appearance, "banana sign." The incidence of newborn neonates with MMC has decreased dramatically in societies in which the diagnosis of MMC on fetal ultrasound is an acceptable reason for abortion [9-11].

The newborn child with MMC should be investigated with spinal ultrasound prior to corrective surgery. Major associated anomalies such as diastematomyelia at a higher level than the MMC should alert the neurosurgeon that a more extensive procedure is necessary in addition to reconstruction of the dural sac and closure of the skin. Neonates who deteriorate following primary closure of the MMC should, for the same reason, undergo urgent myelography.

The patient with MMC may experience neurological deterioration later in life and will then return for neuroradiological investigation. The purpose of the investigation at this time is to detect complications that may be postoperative or represent further development of the malformation. Hence, hydromyelia may develop and give late symptoms. Inclusion tumors, dermoids, or arachnoid cysts may represent postoperative complications. Re-tethering with adhesions of the spinal cord to the dura is always present radiographically and is of questionable significance. In this group of patients it is extremely important to choose the mode of investigation by the expected pathology. MRI is the obvious choice if hydromyelia is suspected but this modality cannot exclude dermoid tumors nor detect compartmentalization of the subarachnoid space with cysts unless very large and expanding. Only myelography and subsequent CT can detect these lesions [12]. Whatever the imaging modality, the pathology is complex and these studies are very difficult to interpret and should be concentrated to institutions specializing in treatment of these patients (Fig. 1).

Closed Spinal Dysraphism

The term "closed spinal dysraphism" includes entities that may cause neurological, urological and orthopedic problems in children and young adults. It is generally agreed that early correction of these

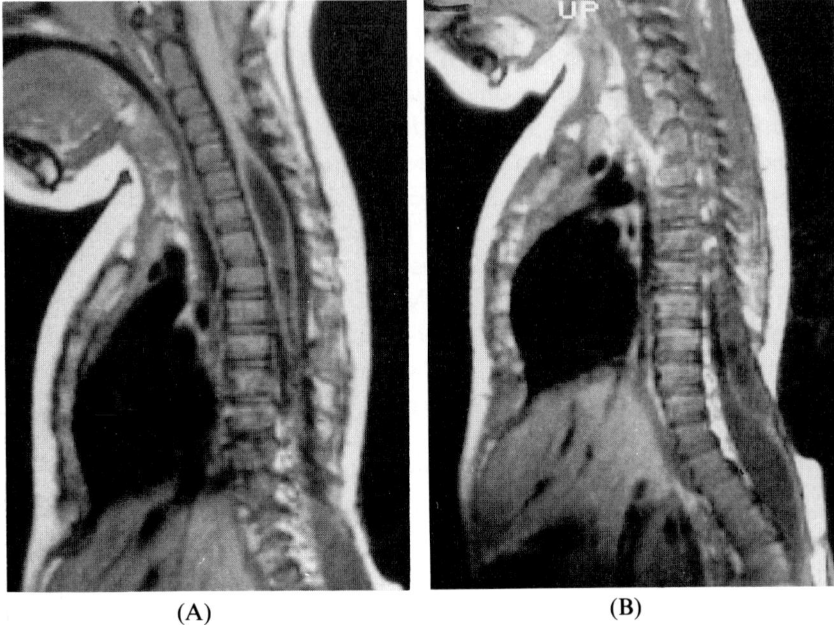

(A)   (B)

Figure 1. *OPEN SPINAL DYSRAPHISM. This 2.5-year-old male, who had surgery for open spinal dysraphism in the neonatal period, presented with increasing symptoms from the arms as well as increased tone in the lower limbs. (A) Sagittal MR image of the cervical spine and upper thoracic spine shows the cerebellar tonsils to be dysplastic and extending down to the level of C4. A large cyst, representing a dilated central canal, hydromyelia, is seen in the spinal cord. (B) Another sagittal image 8 mm from the the image in (a) shows the lower end of the cord. Hydromyelic cyst extends to the end of the cord which continues in a filum. The filum and distal cord is located close to and probably attached to the posterior dura.*

malformations will prevent new symptoms to develop and halt progression of those present. Hence, it is not considered appropriate to delay surgery even if the patient is asymptomatic [8,13,14]. The old term, "spina bifida occulta" is unfortunate as isolated defects in the posterior elements of the lumbo-sacral region are found in 10-20% of the normal population. Although these defects also occur in association with closed spinal dysraphism, the diagnostic significance of this finding is limited and of no use in the work-up of patients suspected of having this malformation syndrome.

The term, "closed spinal dysraphism", implies unbroken skin. However, cutaneous manifestations of an underlying malformation are common. A small area of atrophic skin, hyper-pigmentation, strawberry naevus, abnormal hair growth, subcutaneous lipoma or dermal sinus are all findings that should result in primary referral to a neurosurgeon who should organize the radiological evaluation as it should be done in close cooperation with the attending neurosurgeon. Once the suspicion of closed spinal dysraphism has been raised, a normal neurologic examination does not preclude neuroradiological investigation. Such an investigation must either fully exclude a malformation or define all elements of the malformation. Plain films of the spine are of no help in this situation and should be avoided to minimize radiation. Neurosonography may show some components of a malformation but can never exclude an abnormality. However, it is a harmless investigation and the results can be very useful in the planning of further neuroradiological studies (Fig. 2). The limitations of MRI has been outlined above and if performed, has to be very time consuming as it is very difficult to exclude a malformation without an extensive examination. An investigation in this situation must have a very high sensitivity and specificity, at this time best fulfilled by myelography combined with CT. Recent MR literature has proposed MR to be superior but the authors have failed to prove this as the rate of false negative examinations remains unknown [7].

The myelogram must be carefully executed when closed spinal dysraphism is suspected. Patient cooperation is extremely important and general anesthesia is preferred in children. The contrast dose and volume must be adapted to the volume of the subarachnoid space. Films of the spine should include the entire spine and be performed both prone and supine. However, it is not necessary to exclude tonsillar herniation as an associated Arnold Chilari II malformation is extremely uncommon. The patient is transferred to the CT scanner without unnecessary delay when filming is complete. CT is limited to areas of pathology but the examination must visualize the pathology in every detail. The CT scanning is necessary even if the regular films show no abnormalities. The CT scan should in this situation include conus, cauda equina and include the distal end of the dural sac. Slice thickness should not exceed 5 mm but the inter-scan distance can be increased to opti-

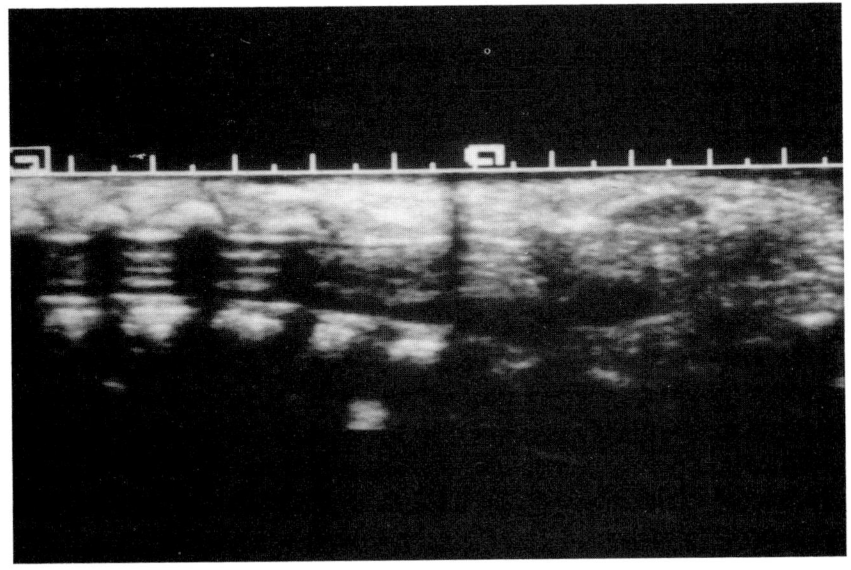

(A)

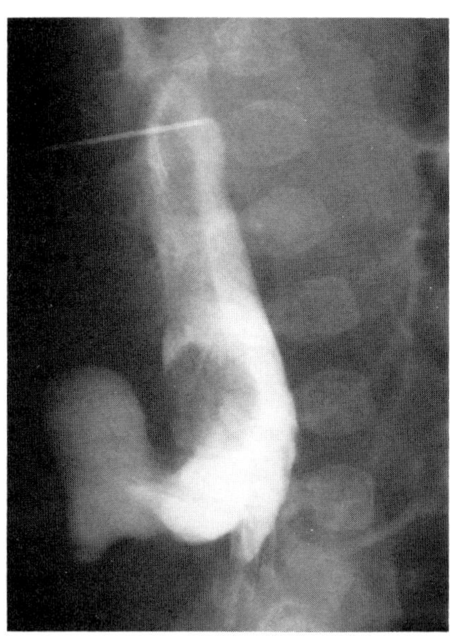

(B)

mize the number of scans and hence the radiation dose. Best result is achieved when magnification and bone algorithm is used for image reconstruction. Images should be documented using wide window and with frequent evaluation of tissue density in order not to overlook abnormal deposits of fat in the spinal canal [15] (Figs. 3,4).

The entity of closed spinal dysraphism include many components of developmental pathology. The most recent theory of etiology and pathogenesis speculate in focal damage to the spine and its content during early fetal life. The repair process may include various mesodermal components such as elastic or fibrotic bands with lipo-matous tissue tethering the cord. Further growth of these abnormal or damaged mesodermal components will result in a low position of the cord which will remain low in position even if the adhesions are released [16]. This theory further explains the variation of patho-logical findings in the syndrome of closed spinal dysraphism. The radiologist must be aware of this and interpret the studies with great suspicion and care. Several components can be present in the same case and can be found outside the immediate geographic vicinity.

The adhesions between cord and dural sac can be caused by a lumbo-sacral lipoma which may be in continuity with filum termi-nale (Fig. 5), *lipo-myeloschisis* or a thickened fibrotic filum with or

---

Figure 2. *CLOSED SPINAL DYSRAPHISM. This 3-months-old male presented at birth with a lipoma over the lower back. Neurological exam is normal. Myelography followed by CT provides a detailed description of the malformation allowing the surgeon to proceed with surgery without encountering unexpected features of the anomaly. (A) A spinal ultrasound done at two days of age show a low lying cord which is continuous in its lower end with hyperechoic tissue, representing lipoma. (B) A lateral view from the myelogram performed at three months of age shows the low cord and an attached mass, lipoma, in the subarachnoid space. Note how the nerve roots appear to exit the cord outside the spinal canal close to a meningocele and have a horizontal course. However, the roots are always located in the subarachnoid space and do not go through the lipoma which is located extradurally. (C) A CT scan at the level of the lipoma shows how the lipoma is located in the left aspect of the spinal canal and how the placode has rotated 90° facing the remaining narrow subarachnoid space in the right aspect of the spinal canal.*

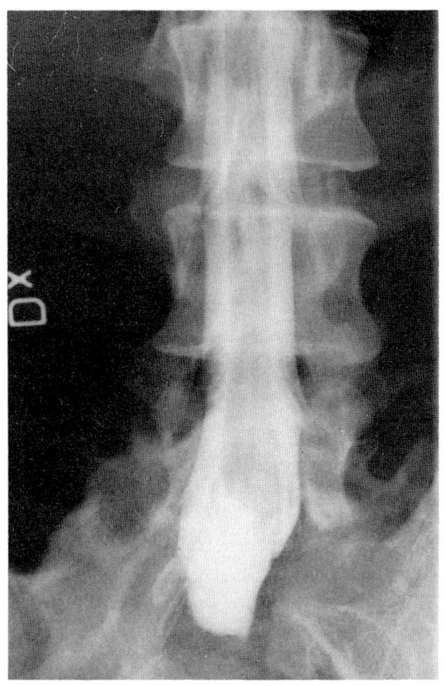

(A)

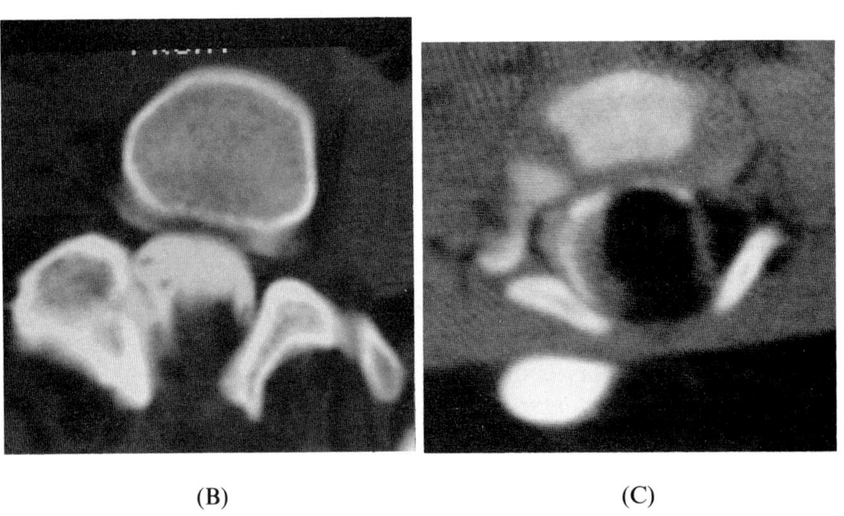

(B)   (C)

without lipoma [15] (Fig. 3). *Diastematomyelia* may be caused by a bony spur but more commonly a aberrant fibrotic band may split and tether the cord but not split the dural sac [17]. Fibrous bands anywhere in the subarachnoid space may attach to the dura while a dermal sinus in other situations may provide the tethering elements.

Terminal myelo-cystocele represents an uncommon form of spinal dysraphism. The pathology of this lesion includes closed spinal dysraphism with a meningocele continuous with the subarachnoid space. A low lying, hydromyelic spinal cord extends through the meningocele into a terminal cyst which is continuous with the hydromyelic cavity and lined by ependyma. This malformation can be diagnosed using spinal ultrasound as gentle compression of the terminal cyst will cause simultaneous dilatation of the hydromyelic cavity [18].

Figure 3. *CLOSED SPINAL DYSRAPHISM. This 16-year-old female had surgery at 21 months of age for "lipo-myelomeningocele." She now presents with scoliosis and with a smaller left leg and foot. (A) An AP supine view of the lower spine show a low cord ending at the level of L5-S1. Note the horizontal course of the lumbar nerve roots as the exit almost at the level of their origin from the spinal cord. Also note that the lumbar roots have several rootlets, an appearance normally found in the cervical spine. There was no evidence of a Chiari II malformation. (B) A CT scan obtained at the level of L5. Note the spina bifida and how the cord has formed a placode directly attached to the subcutaneous tissue posteriorly. A small amount of fat can be seen in the placode. The rootlets exit the placode from its ventral surface into the subarachnoid space. Four rootlets can be identified and represent the two dorsal and two ventral roots at this level.*

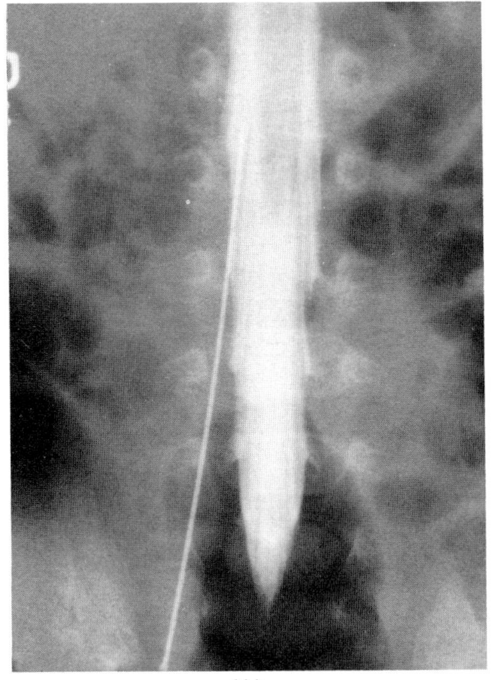

(A)

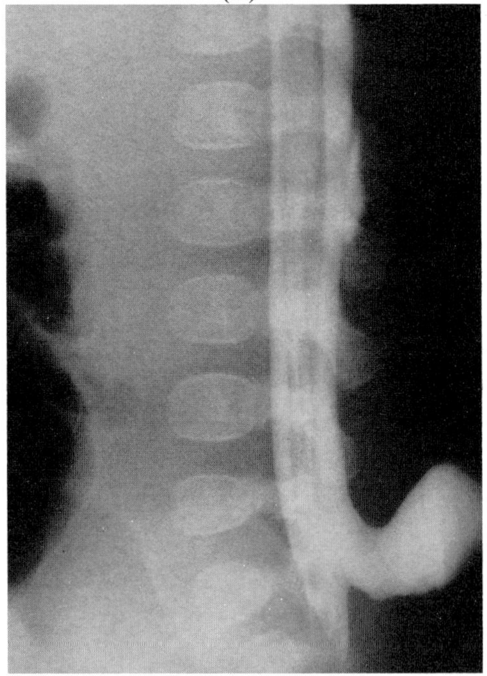

(B)

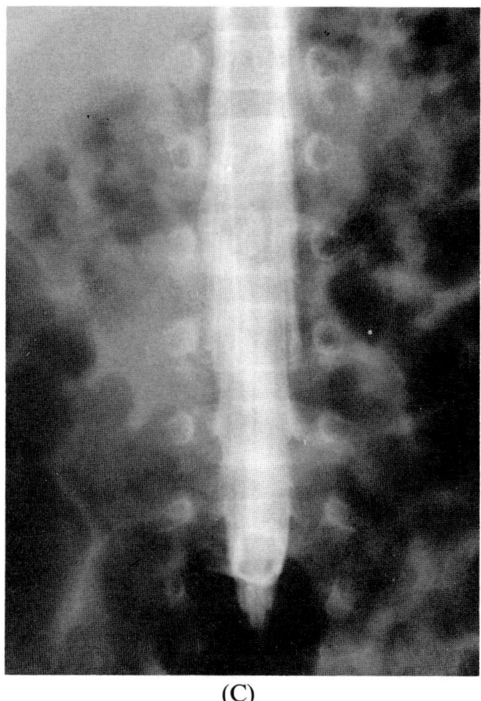

(C)

Figure 4. *CLOSED SPINAL DYSRAPHISM (MENINGOCELE). This 1-month-old girl was born with a soft round lump in the midline over the lower lumbar spine. (A) The lumbar puncture should be performed off the midline under fluoroscopic control to avoid puncture of a low lying cord. The puncture in this case was performed at the l2-3 level and the conus ended at the L3-4 level, too low to be normal. (B) Lateral view of the lumbar spine shows contrast but no nervous tissue in the meningocele. Note the fibrous band (arrow) that tethers the dural sac. This band is found between the lamina in the most cranial dysraphic arch, in this case S1. (C) Supine AP view shows the low position of conus medullaris and contrast in the neck of the meningocele.*

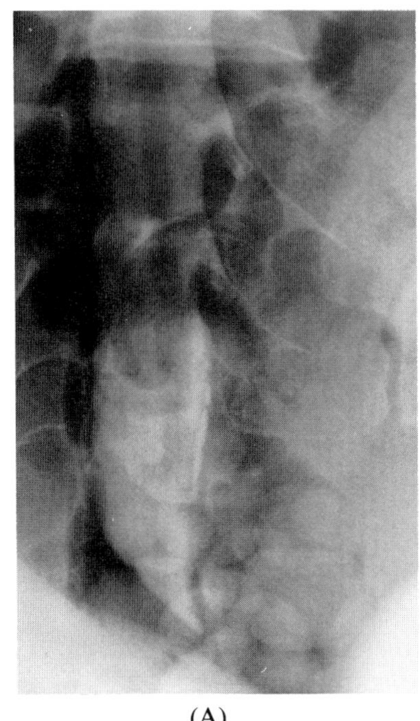

(A)

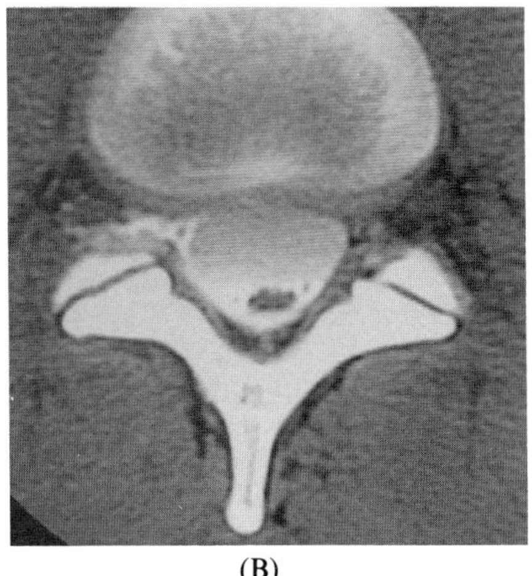

(B)

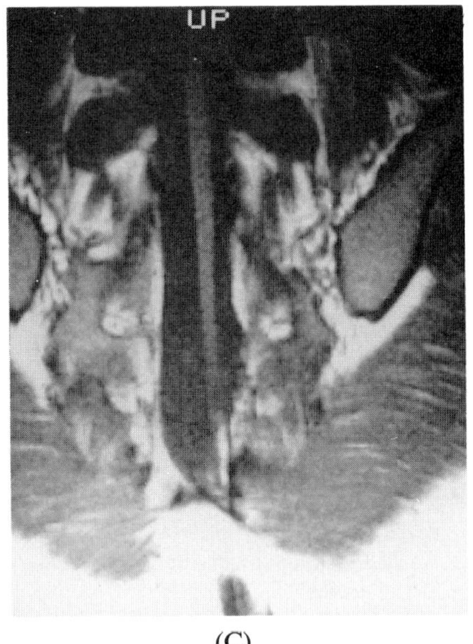

(C)

Figure 5. *CLOSED SPINAL DYSRAPHISM. This 20-year-old male has had a "pit" over the lower back since birth. He is now complaining of progressive numbness and some weakness in the left foot. No other neurological symptoms or findings. (A) Myelography showed a thin cord attached to the dural sac in the lower sacral spine. (B) The subsequent CT scan proved that nerve roots did exit from the cord at the level of L5. (C) A coronal image from the MRI study showed in addition a minute lipoma at the insertion of the cord in the distal sac. Despite multiple imaging sequences, it was not possible to identify the nerve roots with any certainty, and MR could not identify the level of the transition from cord to a thickened filum terminale.*

References

1. Nadich TP, Radkowski MA, Britton J. Real-time sonographic display of caudal spinal anomalies. Neuroradiology 1986;28:512-527.
2. Wippold FJ, Citrin C, Barkovich AJ, Sherman JS. Evaluation of MR in spinal dysraphism with lipoma: comparison with metrizamide computed tomography. Pediatr Radiol 1987;17:184-188.
3. Tortori-Donati P, Cama A, Rosa ML, Andreussi L, Taccone A. Occult spinal dysraphism: neuroradiological study. Neuroradiology 1990;31:512-522.
4. Merx JL, Bakker-Niezen SH, Thijssen HOM, Walder HAD. The tethered spinal cord syndrome: a correlation of radiological features and preoperative findings in 30 patients. Neuroradiology 1989;31:63-70.
5. Scatliff JH, Kendall BE, Kingsley DPE, Britton J, Grant DN, Hayward RD. Closed spinal dysraphism: analysis of clinical, radiological and surgical findings in 104 consecutive patients. AJNR 1989;10:269-277.
6. Barkovich AJ, Edwards MSB, Cogen PH. MR Evaluation of Spinal Dermal Sinus Tract in Children. AJNR 1991;12:123-129.
7. Kuharik MA, Edwards MK, Grossman CB. Magnetic resonance evaluation of pediatric spinal dysraphism. Pediat Neurosci 1985-86;12:213-218.
8. Defects of the neural tube I: fetal and Neonatal Neurology and Neurosurgery. Churchill Livingstone, Edinburgh 1988;265-300.
9. Nyberg DA, Mack LA, Hirsch J, Pagon RO, Shepard TH. Fetal hydrocephalus: sonographic detection and clinical significance of associated anomalies. Radiology 1987;163:187-191.
10. Filley RA. The "lemon" sign: a clinical perspective. Radiology 1985;167:573-575.
11. Garel L, Boisvert J, Filitrault D, Grignon A, Perreault G, Patriquin H. Fetal sonography: 1. Neural tube defects. Pediatr Radiol 1989;19:157-162.
12. Nelson MD, Bracchi M, Naidich TP, McLone DG. The natural history of repaired meylomeningocele. RadioGraphics 1988;8:695-706.
13. Hoffman HJ, Taecholarn C, Hendrick EB, Humphreys RP. Management of lipomyelomeningoceles. J Neurosurg 1985;62:1-8.
14. Pierre-Kahn A, Lacombe J, Pichon J, Giudicelli Y, Renier D, Sainte-Rose C, Perrigot M, Hirch J-F. Intraspinal lipomas with spina bifida: prognosis and treatment in 73 cases. J Neurosurg 1986;65:756-761.

15. Naidich TP, McLone DG, Mutluer S. A new understanding of dorsal dysraphism with lipoma (lipomyeloschesis): radiologic evaluation and surgical correction. AJR 1983;140:1065-1078.
16. Sarwar M, Virapongse C, Bhimani S. Primary tethered cord syndrome: a new hypothesis of its origin. AJNR 1984;5:235-242.
17. Scotti G, Musgrave MA, Harwood-Nash DC, Fitz CR, Chuang SH. Diastematomyelia in Children: metrizamide and CT metrizamide myelography. AJNR 1980;1:403-410.
18. McLone DG, Naidich TP. Terminal myelocystocele. Neurosurgery 1985;16:36-43.

Lumbar Spinal Stenosis

Michael S. Huckman

*Rush-Presbyterian University and St. Luke's Medical Center,
Chicago, Illinois, USA*

Introduction

Lumbar spinal stenosis (LSS) was first described by Verbiest [1] who recognized that there could be compression of nerve roots in the lumbar spinal canal in the absence of neoplasm and in the absence of herniated disc. It may involve the central spinal canal, and/or the lateral recesses and foramina. It becomes clinically significant when nerve entrapment results in leg pain or sensory or motor changes. The diagnosis therefore depends on a *combination* of clinical signs and symptoms in the presence of radiographic evidence of narrowing of one or more of the above areas of the lumbar canal.

Lumbar spinal stenosis (LSS) was classified by Nelson as being of two major types: primary or secondary. The *primary* type is due to congenital narrowing of the canal with reduced sagittal diameter due to short pedicles, decreased coronal diameter due to reduced interpediculate distances or a combination of the two as occurs in achondroplasia. *Secondary* refers to the acquired forms of LSS and on occasion may be superimposed on primary LSS [2]. The following etiologic classification of LSS is loosely based on that of Nelson.

Congenital
    A.   Idiopathic congenital narrow canal
    B.   Achondroplasia
    C.   Osteopetrosis

"""

Acquired

A. Degeneration
- Central portion of spinal canal
- Peripheral portion of canal, lateral recesses, and nerve root canals
- Degenerative spondylolisthesis

B. Combined (any combination of congenital, developmental or degenerative stenosis

C. Iatrogenic
- Post-laminectomy
- Post-fusion
- Post chemonucleolysis

D. Post-traumatic

E. Miscellaneous causes
- Paget Disease
- Fluorosis
- Acromegaly
- Vertebral hemangioma
- Osteomalacia
- Ankylosing Spondylitis
- Synovial cyst
- Subdural or epidural fluid collections (empyema or hematoma)

Central Spinal Stenosis (CSS)

LSS may be central or lateral or the two may occur together. Any of these may be present at single or multiple levels. The central lumbar spinal canal is normally round or ovoid in its upper portion and becomes triangular or even trefoil in its lowest portion. The canal shape is determined by the interfacet distance and the pedicle length. In males, the lumbar canal is usually narrowest at L3-4 and L4-5 and in females it is narrowest at L5-S1 [3,4]. Changes in the three-joint complex further influence the canal size and shape [4,5]. These joints, which are present at each vertebral level, are the two posterior facet joints and the intervertebral disc. Lesions which affect one of these joints also affect the others. A recent study has shown that disc degeneration almost invariably precedes facet joint degeneration. This study was conducted by looking at the disc integrity with sagittal T2 weighted MR scans and at the facet joints with wide window CT scans in a large cohort of patients who had both examinations prior to surgery [5]. The congenitally narrow canal alone is rarely symptomatic, but comprise of such a canal by disc prolapse, ligamentum flavum hypertrophy, pedicle hypertrophy, degenerative hypertrophy of the articular facets, or combinations of these factors may be enough to cause the clinical syndrome of spinal stenosis.

According to Kirkaldy-Willis [6] central stenosis is most often the result of degenerative disease of the articular facets which in turn is due to aging and repeated minor trauma. This may occur with or without a previously congenitally narrowed canal. Osteophytes arising on the superior facets tend to compromise the lateral recess and the intervertebral foramen and their contents. Osteophytes of the inferior facets indent the dura from behind, narrow the interlaminar angle and lead to central stenosis. Besides osteophyte formation, there is often accompanying reactive profileration of capsular and soft tissues including the ligamentum flavum which further narrows the lateral recesses, foramina, and central spinal canal. The thickening of the ligamentum flavum may not be an actual "hypertrophy", but may rather be thickening of the ligament by virtue of the shortening of its antero-posterior dimension secondary to narrowing of the apophyseal joint space (V. Haughton, personal communication). CSS usually occurs at L4-5 and spreads to produce stenosis at levels above and below [6].

Symptoms of Central Spinal Stenosis

Patients with CSS are often misdiagnosed and may suffer for years often being considered malingerers. The usual patient is a male in the third to fourth decade [3] who has had minor back pain for many years which is aggravated by standing and activity and alleviated by sitting or crouching. In cases with congenital stenosis, symptoms may begin much earlier [7]. The symptoms are those of vascular claudication, but in addition there is numbness, tingling, and weakness. Physical examination usually shows limited spine motion with aggravation of pain on extension [3,4,7].

The claudicant syndrome of CSS is due to compression of spinal arteries and interference with the blood supply to the roots of the cauda equina [8]. According to Cailliet [9], this is felt to be due to increased CSF pressure behind the obstruction which in turn may compress the venules of the cauda equina with resultant ischemia. He states that the symptoms usually follow the cycle of exercise, pain, rest, and relief. Aortoiliac claudication (AoIC) causes pain in hips, thighs, and buttocks and it is "aching," "squeezing" or "cramping" but rarely causes weakness. Neurogenic claudication (NeuC) is more likely to affect the lumbar spine and buttocks and it may be "tingling" but not "cramping" and may be associated with weakness. AoIC begins after walking a long distance; NeuC begins after walking up an incline. Relief from AoIC comes quickly after the cessation of walking; relief from NeuC comes only after sitting and assuming a flexed trunk posture. Peripheral pulses may disappear after walking in the patient with vascular compromise, and while the leg may be pale, there are usually no residual neurologic findings. However in NeuC there may be persistent numbness, absent ankle jerk, and pain on straight leg raising [9].

Radiographic Confirmation Of Central Spinal Stenosis

Hinck et al. [10,11] measured the normal sagittal and interpediculate diameters of the spinal canal at various levels in adults and children. These measures were done on plain radiographs. However, because of the shape of the spinal canal in cross section, the value of such measures is questionable. One may have a normal sagittal and a normal interpediculate measure and still have significant spinal stenosis because of the "trefoil" appearance of the degeneratively narrowed canal.

A number of linear measures may be made on the CT scan which, with the proper clinical syndrome, can confirm a diagnosis of CSS. The normal mid-sagittal bony diameter of the spinal canal at L1 and L5 ranges from 13.8 to 20.4 mm and at the intermediate levels measures 13.4 to 18.8 mm. (One must be careful to do bony measures on CT at wide window widths (1500+) as the bony diameters of the canal may appear less than they actually are when measured at narrow window widths.) Ullrich et al. [12] did extensive measures of normal and stenotic spinal canals and reported that a sagittal diameter in the lumbar canal of less than 11.5 mm was indicative of stenosis. They reported that interpediculate distances of less than 16mm at L4-5 and less than 20 mm at L5-S1 were abnormal. The interfacet distance normally measures 2-4 mm and is considered abnormal if it is less than 2 mm. The cross sectional area of the central canal best describes the severity of the stenosis (Fig. 1) Ullrich et al. stated that an area measure of less than 1.45 sq. cm. indicates an abnormal bony canal.

It is known that the ligamentum flavum, when thickened, may increase the severity of CSS. This is a thick yellow elastic ligament which extends the length of the canal. It is attached to the laminae and articular process at each level and on CT is intermediate in density between fat and bone [13]. It normally has a thickness of 2-4 mm and is considered hypertrophied if it is more than 5 mm thick (MH Gado, personal communication) (Fig. 2). We have measured the cross sectional area in a group of normal and stenotic canals *within the ligamentum flavum* and use the following rule of thumb in classifying spinal stenosis on CT:

Normal = area greater than 2.5 sq cm.
Mild spinal stenosis = area of 1.7-2.5 sq cm.
Moderate spinal stenosis = area of 1.0-1.7 sq cm.
Severe spinal stenosis = area less than 1.0 sq cm.

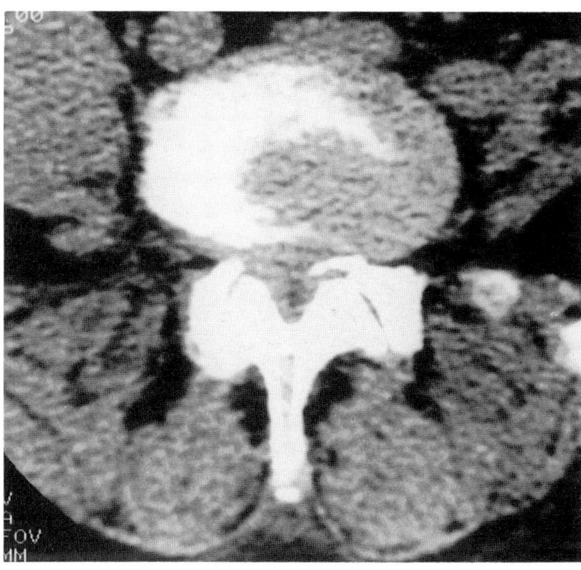

Figure 1. *FACET ARTHROPATHY. Axial CT scan at L4-5 showing severe facet joint arthropathy and severe central spinal stenosis.*

Post myelographic CT scan (CTM) enables a more accurate evaluation of the thickness of the ligamentum flavum, shows the difference between the cross sectional areas of the bony spinal canal and the thecal sac, and may identify nerve roots.

The CT picture of symptomatic CSS shows a narrowed canal, thick ligamentum flavum, decrease in epidural fat, and the presence of degenerated discs and facet joints. The canal loses its oval or triangular shape and becomes more "trefoil" [14] (Fig. 1).

Contrast between soft tissues, such as the disc and the ligamentum flavum and the thecal sac, may be greater on CTM than on conventional CT or MR, and CTM has a role in the evaluation of subtle spinal stenosis [15]. If myelography shows a complete block, enough contrast medium may get by so that evaluation of the level and degree of stenosis of the thecal sac below the obstruction may be accomplished.

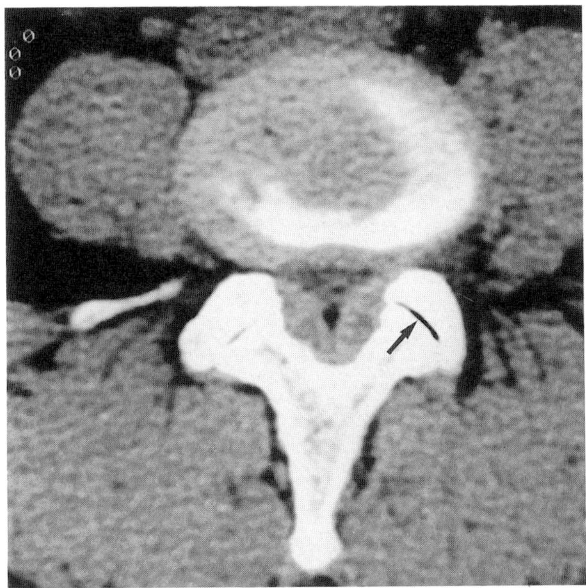

Figure 2. *DISC BULGE AND THICKENED LIGAMENTUM FLAVUM. Axial CT scan showing severe central spinal stenosis with disc bulge and thickened ligamentum flavum. Note vacuum change in the left facet (arrow).*

Stovring et al. [16] described a method of successful myelography after "dry" lumbar puncture. Using a 22 gauge needle, the position of the needle is confirmed by fluoroscopy. Even though there is no backflow of cerebrospinal fluid, the contrast medium is injected under fluoroscopic guidance to be certain that the injection is intrathecal. Because the canal is stenotic, it is often not necessary to use the full standard dose of contrast material to obtain optimal visualization of the thecal sac. If patients experience a sensation of low back pressure radiating into the legs, the injection rate should be slowed.

A high grade obstruction to the flow of contrast material in patients with spinal stenosis may be overcome during myelography by a maneuver described by Kapila and Chakeres [17]. When the stenosis is confirmed, the needle is removed and the patient is asked to sit on the edge of the horizontal myelographic table for about one minute with elbows on knees. The patient is then repositioned prone on the table and frequently the contrast material will have passed the obstruction. This maneuver was attempted based on the knowledge that pain in patients with LSS is often relieved by flexion and aggravated by lordosis. This is presumed to be due to stretching and thinning of the ligamentum flavum and decreasing the annular bulge of the disc, phenomena which occur during flexion [17].

According to Modic et al. [18] the MR scan shows narrowing of the thecal sac, lateral recesses and foramina and, on T1 weighted sagittal scan, decreased fat in the "fat window" (Fig. 3) and decreased fat in the interlaminar angle (Fig. 4) on the axial acquisition. While the soft tissues are well seen by MR, the identification of facet joint disease is still better with CT, although the overall detection of spinal stenosis is equivalent with the two techniques [19].

Degenerative Spondylolisthesis

Degenerative spondylolisthesis (DeSpL) with an intact neural arch usually occurs between the fourth and fifth lumbar vertebrae. It is 2-3 times more common in women than men and four times higher in diabetics than in non diabetics. The symptoms usually begin after the age of 50 and consist of unilateral or bilateral back pain and

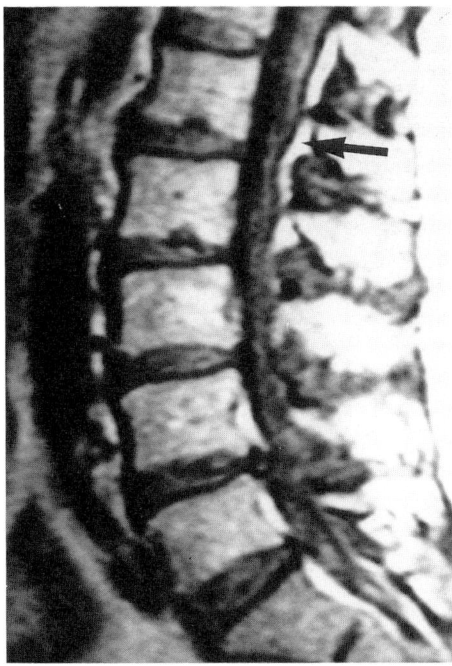

Figure 3. *MR AND LOSS OF FAT WINDOW. Sagittal T1 weighted MR acquisition in a patient with lumbar spinal stenosis. Arrow indicates normal fat window. There is absence of this window at L4-5 and L5-S1 where the thecal sac is narrowed by spinal stenosis.*

sciatica and tingling and numbness in the legs which is relieved by rest [7]. Compression of nerve roots may be due to an associated herniation of the nucleus pulposus or may be due to mobile bone structures impinging on the cauda equina [2]. This occurs when the posterior elements of the vertebra move forward and compress the cauda equina against the body of the vertebra below. Whereas congenital spondylolisthesis is most likely to occur at L5-S1, DeSpL is most likely to occur at L4-5 and is not associated with a defect in the pars interarticularis.

The radiographic diagnosis of DeSpL can be made with myelography, CT (Fig. 5), MR (Fig. 6), and CTM (Fig. 7). In addition to degenerative changes in the articular facets, there may be an associated "vacuum facet" phenomenon [20]. Since there is breakdown of cartilage lining the apophyseal joints, there is anterior

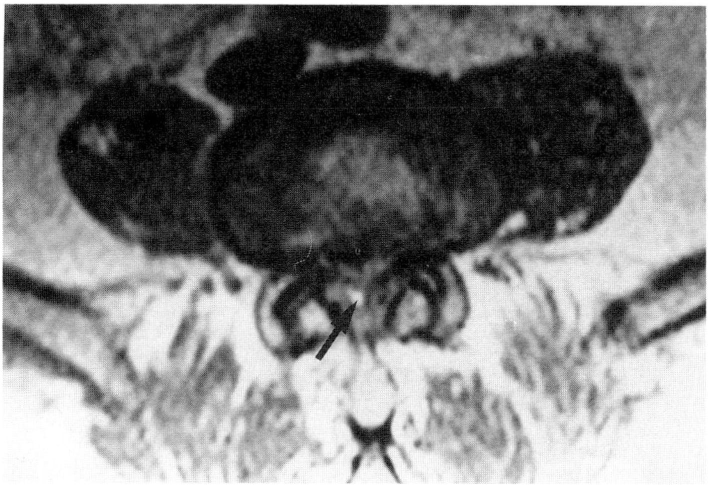

Figure 4. *MR AND LOSS OF INTERLAMINAR FAT. Axial T1 weighted MR scan in spinal stenosis showing diminished fat in the interlaminar angle (arrow).*

subluxation, usually of L4 upon L5, and overriding of the facets. Since the neural arch is intact, there is traction between the opposing facets and therefore a vacuum phenomenon in the facet joints and occasionally in the associated intervertebral disc [20] (Fig. 5). It is our experience that it is often possible to see, in an axial CT, the posterior margins of both the upper and lower vertebral bodies in the same section because of the subluxation and the narrowed disc space (Fig. 7). The mobility of the bony elements also results in foraminal narrowing. Axial and sagittal CT and MR sections show diminished epidural fat and severe narrowing of the thecal sac.

The stenosis of the sac may be so severe that there may be tortuous and elongated nerve roots above the narrowing on myelography [21,22,23] (Fig. 8). deTribolet and Campiche [24] pointed out that these have a strong correlation with the presence of neurogenic claudication. They believe they are due to chronic compression which prevents their free movements in the thecal sac, stretching the roots and finally producing a permanent elongation [24]. Severe stenosis secondary to DeSpL may cause complete block which can be decompressed by the flexion maneuver described above [17].

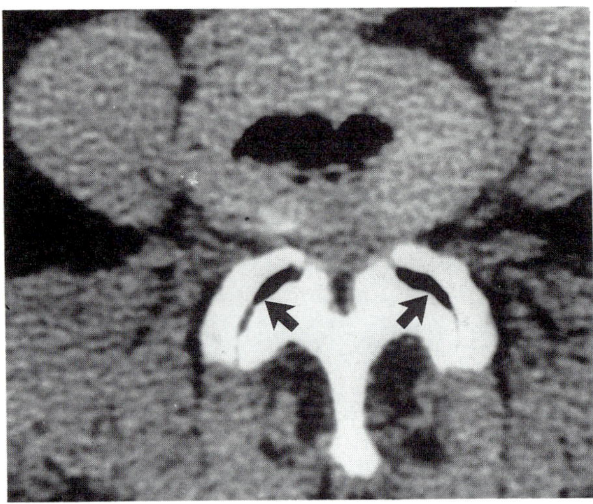

Figure 5. *SPONDYLOLISTHESIS AND CT. Axial CT at L4-5 showing degenerative spondylolisthesis with associated vacuum disc and vacuum facet changes bilaterally (arrows).*

Miscellaneous Causes of Central Spinal Stenosis

Spinal stenosis may occur just above the level of an old spinal fusion because of the decreased mobility at the fused level and increased mobility above it (Fig. 9). Quencer et al. [25] noted that, of 164 patients with persistent or recurrent low back pain after spinal fusion, 43% had bony spinal stenosis on CT examination.

Acromegaly may be associated with severe backache, spurs, and hypertrophy of the ligamentum flavum [26]. This growth abnormality may aggravate an already developmentally small canal.

In Paget disease of bone, there are widened medullary spaces and enlarged bony contours to the vertebral bodies and pedicles. Back pain in this disease is due to expansion of the bodies and neural arches in one or many vertebrae. Spinal stenosis is present in about 55% of patients with Paget disease who also have associated back pain which is usually lumbar (Fig. 10). In 80% of these, the narrowing is in the sagittal plane. Better than 90% of patients with Paget disease and back pain have facet joint arthropathy [27].

Epidural lipomatosis is characterized by increased extradural fat in the spinal canal causing compression of the spinal cord and

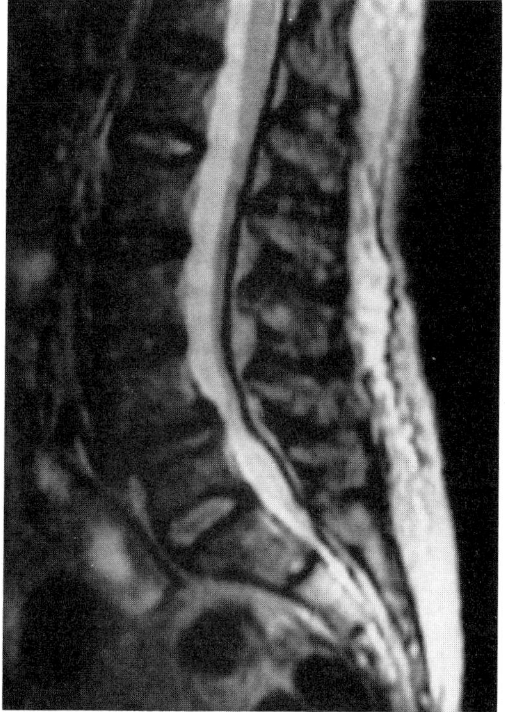

Figure 6. *SPONDYLOLISTHESIS AND MR. T2 weighted sagittal MR scan showing first degree degenerative spondylolisthesis at L4-5 with severe spinal stenosis.*

thecal sac with significant neurologic deficits [28,29]. Patients may present with neurogenic claudication, and paresthesias [28,29]. The syndrome may be the result of endogenous or exogenous steroids. Russell et al. [29] report a cross sectional triangular appearance to the thecal sac due to the compression by fat (Fig. 11). On occasion, the symptoms may be serious enough to justify surgical decompression [29]. At surgery, the fat is unencapsulated normal adipose tissue, not lipoma [28]. The vast majority of cases occur in the thoracic area [28]. Iatrogenic epidural "lipomatosis" may cause obstruction post operatively (Fig. 12).

Synovial cysts (SyCy) are filled with clear mucinous fluid and arise from the lumbar facet joints. They are felt to arise from a herniation of the synovial lining of the facet joint [30]. They show sclerosis and narrowing of the facet joint and dorsal and lateral defects in the thecal sac [30] and are a frequent accompaniment of

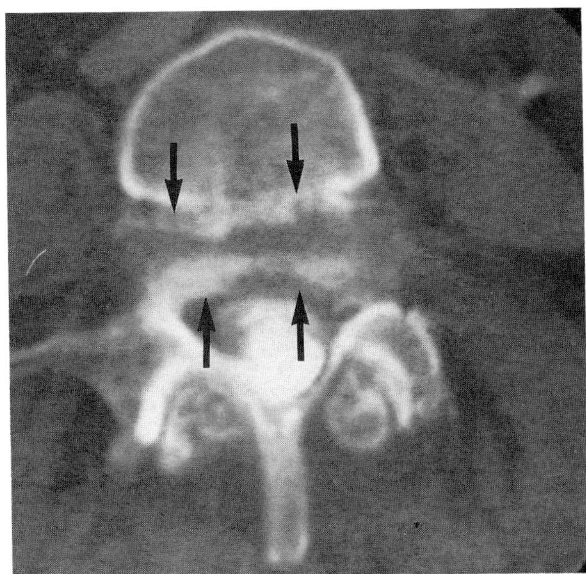

Figure 7. *SPONDYLOLISTHESIS AND CTM. Axial CTM at L4-5 in a patient with degenerative spondylolisthesis. Note that the backs of adjacent vertebral bodies are seen in a single section (arrows).*

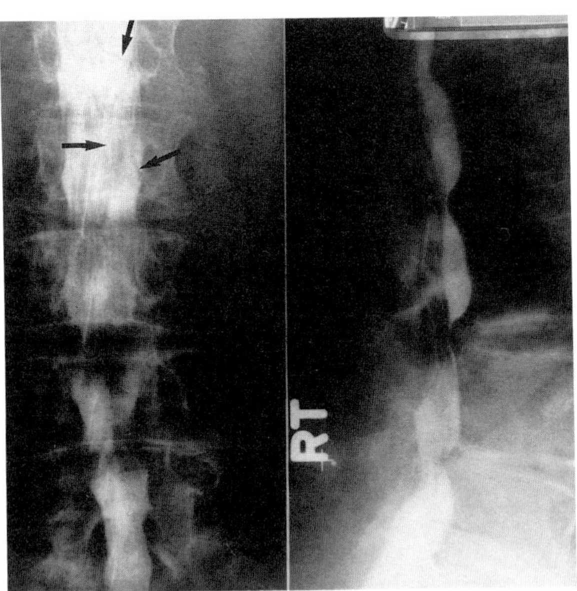

Figure 8. *SPONDYLOLISTHESIS AND MYELOGRAPHY. Myelogram showing degenerative spondylolisthesis at L3-4. Note the tortuous roots of the cauda equina seen above the level of stenosis (arrows).*

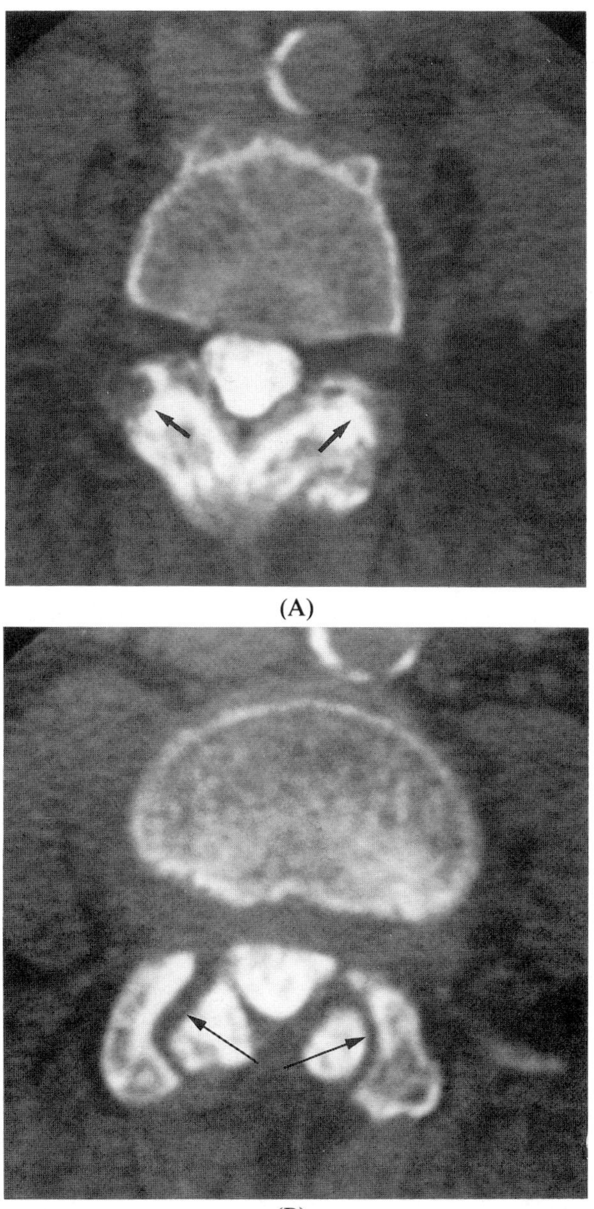

(A)

(B)

Figure 9. *SPONDYLOLISTHESIS FOLLOWING FUSION. Degenerative spondylolisthesis following fusion. (A) CT myelogram at L5-S1 demonstrates a fusion of the facet joints (arrows). Spinal canal appears normal. (B) Level above fusion. Because of decreased mobility at the fused level, there is increased mobility at this level with widening of the facet joints (arrows) and spondylolisthesis.*

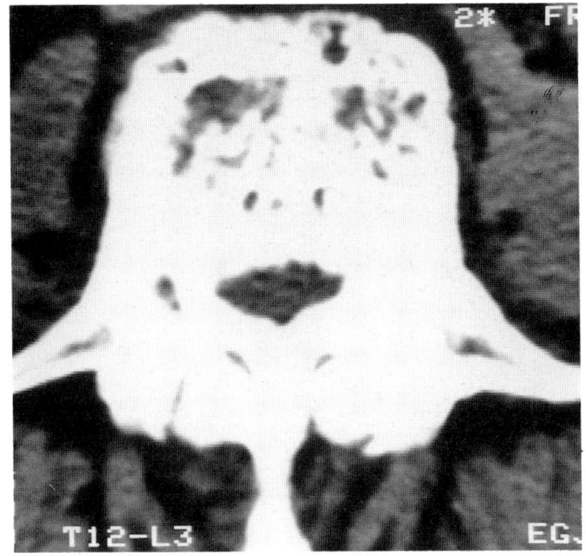

(A)

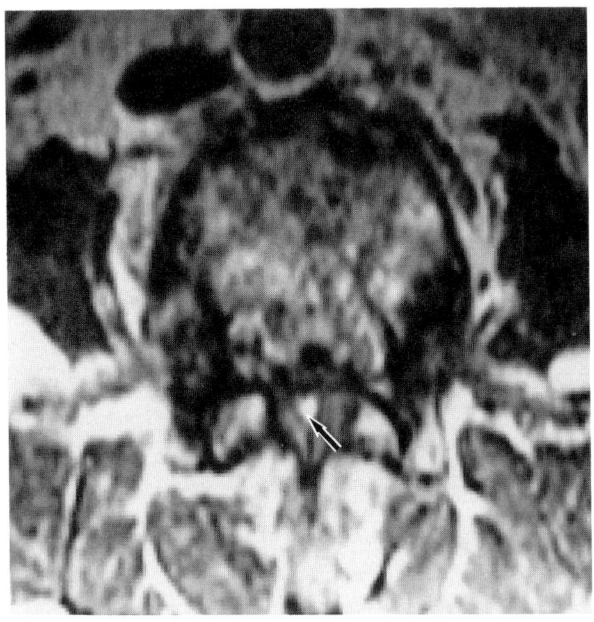

(B)

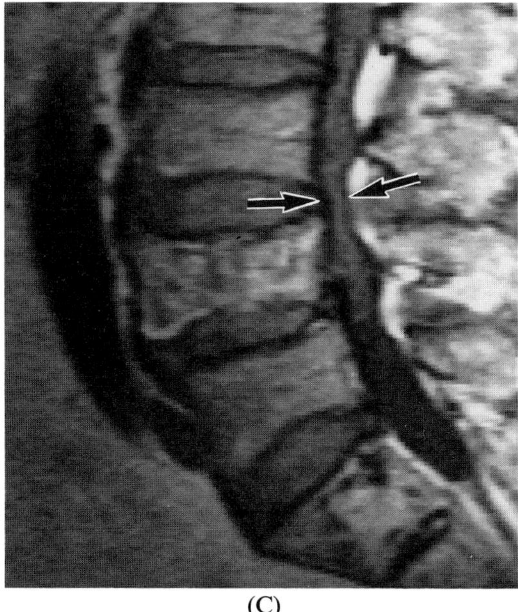

(C)

Figure 10. *PAGET'S DISEASE. (A) CT shows thickened medullary spaces and a narrowed spinal canal. (B) Axial T1 weighted MR scan in Paget's disease showing spinal stenosis with decreased fat in the interlaminar angle (arrow). (C) Sagittal T1 weighted scan in Paget's disease. Widening of the medullary spaces of L4 caused narrowing of the spinal canal at that level (arrows).*

degenerative spondylolisthesis. They are most common at the L4-5 intervertebral disc level [30]. The main symptom of SyCy is pain without motor, sensory or deep tendon reflex change and is felt to reflect the underlying facet joint disease rather than compression of the thecal sac or nerve roots [31]. It appears on CT as a cystic structure adjacent to a degenerated facet joint with calcification in the cyst wall and is usually seen at L4-5 [31] (Fig. 13). CT guided insertion of a needle in the facet joint with opacification of the cyst and subsequent injection of corticosteroids may relieve the symptoms and obviate the need for major surgery [32]. Four excellent descriptions of the MR findings in SyCy [33,34,35,36] point out the variable appearance on MR depending on the contents of the cyst. Awwad et al. [36] state that the true SyCy with serous fluid is

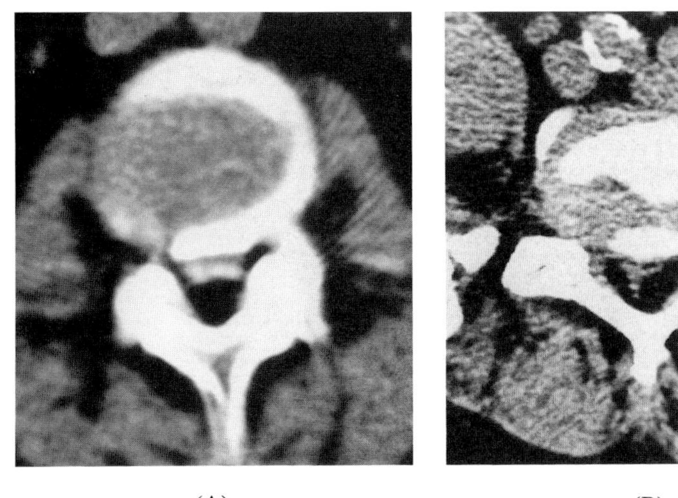

(A) (B)

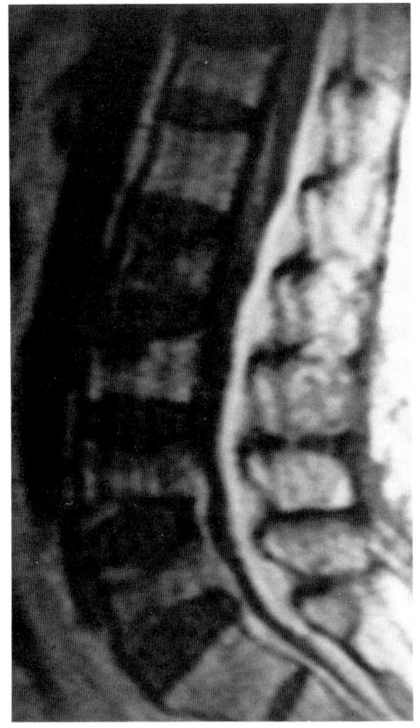

(C)

isointense on T1WI and hyperintense on T2WI. The more viscous or bloody the fluid, the higher is the intensity on all pulse sequences [36].

Spinal stenosis may occur secondary to subdural empyema or hematoma, calcified ligamentum flavum, hemangioma, and traumatic or surgical foreign body.

Lateral Recess Stenosis

The lateral recess is that part of the neural canal which constitutes the nerve root tunnel [37]. It is bordered anteriorly by the posterior surface of the vertebral body and disc, laterally by the pedicle, and posteriorly by the lamina, pars interarticularis, and the superior articular facet [38]. The depth of the lateral recess is measured between the most anterior portion of the superior articular facet and the anterior border of the spinal canal at the superior margin of the pedicle [38]. According to Mikhael et al. [38]:

- lateral recess < *or + to 3 mm* is *stenosed*
- lateral recess *between 3 and 5 mm* is *suggestive* of stenosis
- lateral recess > *than 5 mm excludes* the lateral recess syndrome

The lateral recess syndrome is characterized by intense unilateral sciatic pain, mild neurologic deficit, negative straight leg raising, and Valsalva tests, and slow progression of symptoms. Pain is usually intermittent and is relieved by sitting or squatting [38,39].

While the myelogram is usually normal, CT and MR may show enlargement of the superior articular facet with narrowing of the lateral recess (Figs. 21, 22). As a result, the nerve root in the recess

---

Figure 11. *LUMBAR LIPOMATOSIS. (A) CT myelogram shows narrowed canal due to low density of fat behind the thecal sac. (B) CT myelogram shows a narrowed thecal sac due to surrounding low density fat at L5-S1. (C) Sagittal T1 weighted MR scans show a "string-like" thecal sac compressed by surrounding high intensity fat due to lipomatosis.*

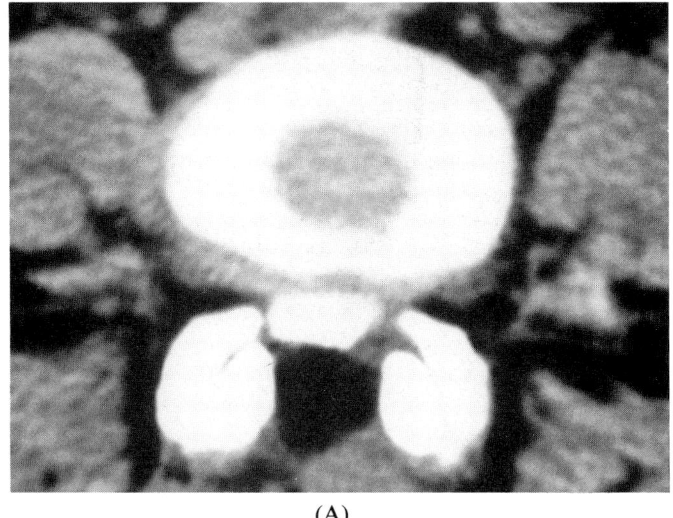

(A)

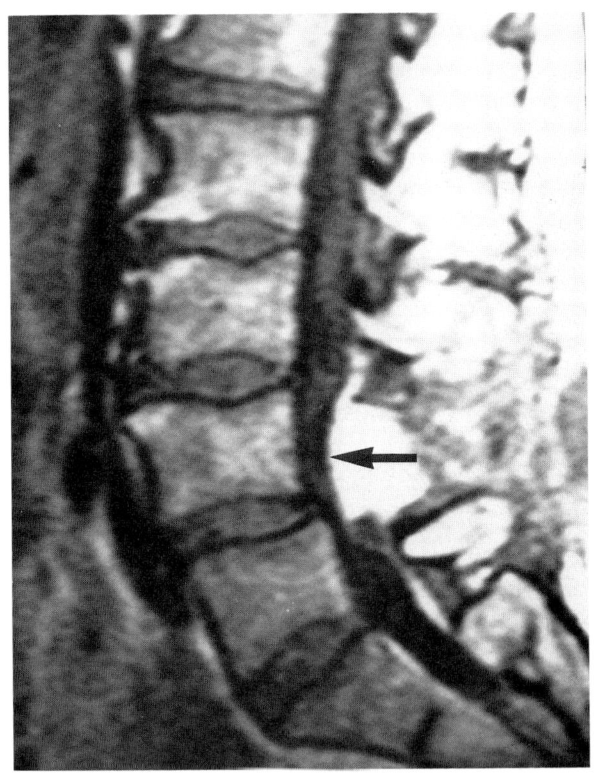

(B)

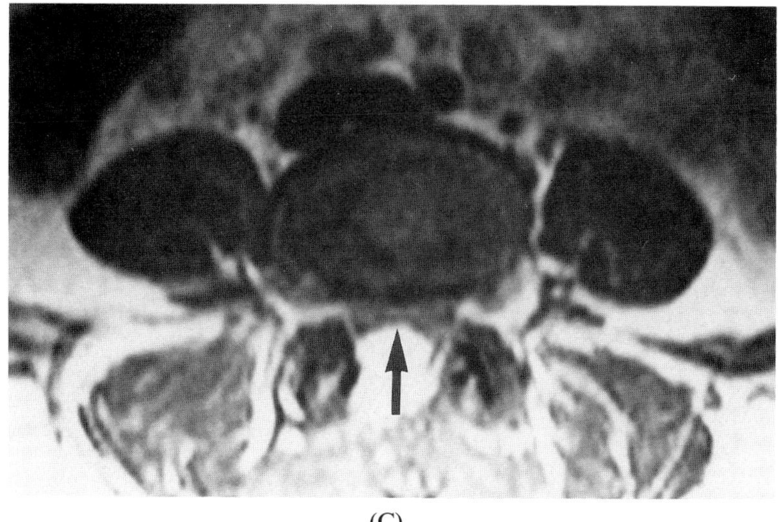

(C)

Figure 12. *"IATROGENIC" LIPOMATOSIS. (A) Post laminectomy CT myelogram shows the presence of a low density fat plug behind and compressing the thecal sac. The plug was inserted at the time of laminectomy. (B, C) Sagittal and axial T1 weighted MR scans show the high intensity fat plug causing spinal stenosis at L4-5 (arrows).*

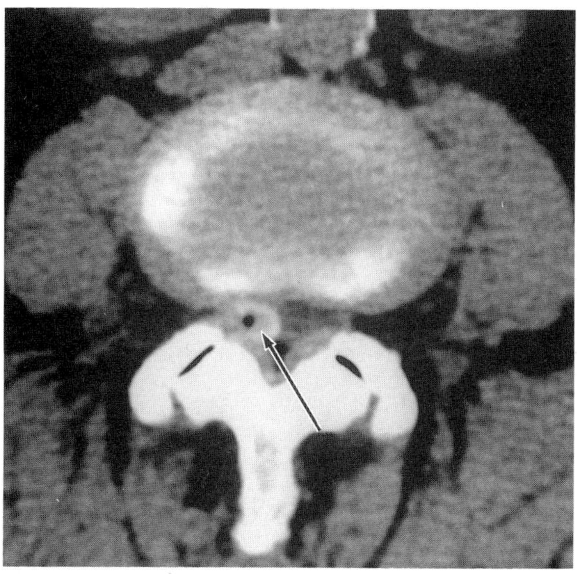

Figure 13. *SYNOVIAL CYST. Axial CT showing right-sided synovial cyst at L4-5 (arrow). Note calcified wall and bilateral facet vacuum changes and the presence of gas within the cyst.*

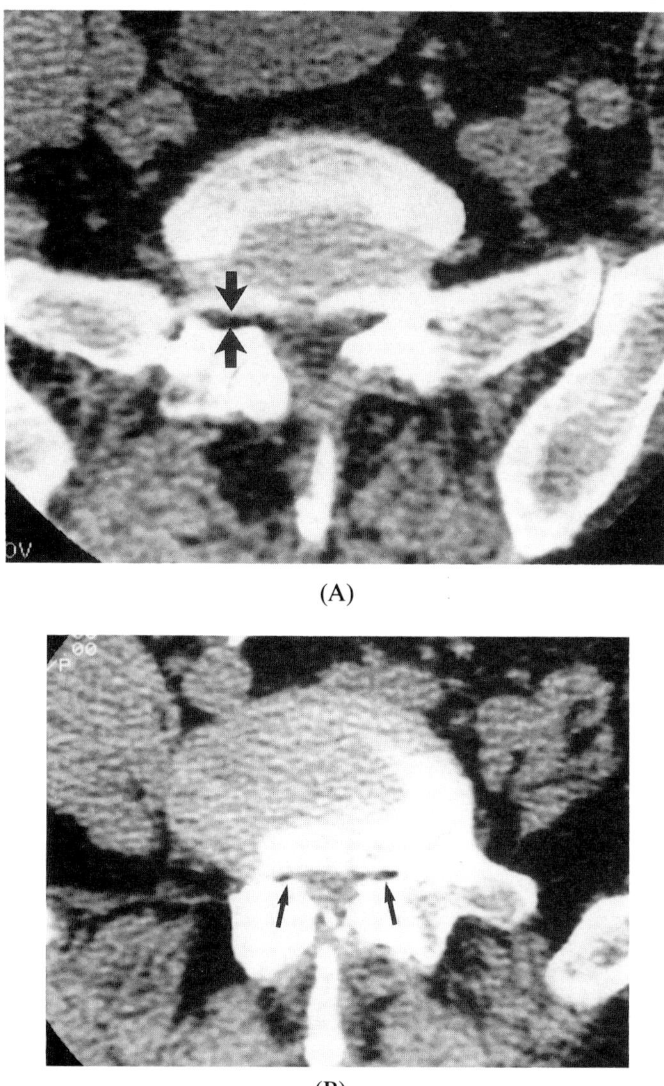

(A)

(B)

Figure 14. *LATERAL RECESS STENOSIS. (A) CT scan at L5-S1 shows bilateral lateral recess stenosis more marked on the right (arrows). (B) Bilateral lateral recess stenosis at L4-5 (arrows) with central spinal stenosis seen on lumbar CT scan.*

is compressed by the disc and the apophyseal joint. These changes may be appreciated by CT, CTM, and MR.

Nerve Root Entrapment

Nerve root entrapment [40] occurs lateral to the lateral recess in the intervertebral foramen. The foramen is best visualized from the lateral aspect where it can be seen to be bounded superiorly and inferiorly by the pedicles, anteriorly by the vertebral body and disc, and posteriorly by the facet joint. On CT and MR, visualization of fat and a discreet root shadow help to evaluate the patency of the intervertebral foramen. Criteria for severity of *nerve root entrapment in the foramen* are:

Mild =   mildly decreased foramen size, root and fat are seen

Moderate =   markedly decreased foramen size, small amount of fat in foramen

Marked =   almost completely obscured foramen, no fat seen

Severe =   foramen cannot be identified

CT vs. MR in Evaluation of Spinal Stenosis

MR seems as accurate as CT in demonstrating the level and degree of spinal stenosis, especially where there is marked narrowing of the thecal sac so that the contrast material injected at myelography does not extend below the level of the block. If only a small amount of contrast passes the block, CTM will usually provide an adequate picture. Even if it does not get by the block, MR with T2W1 can show the thecal sac above or below the block.

Facet disease is less well evaluated with MR than with CT [19]. The decision as to which instrument to use to evaluate neurogenic claudication and sciatica depends on the availability of equipment and the experience of the radiologist with that particular instrument.

References

1. Verbiest HA. Radicular syndrome from developmental narrowing of the lumbar vertebral canal. J Bone Joint Surg 1954;36B:230-241.
2. Nelson MA. Surgery of the spine. In: Jayson M, ed. The lumbar spine and back pain. London: Sector Publishing Ltd., 1976:367-394.
3. Baddeley H. Radiology of lumbar spinal stenosis. In: Jayson M, ed. Spine and back pain. London: Sector Publishing Ltd., 1976;151-171.
4. Rothman RH, Simeone FA. The Spine. 2nd ed. Philadelphia: W.B. Saunders Company, 1982;518-521.
5. Butler D, Trafimow JH, Andersson GBJ, et al. Discs degenerate before facets. Spine 1990;15:111-113.
6. Kirkaldy-Willis WH. Pathology and pathogenesis of lumbar spinal stenosis. In: Symposium on the lumbar spine, Brown FW, ed. American Academy of Orthopedic Surgeons, 1978:16-20.
7. Frymoyer JW. Back Pain and sciatica. N Engl J Med 1988;318:291-300.
8. Dixon AS. Diagnosis of low back pain-sorting the complainers. In: The lumbar spine and back pain, Jayson M, ed. London: Sector Publishing Ltd., 1976:77-92.
9. Cailliet R. Low back pain syndrome. 3rd ed. Philadelphia: FA Davis Company, 1981:180-183.
10. Hinck VC, Hopkins CE, Clark WM. Sagittal diameter of the lumbar spinal canal in children and adults. Radiology 1965;85:929-937.
11. Hinck VC, Clark WM Jr, Hopkins CE. Normal interpediculate distances (minimum and maximum) in children and adults. AJR 1966;97:141-153.
12. Ulrich CG, Binet EF, Sanecki MG, Kieffer SA. Quantitative assessment of the lumbar spinal canal by computed tomography. Radiology 1980;134:137-143.
13. Haughton VM, Syvertsen A, Williams AL. Soft-tissue anatomy within the spinal canal as seen on computed tomography. Radiology 1980;134:649-655.
14. Lee BCP, Kazam E, Newman AD. Computed tomography of the spine and spinal cord. Radiology 1978;128:95-102.
15. Raininko R. The value of CT after total block on myelography: experience with 25 patients. Fortschr Roentgenstr 1983;138:61-65.
16. Stovring J, Saksanen SJ, Fernando LT, Robertson GH. Successful myelography after dry spinal puncture. Radiology 1982;143:265-266.
17. Kapila A, Chakeres DW. Flexed sitting maneuver for complete lumbar myelography in patients with severe spinal stenosis ana apparent block. Radiology 1986;160:265-267.
18. Modic MT, Masaryk T, Boumphrey F, et al. Lumbar herniated disk disease and canal stenosis: prospective evaluation by surface coil MR, CT, and myelography. AJNR 1986;7:709-717.
19. Haughton VM. MR imaging of the spine. Radiology 1988;166:297-301.
20. Lefkowitz DM, Quencer RM. Vacuum facet phenomenon: a computed tomographic sign of degenerative spondylolisthesis. Radiology 1982;144:562.
21. Cronqvist S, Thulin CA. Significance of tortuous filling defects at lumbar myelography. Acta Radiol Diagn 1979;20:561-568.
22. Duncan AW, Kido DK. Serpentine Cauda equina nerve roots. Radiology 1981;139:109-111.
23. Hacker DA, Latchaw RE, Yock DH, et al. Redundant lumbar nerve root syndrome: myelographic features. Radiology 1982;143:457-461.
24. de Tribolet N, Campiche R. Redundant nerve roots of the cauda equina-a rare disease? Eur Neurol 1982;21:169-174.

25. Quencer RM, Murtagh FR, Post MJD, et al. Postoperative bony stenosis of the lumbar spinal canal: evaluation of 164 symptomatic patients with axial radiography. AJR 1978;131:1059-1064.
26. Gelman MI. Cauda equina compression in acromegaly. Radiology 1974;112:357-360.
27. Zlatkin MB, Lander PH, Hadjipavlou AG, Levine JS. Paget disease of the spine: CT with clinical correlation. Radiology 1986;160:155-159.
28. Quint DJ, Boulos RS, Sanders WP, et al. Epidural lipomatosis. Radiology 1988;169:485-490.
29. Russell NA, Belanger G, Benoit BG, et al. Spinal epidural lipomatosis: a complication of glucocorticoid therapy. Can J Neurol Sci 1984;11:383-386.
30. Bhushan C, Hodges FJ, Wityk JJ. Synovial cyst (ganglion) of the lumbar spine simulating extradural mass. Neuroradiology 1979;18:263-268.
31. Hemminghytt S, Daniels DL, Williams AL, Haughton VM. Intraspinal synovial cysts: natural history and diagnosis by CT. Radiology 1982;145:375-376.
32. Bjorkengren AG, Kurz LT, Resnick D, et al. Symptomatic intraspinal synovial cysts: opacification and treatment by percutaneous injection. AJR 1987;149:105-107.
33. Liu SS, Williams KD, Drayer BP, et al. Synovial cysts of the lumbosacral spine: diagnosis by MR imaging. AJNR 1989;10:1239-1242.
34. Jackson DE, Atlas SW, Mani JR, Norman D. Intraspinal synovial cysts: MR imaging. Radiology 1989;170:527-530.
35. Silbergleit R, Gebarski SS, Brunberg JA, et al. Lumbar synovial cysts: correlation of myelographic, CT, MR, and pathologic findings. AJNR 1990;11:777-779.
36. Awwad EE, Martin DS, Smith KR, Bucholz RD. MR Imaging of lumbar juxtaarticular cysts. J Comput Assist Tomogr 1990;14:415-417.
37. Crock HV. Normal and pathological anatomy of the lumbar spinal nerve rood canals. J Bone Joint Surg 1981;63-B:487-490.
38. Mikhael MA, Ciric I, Tarkington JA, et al. Neuroradiological evaluation of lateral recess syndrome. Radiology 1981;140:97-107.
39. Choudhury AR, Taylor JC. Occult lumbar spinal stenosis. J Neurol Neurosurg Psychiatr 1977;40:506-510.
40. Risius B, Modic MT, Hardy RW, et al. Sector computed tomographic spine scanning in the diagnosis of lumbar nerve root entrapment. Radiology 1982;143:109-114.

Degenerative Disc Disease

Paul E. Berger

Long Beach Memorial Medical Center, Long Beach, California, USA

Introduction

Degenerative disc disease is an extremely common and complex clinical, anatomic and pathologic entity. As such, the variable radiologic findings are also complex.

It is helpful to think of the intervertebral disc as part of a tri-joint complex, composed of the cartilaginous disc and the apophyseal (facet) joints. Pathologic changes in these and the associated ligamentous structures may result in a broad spectrum of radiologic findings.

The disc is composed of a central nucleus pulposus surrounded by a peripheral portion, the annulus fibrosus. The nucleus pulposus is soft and gelatinous in young individuals [1, 2], but with aging it is gradually replaced by fibrocartilage becoming amorphous and discolored and it is difficult to distinguish from the remainder of the intervertebral disc.

A radial tear of the annulus may be a primary event in disc degeneration [3]. When a radial tear develops in the annulus there is shrinkage and disorganization of fibro-cartilage in the nucleus pulposus and replacement of the disc by dense fibrous tissue [2].

Nomenclature

The term *herniation* refers to a *broad spectrum* of imaging findings from very mild to very severe disc abnormalities. To our surgical colleagues and in a medical/legal sense, use of this term may have strong clinical connotations which could result in inappropriate care.

With this in mind it is recommended that the term *herniation* be dropped in favor of a more precise and descriptive terminology. It is hoped that this will be a means of improving communications with other physicians with resultant improvement in patient management.

The following terminology is suggested:

"Bulging" disc: a *generalized*, symmetric, broad based circumferential extension of disc material beyond the confines of the vertebral body. This is commonly associated with the loss of disc height.

Disc "protrusion": a *focal* contour abnormality. This can be shown on magnetic resonance imaging to be contained within the annular/ligamentous complex.

Disc "Extrusion": a *larger focal extension* of disc material into the spinal canal or neural foramen which may have a narrow connection to the parent disc and can be demonstrated on magnetic resonance imaging to extend beyond the confine of the annular-ligamentous complex, but is still connected to the parent disc by a pedicle.

"Sequestered" disc: an extruded disc fragment which has migrated away and is separate from the parent disc.

In addition to the above nomenclature it is helpful for some grading system to be used so as to aid in defining the size or degree of the abnormality. A descriptive terminology such as slight, moderate, moderately-severe and severe is suggested but alternatively, measurements can be used.

Radiologic Evaluation

Radiologic evaluation of degenerative disc disease has undergone increasing levels of sophistication with the advent of the newer imaging technologies.

Plain radiographs will permit a global overview of the lumbosacral spine and should be the first test performed. This will permit observation of degenerative changes that effect the disc spaces, facet joints and vertebral bodies (Fig. 1). Oblique films may be

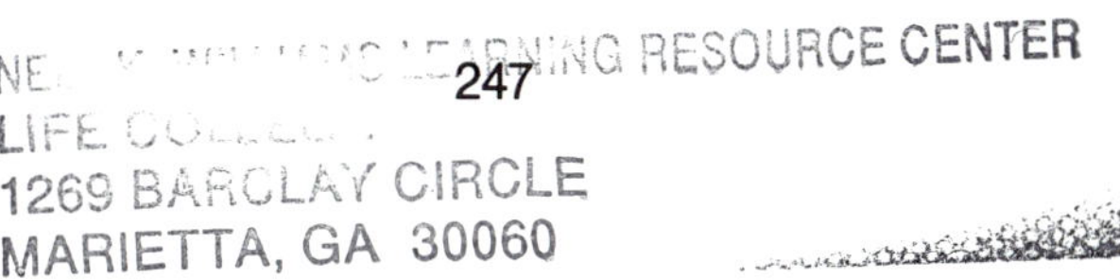

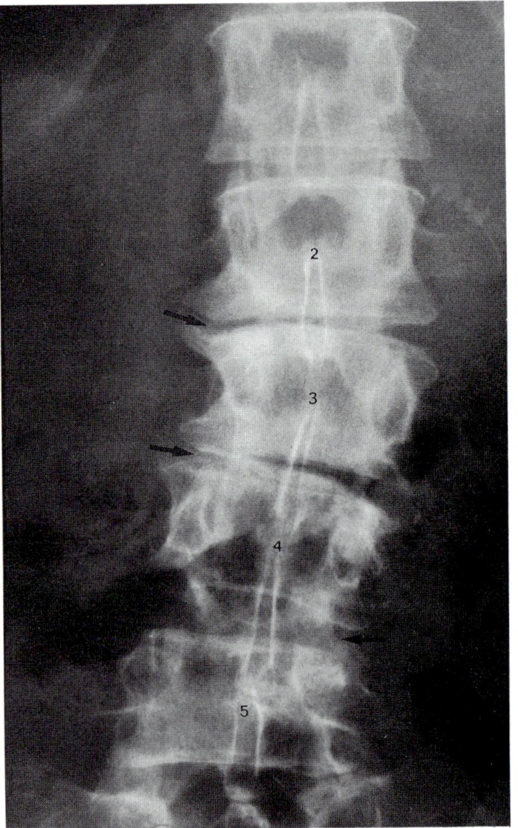

Figure 1. *DEGENERATIVE DISC DISEASE. Plain A-P radiograph in a 65-year-old woman with back pain, demonstrates degenerative changes involving the discs at L2-3 and L3-4 and L4-5 (arrows) and mild generalized rotoscoliosis.*

helpful in evaluation of the facet joints as well as delineating fractures of the pars interarticularis when present. Not routinely performed, but recommended in older patients and patients suspected of having spinal instability, are flexion/extension lateral views of the lumbosacral spine (Fig. 2). This can be very helpful in diagnosing spondylolisthesis, i.e. a subluxation of one vertebral body on another. In younger patients and when present at the L5-S1 level this is usually due to bilateral fractures of the pars interarticularis of L5. In older patients and when present at L4-5 this is most commonly due to degenerative changes involving the disc, apophyseal (facet) joints and the associated ligamentous structures.

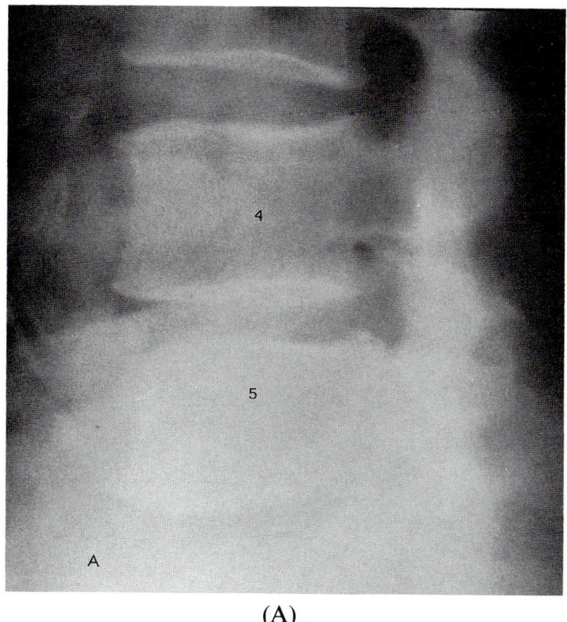

(A)

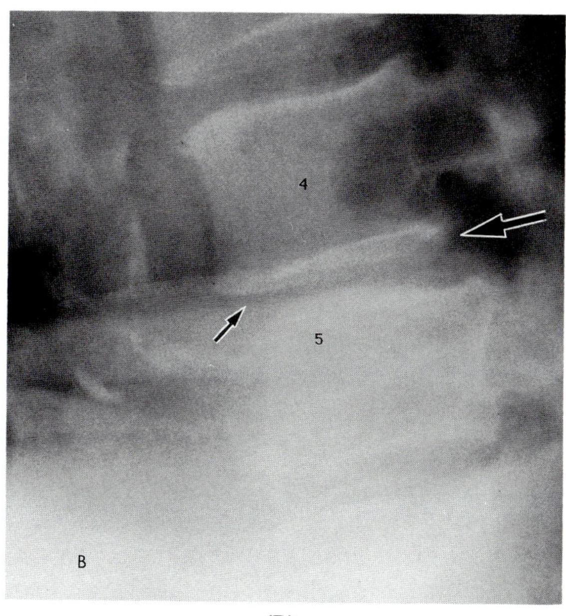

(B)

Figure 2. DEGENERATIVE SPONDYLOLISTHESIS. *Extension* (A) *and flexion* (B) *lateral radiographs demonstrates anterior subluxation of L4 (large arrow) and narrowing of anterior L4-5 disc space, during flexion (small arrow).*

Osteophyte off the anterior aspects of the lumbar spine show a definite association with loss of disc substance. Two types of osteophyte have been described, traction osteophyte which are horizontally oriented bone excrescences from the anterior margins of two adjacent vertebral bodies, and claw osteophytes in which the outgrowth is triangular and curved at its tip. It was thought that traction osteophytes in particular were associated with spinal instability but more recent work suggests that both these osteophytes represent different states of the same pathologic process, with the traction osteophyte progressing to a claw osteophyte [4].

Myelography

Myelography has been a good method for evaluating patients with degenerative disc disease. It provides an overview of the neural elements within the lumbosacral canal. Myelography can show direct compression and cut-off of the nerve roots. A potential advantage of myelography over other imaging techniques is the ability to examine the contrast filled thecal sac and nerve roots with the patient upright during weight bearing (i.e. the position in which the patient usually is clinically symptomatic). Also filming the patient in lateral flexion and extension may show the dynamic effects of instability on the thecal sac and nerve roots. Disadvantages include the fact that myelography is invasive with risks and complications, and does not provide the exquisite detail of the bony and ligamentous spinal canal offered by the newer imaging modalities.

Computer Tomography

Computer Tomography (CT) provides superb cross sectional images of the osseous spine with unsurpassed detail when compared with any other modality. Reformatting in the sagittal and coronal planes adds to the utility of this modality [5]. Excellent images of the spinal canal content, ligaments and paraspinal musculature are also obtained. Because it is non-invasive it has the ability to provide exquisite osseous anatomy as well as demonstrate the thecal sac and exiting nerve roots, CT became a primary imaging modality for evaluating patients with degenerative disc disease.

At any given disc space in the lumbar spine two nerves on each side must be evaluated: (1) the nerve *exiting* under the pedicle of the level above the disc, (2) the nerve *traversing* the disc space in the lateral aspect of the central spinal canal; which is anatomically the *subarticular recess* at the level of the facet joint and disc space. (Note: this area is often referred to as the lateral recess, but the lateral recess is actually the lateral aspect of the central spinal canal at the level of the pedicle.)

It is very helpful to the surgeon to clearly state the exact location of impingement on the nerve by either the disc or osseous impingement. These are categorized as: (1) central (Fig. 3); (2) paracentral, usually impinging upon the traversing nerve root in the subarticular recess (Fig. 4); (3) lateral (foraminal), usually impinging on the exiting preganglionic nerve root and ganglion (Fig. 5); (4) far lateral (extraforaminal), usually impinging upon the post ganglionic spinal nerve.

Comparisons of CT with myelography in the evaluation of lumbar disc herniation show CT to be somewhat less sensitive but more specific [6]. When compared to surgical findings CT has shown an accuracy from 83-93% [7,8]. On CT the disc may be seen to show a generalized bulging, but considered more clinically significant is a *focal* extension of the disc margin beyond the vertebral margin, with resulting epidural fat, nerve root, or thecal sac displacement.

Pseudodiscs, that is a finding which simulates disc bulge or protrusion, may be caused by scoliosis, conjoined nerve roots and partial volume averaging. In these cases reformatting in the sagittal plane can help provide the correct diagnosis and aid in avoiding these pitfalls.

CT may also be extremely valuable in the diagnosis of lumbar spinal stenosis. Criteria for the diagnosis of lumbar stenosis on CT are (1) a distortion or paucity of epidural fat either in the neural foramina, subarticular recess, or posteriorly between the ligamentum flavum, and (2) a diminution in the overall size of the neural foramina, neural canal, and/or thecal sac. This is often due to a combination of findings which include loss of height and/or generalized bulging of the disc, ligamentum flavum hypertrophy or redundancy, and importantly facet hypertrophy, especially the superior articular facet. As with disc abnormalities, reformatting the

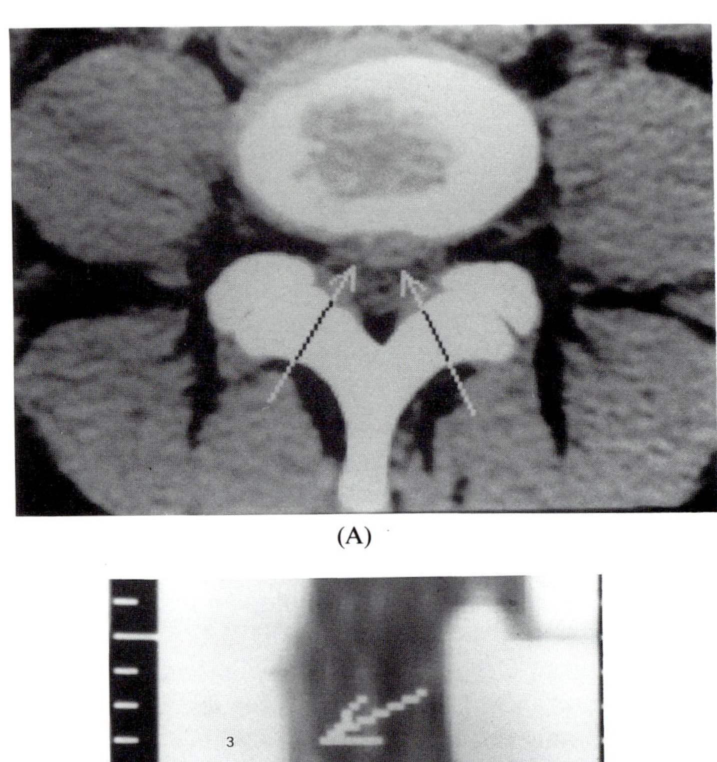

(A)

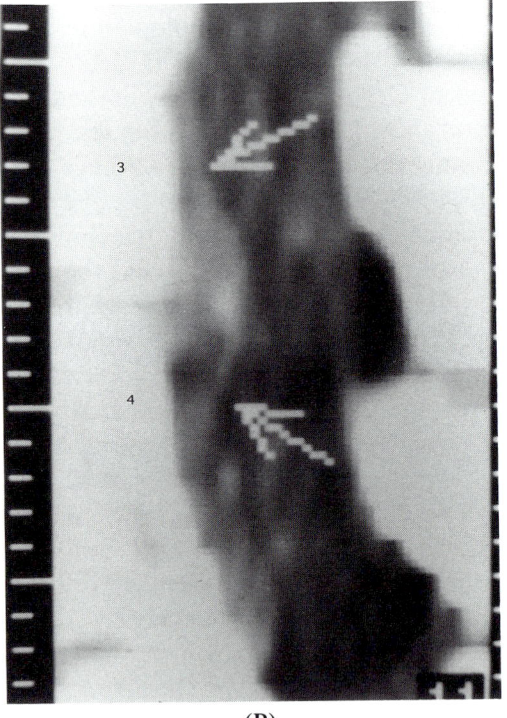

(B)

Figure 3. *CENTRAL DISC PROTRUSION. Transaxial* (A) *and sagittal reformatted image* (B) *demonstrates focal central disc protrusion (arrows A) and posteriorly displaced posterior longitudinal ligament (arrows B).*

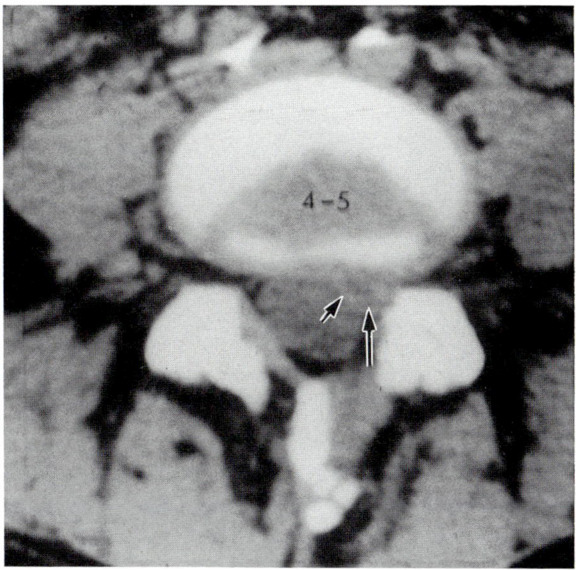

Figure 4. *PARACENTRAL DISC PROTRUSION. Asymmetry of fat planes and slight increased density helps demonstrate focal disc protrusion (arrows).*

images in the sagittal plane is helpful in demonstrating the degree of neural foramen stenosis (Fig. 6).

Other osseous abnormalities such as fractures of the pars intra-articularis may be well demonstrated on CT. Occasionally, these may be bilateral and quite symmetrical simulating facet joints on transaxial imaging. Again, reformations in the sagittal plane are of value in making the diagnosis (Fig. 7).

Two interesting studies have been performed evaluating the effect of axial loading and posture (flexion/extension) on CT findings. In one study [9] axial loading as would be produced by weight bearing was shown to diminish the diameters and cross-sectional areas of the spinal canal and neural foramina but did not result in displacement, distortion, or compression of nerve roots. In another study of CT examination of the spinal canal in flexion and extension [10] there was bulging of the disc toward degenerated hypertrophic facets in extension, resulting in a pincers mechanism at the anterolateral angles of the spinal canal with the risk of bilateral root compression. In addition there was also a posterior (dorsal) indentation of the thecal sac because of thickening of the ligamentum flavum and anterior movement of the dorsal fat pad.

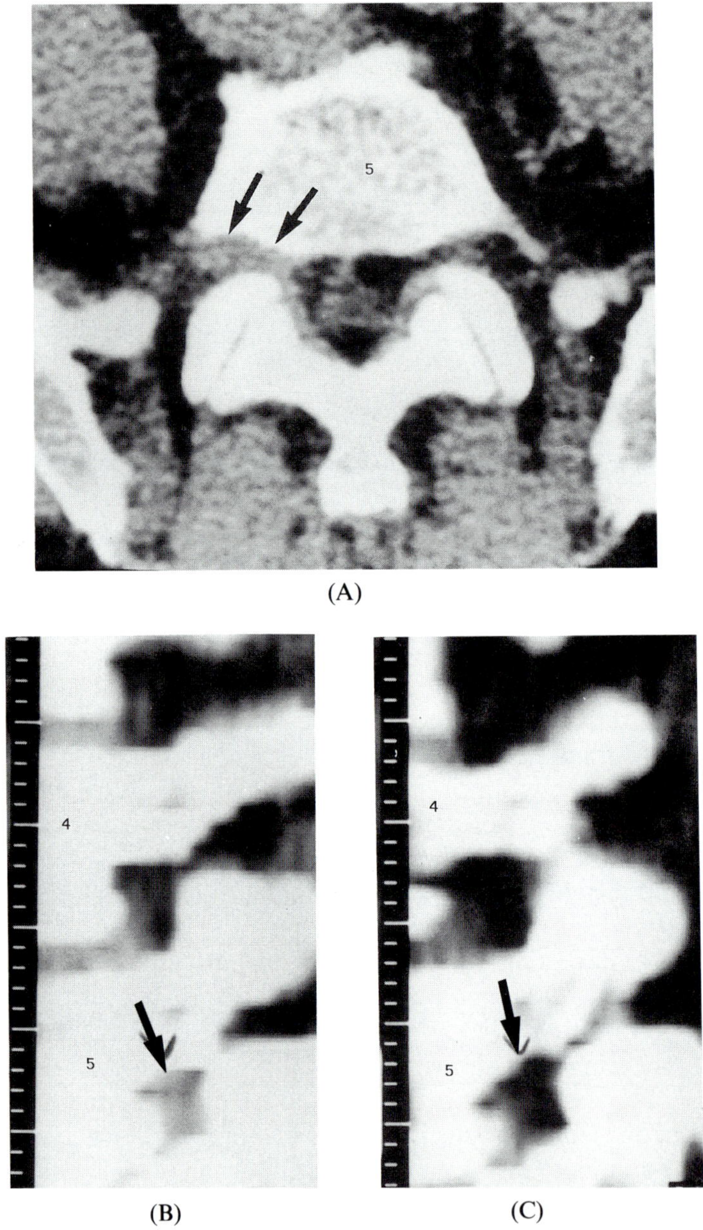

(A)

(B)   (C)

Figure 5. *FORAMINAL DISC PROTRUSION. Transaxial CT demonstrates area of increased density within the right L5-S1 neural foramen (arrows) displacing normal fat in this region. This finding can be confirmed on the sagittal reformatted images (B, C) showing increased density in right neural foramen (B) compared with left (C).*

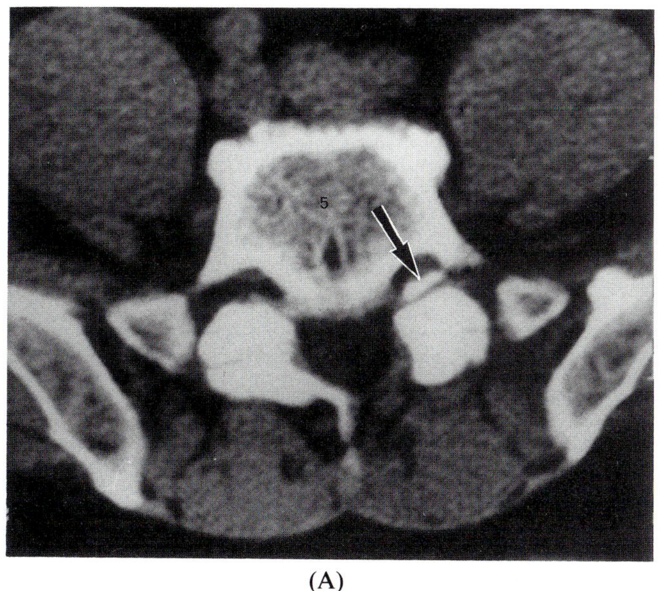

(A)

(B)

Figure 6. *NEURAL FORAMINAL STENOSIS, MILD. (A) Transaxial CT demonstrates small osseous density (arrow) which can be seen on sagittal reformatted image (B) as a hypertrophic spur (large arrow) off the inferior endplate of L5 resulting in mild narrowing of the neural foramen.*

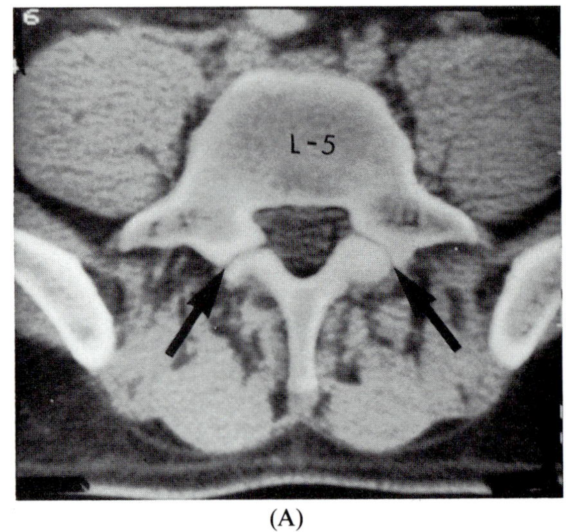

(A)

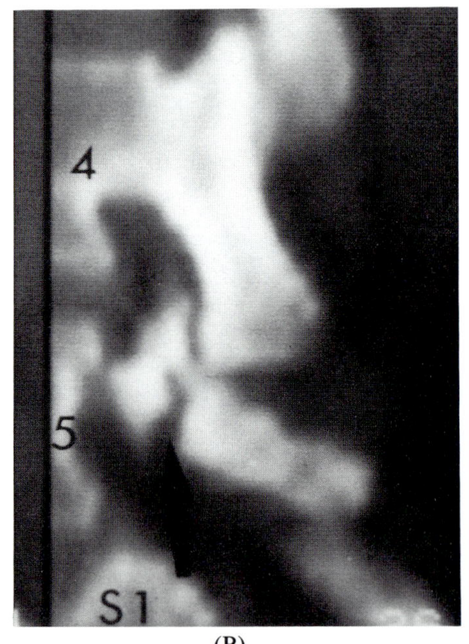

(B)

Figure 7. *PARS INTRAARTICULARIS FRACTURES, BILATERAL.* (A) *Transaxial CT demonstrates bilateral, symmetrical defect (arrows) which simulate facet joints. Sagittal reformatted image* (B) *demonstrates fracture in pars intraarticularis (arrow).*

This mechanism was thought to be the cause of neurogenic claudication and posture dependent sciatica.

Intrathecally enhanced CT, i.e. CT scanning following myelography or following a low dose of contrast material (3 - 5 cc) is a superb examination and can combine the overview offered from myelography with exquisite detail of both osseous and intraspinal neural anatomy [11]. It may be the test of choice in the evaluation of possible arachnoiditis (Fig. 8), in patients with complex degenerative abnormalities, patients with multiple previous operations, and can be very helpful when previous examinations have been equivocal (Fig. 9). Its main drawback is that it is invasive, requiring a spinal tap and the risks associated with it and intrathecal contrast material.

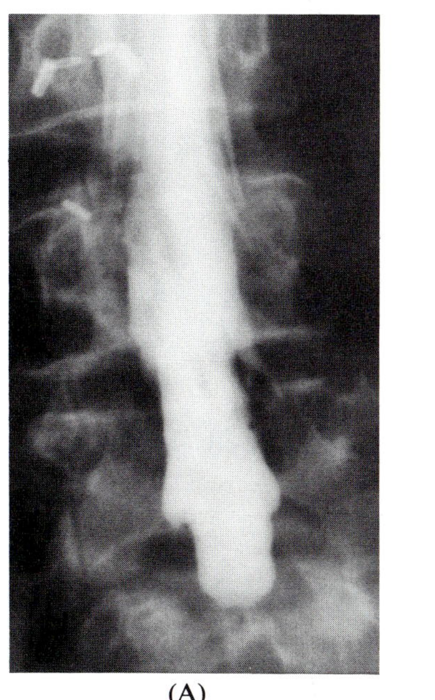

(A)

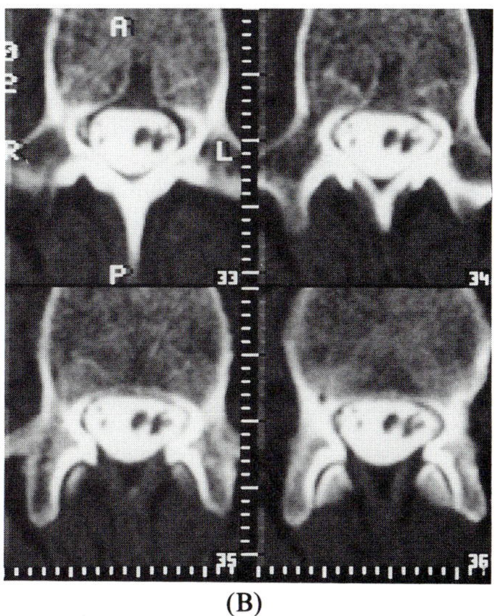

(B)

Figure 8. *ARACHNOIDITIS.* (A) *Myelogram which demonstrates irregular thecal sac with poor delineation of nerve roots from L4 distally. This could be due to arachnoiditis or epidural fibrosis.* (B) *Intrathecally enhanced CT demonstrates thickening, clumping, and irregularity of nerve roots within the thecal sac, characteristic of arachnoiditis.*

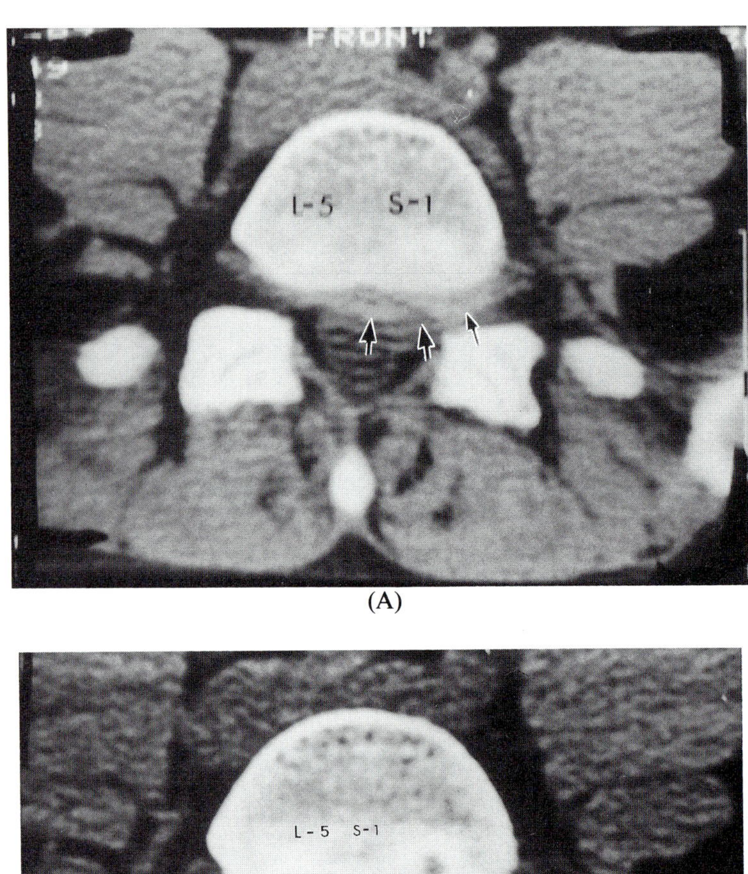

(A)

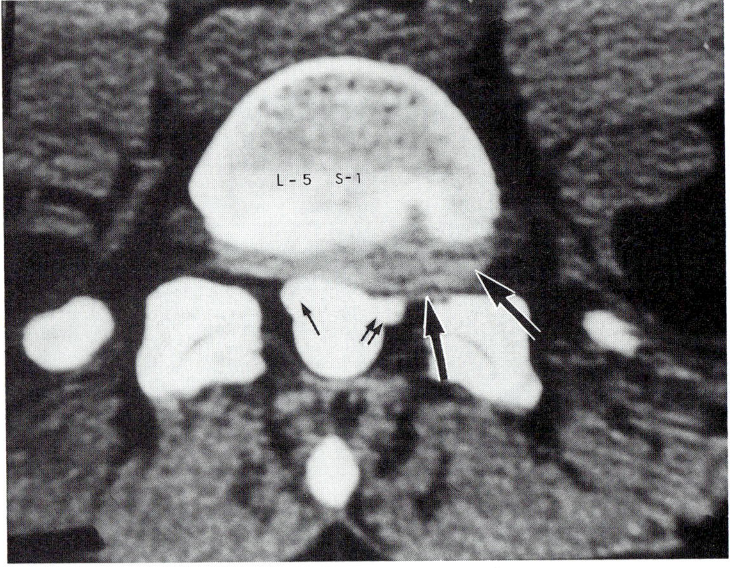

(B)

Figure 9. *FOCAL DISC PROTRUSION WITH NERVE ROOT DIS-PLACEMENT. Transaxial CT (A) at L5-S1 shows a bulging disc (arrows) with inability to definitely identify S1 nerve root. Intrathecally enhanced CT in same patient (B) clearly identifies extradural defect on left side (large arrows) and the S1 nerve root sleeves (small arrows) with posterior displacement of left S1 root (double arrows).*

Magnetic Resonance

Magnetic resonance (MR) imaging, when available is assuming a progressively increasing role as the primary imaging modality in the patient with degenerative disc disease [12,13,14]. MR has several advantages over CT. MR does not use ionizing radiation, images can be obtained in multiple planes, and MR has higher contrast resolution. However MR is more costly, cannot be used on certain patients (e.g. those with cardiac pacemakers) and has inferior spatial resolution. CT provides better bone detail although MR is better at evaluating alterations of bone marrow. MR and CT show similar accuracies in evaluation of lumbar disc nerve root compression and spinal stenosis [7].

MR provides visualization of the entire spectrum of degenerative disc disease from early dehydration to incomplete and complete radial tears, and contained versus extruded disc material (Figs. 10, 11, 12, 13).

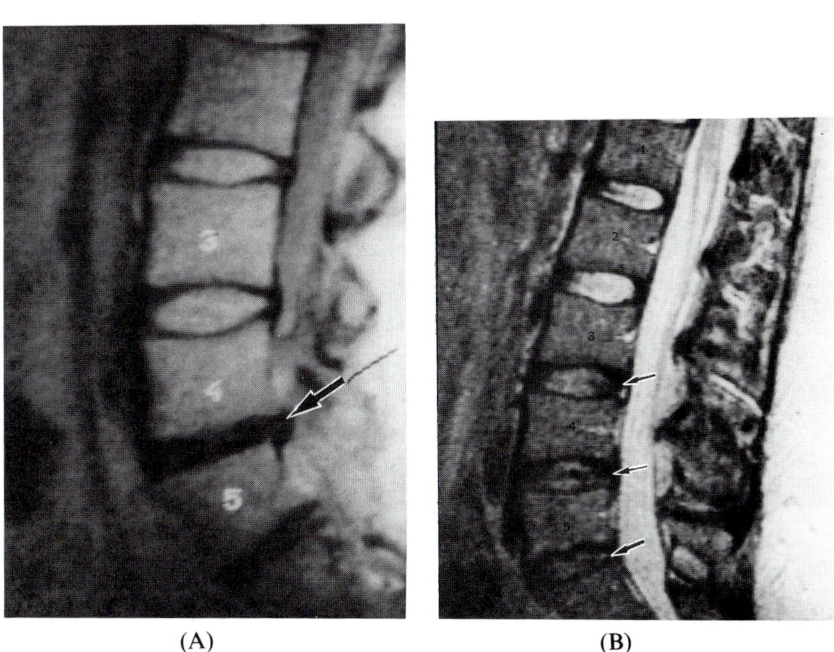

(A)   (B)

Figure 10. *DISC DEGENERATION, MRI. Two patients (A), (B) with disc degeneration (arrow). On T2 weighted images the well hydrated discs are of high intensity (bright) and the degenerated discs are of decreased intensity (dark) (arrows).*

CT cannot distinguish the central nucleus pulposus from the peripheral annulus. T2-weighted spin echo MR sequences are able to differentiate the central bright zone comprised of normally hydrated inner annulus and nucleus, and the outer annulus/posterior longitudinal ligament complex, which is depicted as a sharply defined low signal intensity linear structure forming the posterior margin of the disk. Both epidural fat and the subarachnoid space posterior to it exhibit relatively higher signal, providing excellent inherent contrast (Fig. 10).

The posterior longitudinal ligament anatomically and visually on MR, merges with the outer annular fibers to form a single supportive structure at the level of the disc space. The integrity of the fibers of this structure, even when thinned and bulging is the sine qua non of a "contained" disc abnormality, namely contained by the outer annular fibers and posterior longitudinal ligament (Fig. 11). Complete disruption of this complex is required for a "non-contained" extrusion of disc material (Figs. 12, 13).

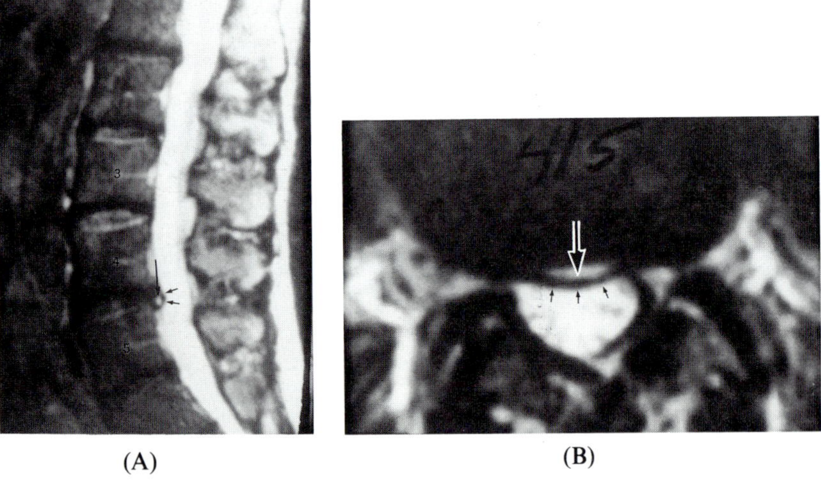

(A)   (B)

Figure 11. *FOCAL DISC PROTRUSION WITH INTACT POSTERIOR LONGITUDINAL LIGAMENT ("CONTAINED DISC"). Sagittal (A) and transaxial (B) T2-weighted images showing protrusion of high intensity disc material (annular tear) (long arrows) with intact posterior longitudinal ligament (small arrows).*

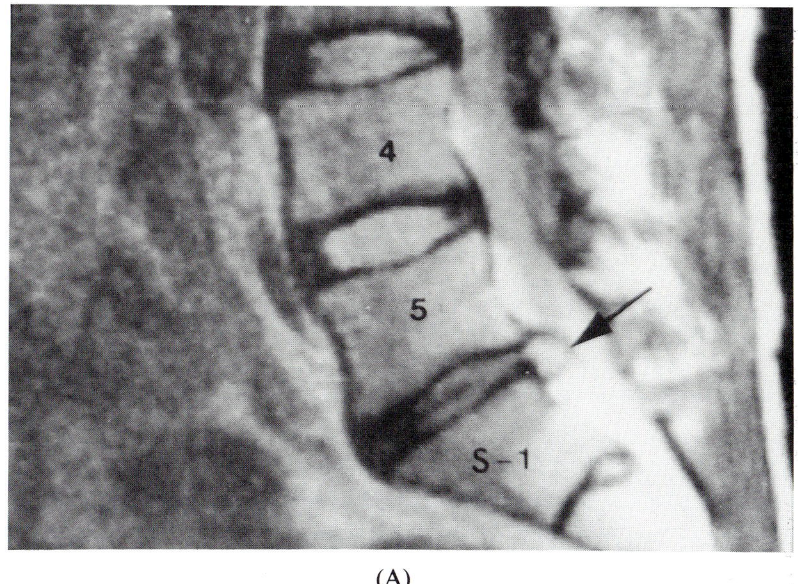

(A)

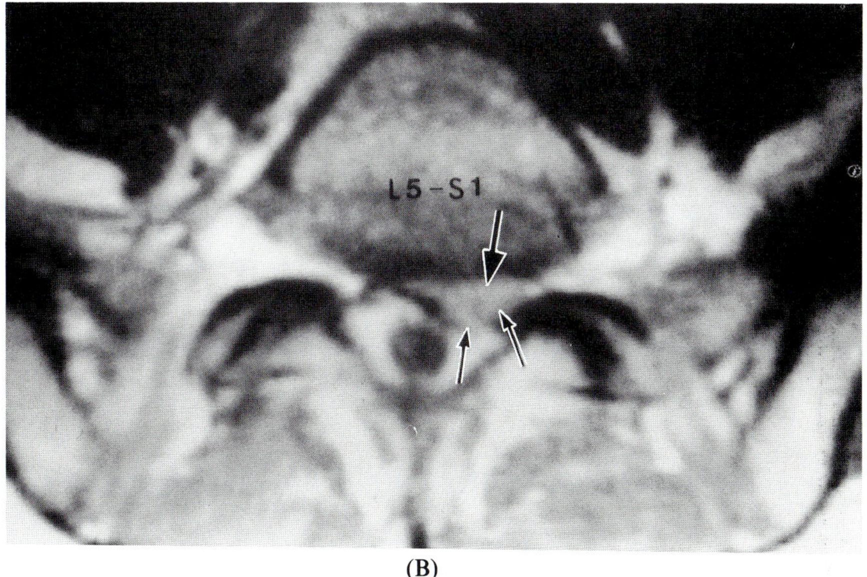

(B)

Figure 12. *EXTRUDED DISC MATERIAL ("NON-CONTAINED DISC"). Sagittal (A) and transaxial (B) images demonstrating high intensity disc material protruding posteriorly on left. The posterior longitudinal ligament is not intact (B, small arrows).*

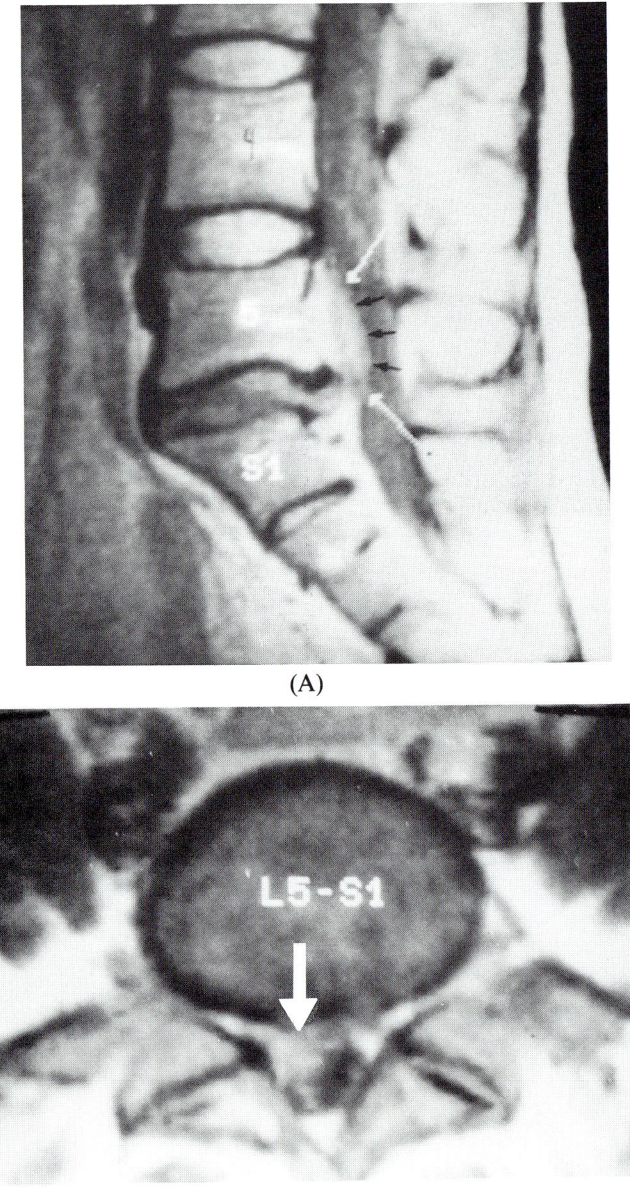

(A)

(B)

Figure 13. *LARGE EXTRUDED DISC. Sagittal* (A) *and transaxial* (B) *images demonstrating large area of increased intensity (arrows) extending from L5-S1 disc space superiorly to the superior aspect of L5. The thecal sac is seen as the area of lower intensity (darker) displaced posteriorly by the extruded disc material.*

Evaluation of the post-operative spine is one of the most challenging endeavors facing the radiologist. The differentiation of post-operative scar (epidural fibrosis) from recurrent or residual disc herniation is an important one to the surgeon. To this end, the procedure of choice is MR imaging prior to and following an intravenous injection of gadopentatate (gadolinium) [15]. In a study of 44 patients at 50 re-operated levels an accuracy of 96% was found in the differentiation of scar, disk, and scar (+) disc [15] (Fig. 14).

Clinical correlation

One note of caution needs to be mentioned. CT scanning and MR imaging are sophisticated imaging modalities capable of demonstrating a broad spectrum of pathologic changes that effect the lumbar spine and its content. However studies have indicated that "abnormal" findings may be demonstrated in at least one third of all asymptomatic individuals, occurring with even higher prevalence as age increases. Thus it is mandatory that findings on these imaging studies must be looked at in light of the patients clinical and neurologic findings such that appropriate treatment regimens may be provided for our patients.

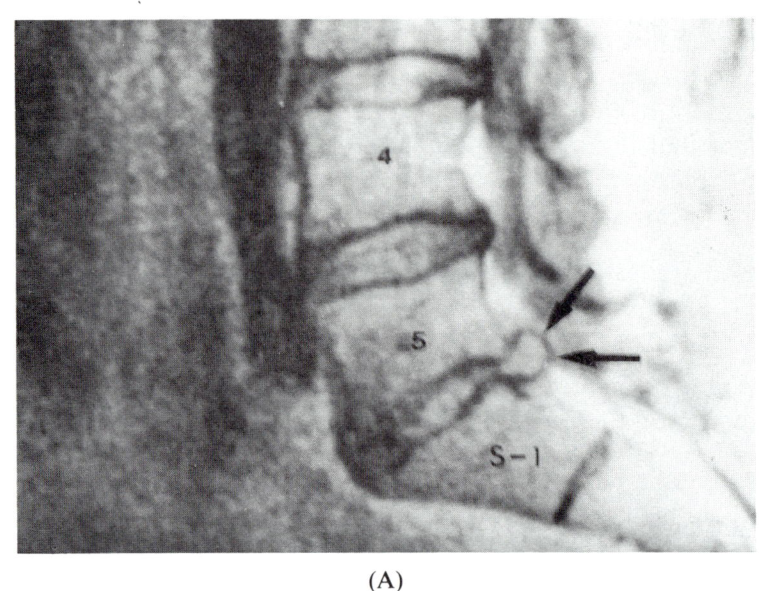

(A)

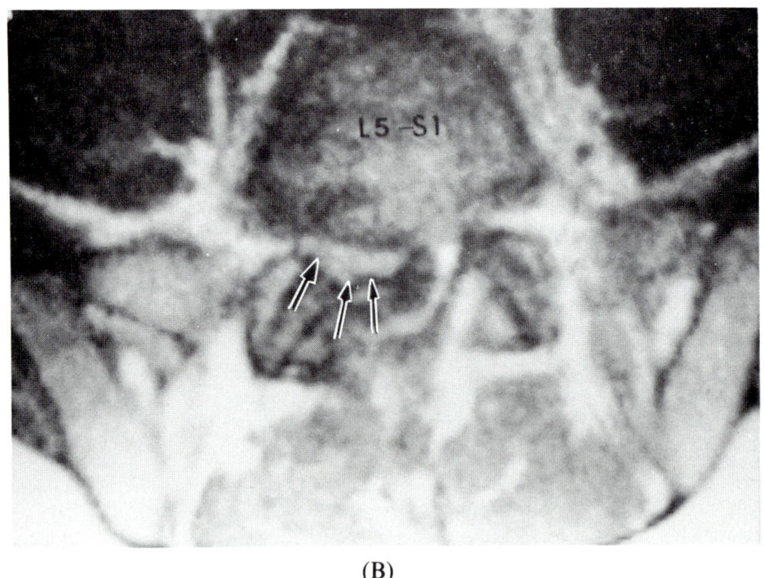

(B)

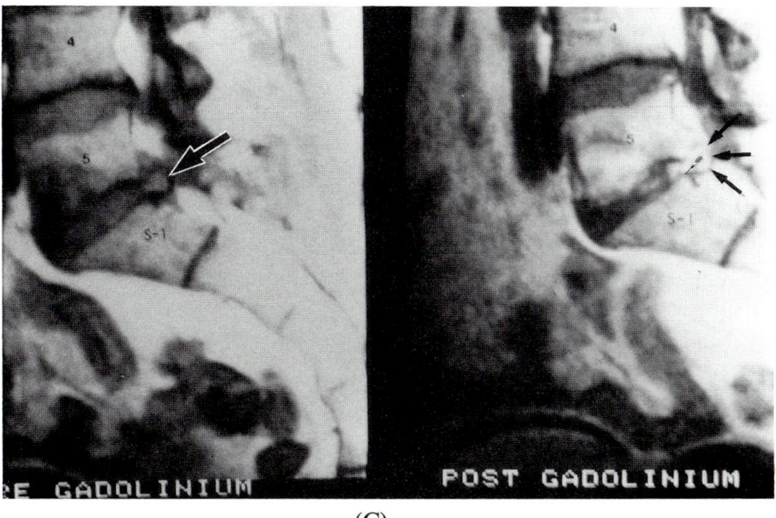

(C)

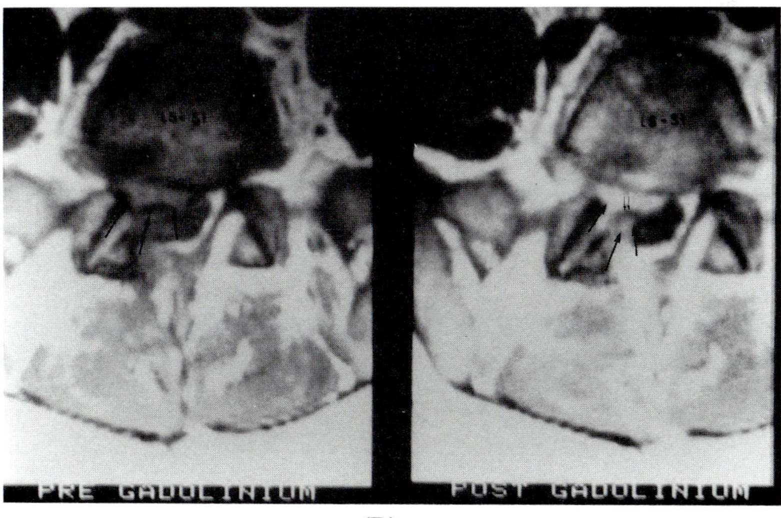

(D)

Figure 14. *DISC VS. SCAR. Patient with previous surgery at L5-S1 has recurrent back pain. Sagittal (A) and transaxial (B) images demonstrate large extradural abnormality (arrows) which appears to be a large recurrent disc protrusion. Pre- and post gadolinium T1 weighted sagittal (C) and transaxial (D) images show low density extradural abnormality on the pre-gadolinium images (arrows) most of which strongly enhances (becomes bright, arrows) on the post-gadolinium images indicative of an epidural scar. A small area of decreased intensity within the scar is seen representing a small disc fragment (small arrows).*

References

1. Resnick D. Degenerative diseases of the vertebral column. Radiology 1985;156:3-14.
2. Yu S, Haughton VM, Sether LA, et al. Criteria for classifying normal and degenerated lumbar intervertebral discs. Radiology 1989;170:523-526.
3. Yu S, Haughton VM, Ho PSP, et al. Progressive and regressive changes in the nucleus pulposus: Part II: the adult. Radiology 1988;169:93-97.
4. Pate D, Goobar J, Resnick D, et al. Traction osteophytes of the lumbar spine: radiologic-pathologic correlation. Radiology 1988;166:843-846.
5. Rothman SLG, Glenn WV Jr. Multiplanar CT of the spine. University Park Press, Baltimore, 1985:1-18.
6. Schipper J, Kardaun J, Braakman R, et al. Lumbar disc herniation: diagnosis with CT or myelography? Radiology 1987;165:227-231.
7. Modic MT, Masaryk T, Boumphrey F, et al. Lumbar herniated disc disease and canal stenosis: prospective evaluation by surface coil MR, CT and myelography. AJR 1986;147:757-765.
8. Firooznia H, Benjamin V, Kricheff II., et al. CT of lumbar spine disc herniation: correlation with surgical findings. AJR 1984;142:587-592.
9. Nowicki BH, Yu S, Reinartz J, et al. Effect of axial loading on neural foramina and nerve roots in the lumbar spine. Radiology 1990;176:433-437.
10. Penning L, Wilmink JT. Posture-dependent bilateral compression of L4 or L5 nerve roots in facet hypertrophy: A dynamic CT-myelographic study. Spine 1987;12:488-500.
11. Dublin AB, McGahan JP, Reid MH. The value of computed tomographic metrizamide myelography in the neuroradiological evaluation of the spine. Radiology 1983;146:79-86.
12. Modic MT, Pavlicek W, Weinstein MA, et al. Magnetic resonance imaging of intervertebral disc disease. Radiology 1984;152:103-111.
13. Edelman RR, Shoukimas GM, Stark DD, et al. High resolution surface-coil imaging of lumbar disc disease. AJR 1985;144:1123-1129.
14. Berger PE, Atkinson MS, Wilson WJ, Wiltse L. High resolution surface coil magnetic resonance imaging of the spine: Normal and pathologic anatomy. Radiographics 1986;6:573-602.
15. Ross JS, Masaryk TJ, Schrader M, et al. MR imaging of the post-operative lumbar spine: assessment with gadopentatate dimeglumine. AJR 1990;155:867-872.

The Specialties of Neuroradiology and Pediatric Radiology

Derek C. Harwood-Nash

The Hospital for Sick Children, Toronto, Ontario, Canada

The two oldest and largest formal specialty persuasions within radiology are pediatric radiology and neuroradiology. There is now a laudable accent on an organ system approach with the one exception being an age oriented group, pediatrics; and on diagnostic imaging appraising all forms of technology. Specific technique or technical oriented groups per se are destined to wither.

Hence it is most appropriate and probably uniquely so, to juxtapose these two senior clinical groups in one educational endeavor such as this with an appropriate overlap in between. Thus may most requirements and expectations be met.

On one hand, the explosion of newer techniques and their resultant sophistication have had a great influence on both neuro and pediatric imaging, probably more so than any other organ or clinical systems. This contribution has been reciprocated by an intense and successful clinical evaluation, utilization and innovation by these two groups. The ease and relative safety of ultrasound, CT, and MRI has availed many patients, adult, and children alike. These very attributes may seduce the unwary radiologist to attempt to image and evaluate such suspect diseases and anomalies, without the necessary training and experience.

Furthermore, it is also necessary for those in neuroradiology to be reasonably knowledgeable of the large mosaic of neurological diseases in the young and the often peculiar and different techniques of investigation and pediatric patient care. Similarly, should the pediatric radiologist have a basic understanding of common afflictions of the pediatric central nervous system and their imaging characteristics and techniques.

Such a broad understanding will also make the general radiologist more competent to the extent of a sufficient recognition of abnormalities; a reasonable understanding of their significance and if necessary leading to suitable referral to someone who has specific specialty training and experience.

These two sets of educational colloquia, pediatric imaging and neuroradiology so combined will be their broad coverage of significant and practical aspects of each, hopefully provide that little extra to elevate radiologists and other interested clinicians be they the experienced, more junior, or student to a respective greater degree of clinical proficiency and diagnostic imaging expertise.

Normal and Abnormal Myelination

Paul E. Berger
*Long Beach Memorial Medical Center, Long Beach,
California, USA*

Introduction

With the addition of magnetic resonance imaging (MRI) to the
diagnostic armamentarium, we are able for the first time, to closely
follow maturation and myelination of the neonatal and infant brain.

An awareness of the chemical properties of myelin and the
effect of these components on the T1 and T2 relaxation times of
the water in the white matter of the brain can help us understand
the role of myelination on the image produced.

Myelin is composed of a bi-layer of lipids (cholesterol and glyco-
lipids) and large proteins [1]. Cholesterol (fat) has a short T1 and
proteins will also decrease the T1 value of water. The result is a
shortening of T1 and therefore an increased intensity (increased
brightness) on a T1 weighted MR image.

Myelin lipids are hydrophobic. Thus when myelination occurs
there is a loss of brain water. This results in a decrease in the T2
value in the white matter and as a result a decreased intensity
(darker) appearance on T2-weighted images.

Thus, myelination will be seen as an area of increased intensity
(brighter) on T1 weighted images and decreased intensity (darker)
on T2-weighted images.

Normal Myelination

Myelination of the brain begins during the fifth fetal month with
the myelination of the cranial nerves and continues throughout life
[2].

At birth, as seen on T1 weighted images, myelination is present in the medulla, dorsal midbrain, cerebellar peduncles, posterior limb of the internal capsule, and ventrolateral thalamus [3,4] (Fig. 1). Maturation proceeds from: (1) central to peripheral, (2) inferior to superior, and (3) posterior to anterior. The cerebellum is myelinated at 3 months of age with an adult appearance on T2 weighted images (Fig. 2).

The pre- and post-central gyri are myelinated at 1 month and maturation of motor tracts is complete by 3 months (Fig. 3).

The pons matures from 3-6 months, with maturation proceeding rostrally along the corticospinal tracts, cerebral peduncles, through the posterior limb of the internal capsule and central portion of the centrum semiovale [4] (Fig. 4).

The optic nerves, tracts, and optic radiations (into the occipital white matter) are myelinated by 3 months and the anterior limb of the internal capsule by 2-3 months. The subcortical white matter matures starting at 3 months in the occipital region and proceeds rostrally to the frontal lobes.

Myelination in the corpus callosum can be a helpful landmark when estimating myelin development. Myelination begins in the splenium (posterior) at 4 months and is complete, involving the genu (anterior) at 6 months (Fig. 5).

T1 vs. T2 Weighted Images

Barkovich et al. [3,4], feel that the early primary process of myelination from about 1-6 months is best evaluated using strongly T1 weighted images (short TR/Short TE). The T1 weighted image will appear adult-like at about 9 months (Fig. 6). T2 weighted images are better at depicting the associated changes of water loss that occur with myelination and may be helpful after 6 months of age. Milestones to look for on both T1 and T2 weighted images are presented in Table 1 and Table 2. Myelination of the frontal white matter is seen as decreased intensity at 14 months of age and the appearance of the brain is adult like on T2 weighted images at 18 months (Fig. 7).

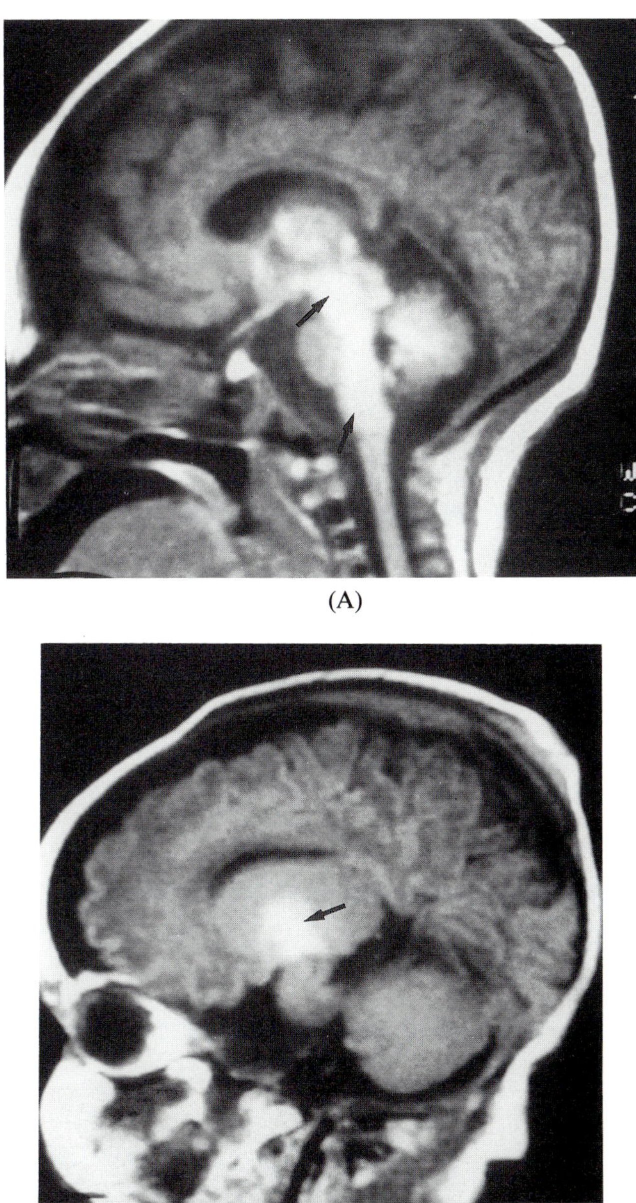

(A)

(B)

Figure 1. *ONE-DAY-OLD BABY. Sagittal T1 weighted images (A, B) (TR 500, TE 15) showing myelination (increased intensity in medulla and dorsal midbrain (A, arrows) and thalamus (arrow, B).*

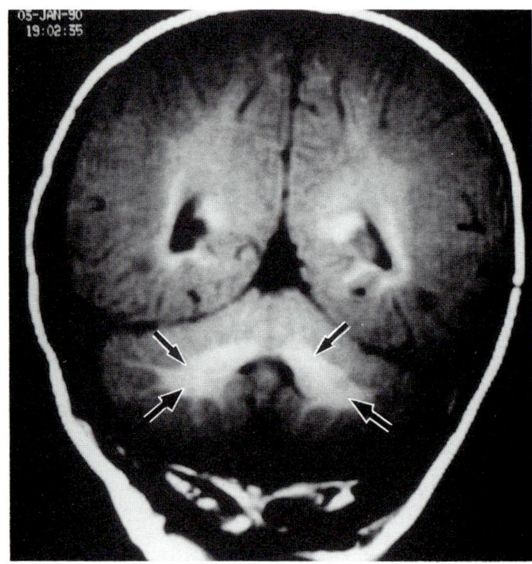

Figure 2. *FOUR-MONTH-OLD BABY. Coronal T1 weighted image(TR 500, TE 15) demonstrating myelinated cerebellar white matter (arrows) which appears as that of an adult.*

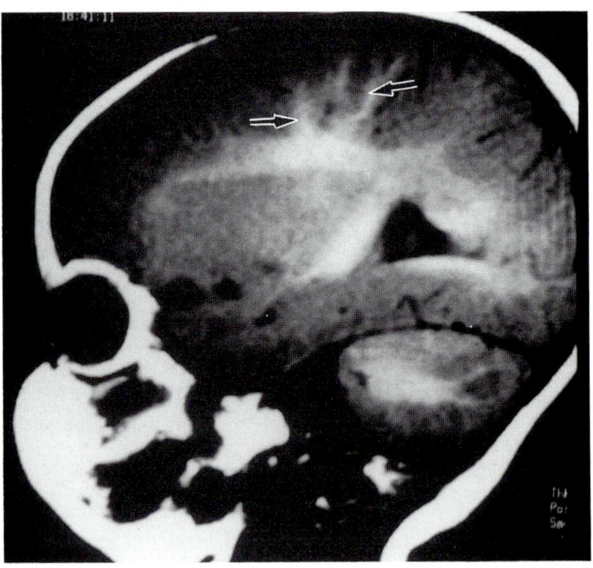

Figure 3. *FOUR MONTH OLD. Sagittal T1 weighted image (TR 500, TE 15) demonstrating myelination of pre- and post central gyri (arrows).*

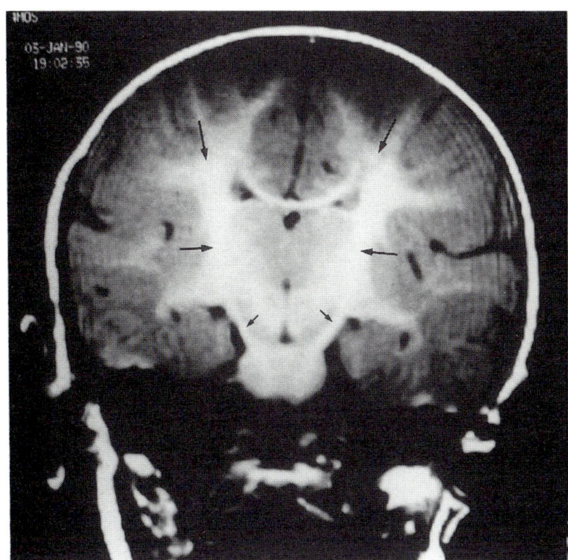

Figure 4. *FOUR MONTH OLD. T1 weighted coronal image (TR 500, TE 15) demonstrating myelination extending from pons, through cerebral peduncles, internal capsule, and centrum semiovale (arrows).*

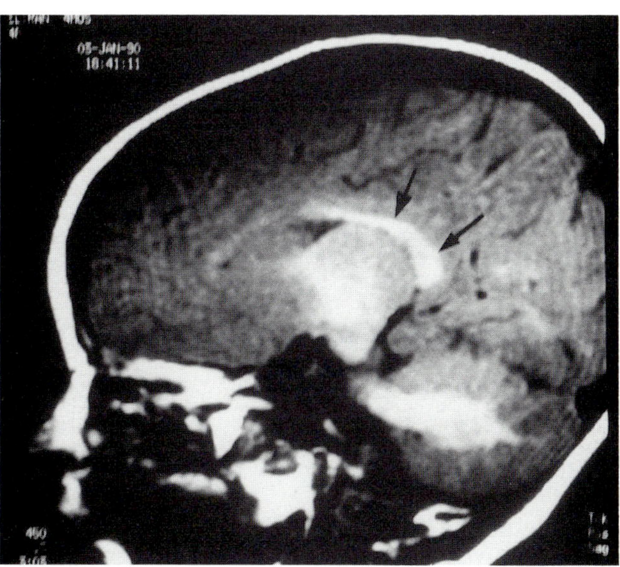

Figure 5. *FOUR MONTH OLD. Sagittal T1 weighted image (TR 500, TE 15) demonstrating myelination of the splenium and posterior body of the corpus callosum (arrows). Note also the myelination of the cerebellar peduncles and thalamus in this baby.*

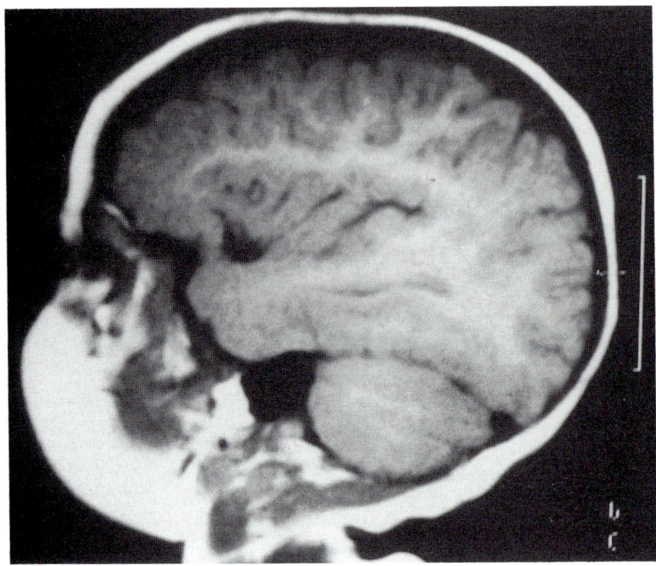

Figure 6. *NINE MONTH OLD. Sagittal T1 weighted image. (TR 500, TE 15). Appearance is similar to that of an adult.*

Table 1.   *Milestones: Normal Myelination (1-6 months) (T1-weighted images at 1.5T). From Barkovich [4]*

Cerebellar white matter	= 3 months
Splenium	= 4 months
Genu	= 6 months

Table 2.   *Milestones: Normal Myelination (T2-weighted images at 1.5T). From Barkovich [4]*

Splenium	= 6 months
Genu	= 8 months
Anterior limb internal capsule	= 11 months
Frontal white matter	= 14 months
Adult patter	= 18 months

Abnormal Myelination

Abnormal myelination as seen on MRI can be divided into two groups. The first group are those patients in whom there is a delay in myelination and the second group are those in whom there has been destruction of brain tissue and myelin (Table 3).

By far the most common cause of a delay or immature myelination is malnutrition [4]. These infants can resume normal myelination and myelination can catch up once nutritional status is improved. In infants and young children who are developmentally delayed and in whom there is no known pathologic diagnosis approximately 10% will show a delay in myelination. Two uncommon causes of delay in myelination are cerebral white matter hypoplasia and Pelizaeus-Merzbacher disease. Cerebral white matter hypoplasia occurs in children who show a delay in achieving normal developmental milestones and have a spastic diplegia. The MR study shows a paucity of cerebral white matter, a thin corpus callosum, and delayed myelination [4]. Pelizaeus-Merzbacher is a rare x-linked leukodystrophy which may present in infancy. The infants or children present with abnormal eye movements, head shaking, cerebellar ataxia, and slow psychomotor development. The symptoms are progressive [5,6]. The MR findings are striking in that there may be only minimal myelin, or complete absence of myelin. The MR study of a child with this disorder may retain the appearance of a newborn due to the absence of myelination.

The second major group of patients with abnormal myelination are those in whom there has been destruction of brain tissue in which myelin is also destroyed (Table 3). In trying to identify the etiology of the abnormal MR scan it is helpful to delineate whether the abnormality involves both gray and white matter, or white matter only. If only white matter is involved one needs to differentiate between diffuse involvement and multifocal abnormalities. In the multifocal group knowing whether the clinical course is acute or subacute will aid in the differential diagnosis (Table 3).

Of a relatively complete list of the entities in Table 3, some features are stated here. The most common cause of abnormality involving both white and gray matter is anoxia. Anoxic injury characteristically involves the frontal and parietal watershed regions

Table 3. *Abnormal myelination*

I. Delay in myelination

    A.   Malnutrition
    B.   Developmental retardation (no pathologic diagnosis)
    C.   Cerebral white matter hypoplasia
    D.   Pelizaeus - Merzbacher disease

II. Destruction of brain tissue (and myelin)

    A.   White and gray matter
        1.   anoxia
        2.   infections
            a. acute disseminated encephalomyelitis
            b. subacute sclerosing panencephalitis
        3.   metabolic disorders
            a. subacute necrotizing encephalomyelitis (Leigh's disease)
            b. mitochondrial cytopathies

    B.   White matter only
        1.   Diffuse
            a. radiation
            b. dysmyelinating disease
                 ● Alexander's disease
                 ● Krabbe's disease
                 ● Adrenoleukodystrophy
                 ● Metachromatic leukodystrophy
        2.   Multifocal
            a. acute
                 ● anoxia
                 ● multiple sclerosis
                 ● infection
            b. subacute
                 ● multiple sclerosis
                 ● radiation
                 ● metabolic disorders
                 ● leukodystrophy
                 ● progressive multifocal leukoencephalopathy
                 ● periventricular leukomalacia

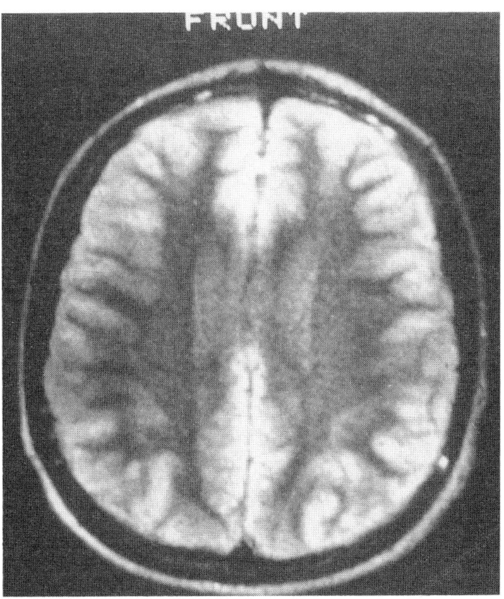

Figure 7. *18 MONTH OLD. Transaxial T2 weighted image (TR 2500/TE 80) Normal adult-like appearance.*

between the circulations of the anterior and middle, and middle and posterior cerebral arteries. The clinical history is one of severe asphyxia. When the foci of abnormalities are multiple and principally involve the region of the corticomedullary junction acute disseminated encephalomyelitis may be the cause (Fig. 8). This is thought to be an immunemediated disorder secondary to a recent viral illness. Metabolic disorders such as Leigh's disease (subacute necrotizing encephalomyelopathy) and mitochondrial encephalomyopathy are uncommon causes of destructive lesions which characteristically demonstrate foci of necrosis in the basal ganglia as well as demyelination in the white matter. In Leigh's disease there is also frequently necrosis in the peri-aqueductal gray matter in the mesencephalon, the cerebral cortex and the spinal cord may be involved (Fig. 9).

When there is diffuse involvement of white matter only, the most likely etiologies would be radiation injury or one of the dysmyelinating disorders. Dysmyelination refers to abnormal formation of myelin and includes uncommon entities such as Alexander's disease, Krabbe's disease, adrenoleukodystrophy and metachromatic leukodystrophy.

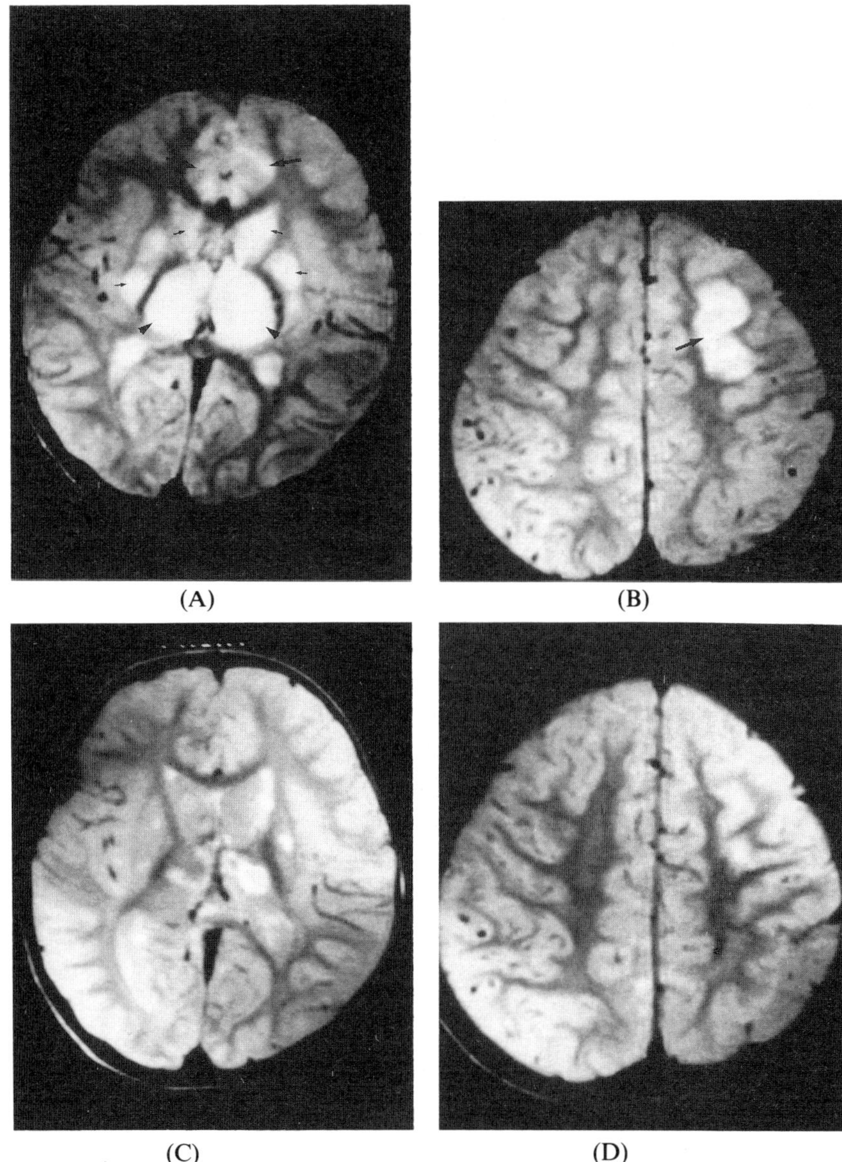

Figure 8. *ACUTE DISSEMINATED ENCEPHALOMYELITIS (ADEM). Six-year-old girl with fever, vomiting, and extreme lethargy. (A, B) Transaxial T weighted images (TR 2500/TE 30) demonstrating bilateral areas of increased intensity in the basal ganglia (small arrows) thalami (arrowheads) and peripheral gray/white matter (large arrows). (C, D) Follow-up study two weeks later following treatment with steroids shows marked improvement in the previously noted areas of encephalitis.*

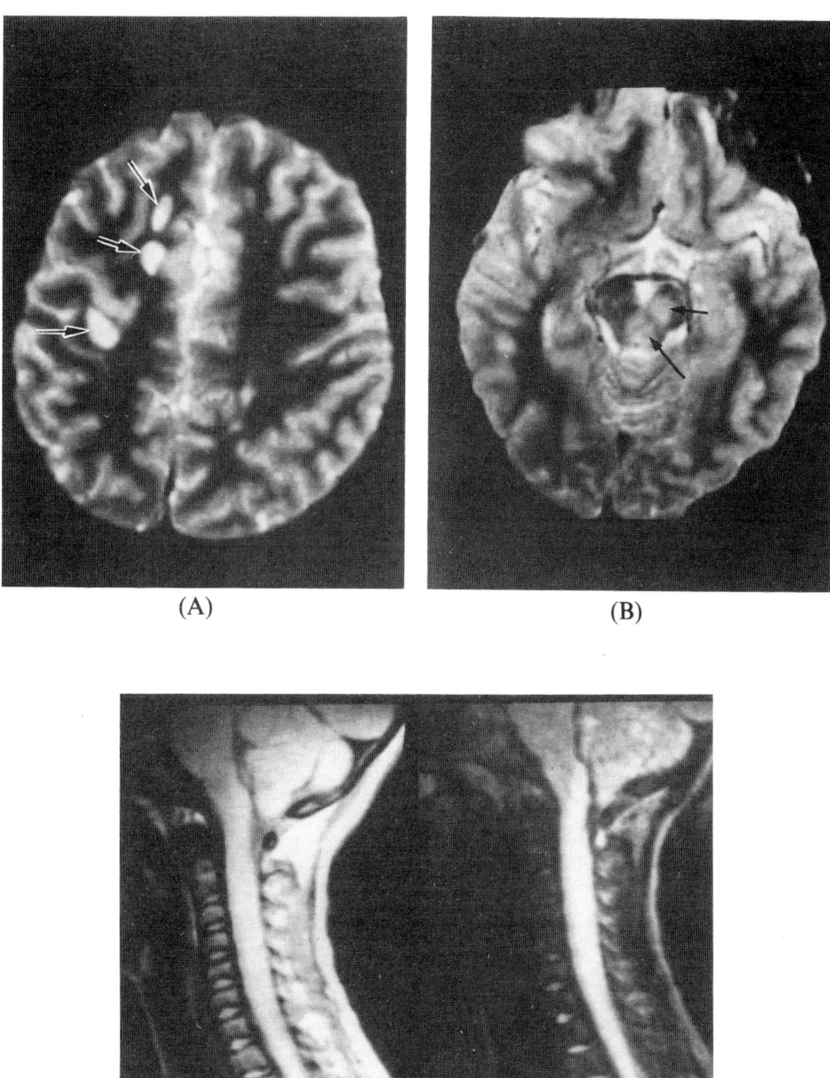

(A)

(B)

(C)

Figure 9. *LEIGH'S DISEASE. Four-year-old boy with headache, stiff neck, and quadriparesis. (A) Transaxial T2 weighted image (TR 2500/TE 80) demonstrating small foci of increased intensity (arrows) in high peripheral white matter. (B) T2 weighted transaxial image at level of brain stem demonstrates abnormal increased signal in periaqueductal mesencephalon and left cerebral peduncle (arrows). (C) Same patient. T2 weighted (TR 2500 TE 30/80) sagittal images through cervical spine showing enlargement and increased intensity of dorsal medulla and entire spinal cord.*

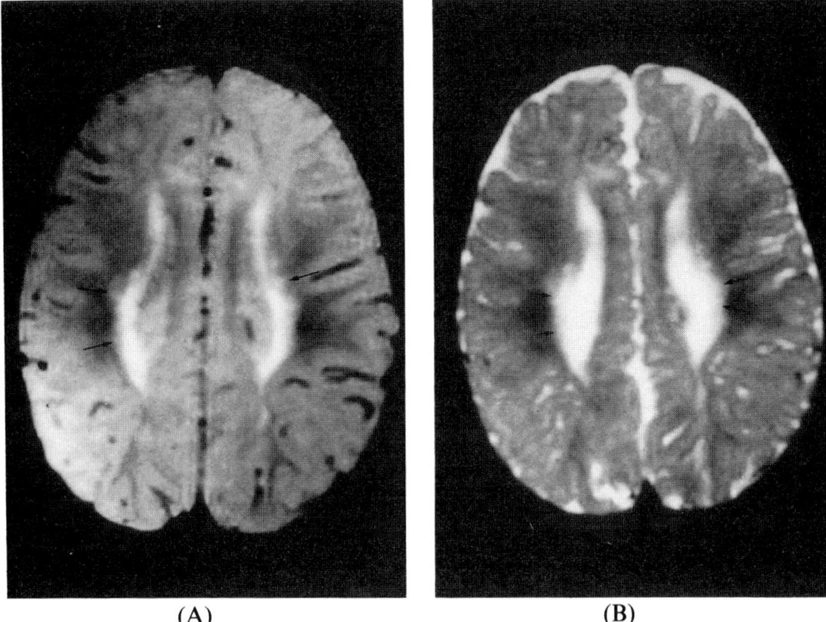

(A)   (B)

Figure 10. *PERIVENTRICULAR LEUKOMALACIA. 20-month-old boy, born prematurely at 28 weeks, now with spastic diplegia. (A, B) Transaxial T2 weighted images (TR 2500 TE30/100) demonstrating small focal areas of increase dintensity in the periventricular white matter (arrows). There is also mild ventricular dilatation and a decrease in the amount of periventricular white matter.*

When multifocal white matter lesions are seen in children the history may be very important to aid in the differential diagnosis (Table 3).

An important entity is periventricular leukomalacia (PVL). Periventricular leukomalacia usually occurs in pre-term infants, and is the result of an hypoxic/ischemic insult that occurs in the watershed zone of arterial supply which in this age group is in the periventricular white matter. Areas most frequently involved are the posterior periventricular white matter at the trigone of the lateral ventricles. Lesions may affect the geniculocalcarine tract and cause visual impairment, or corticospinal tracts in the corona radiata and damage the motor fibers which control the function of the lower limbs and trunk. Thus, the usual clinical sequelae are spastic diplegia or quadriplegia and cortical blindness with relative preservation of cognitive functions. MRI findings include a decrease in the amount of white matter in the periventricular region and centrum semiovale [7]. More severe cases show small cavitated infarcts in the periventricular region. There is often ventriculomegaly. On T2 weighted images abnormal areas of increased signal intensity are seen which may extend superficially beyond the periventricular region (Fig. 10). This most probably represents areas of gliosis [7].

It is clear that MRI provides us with a new opportunity to evaluate both the normal development and heretofore subtle pathologic changes that affect the brain of the infant and child.

References

1. Braun PE. Molecular organization of myelin. In: Morell P, ed. Myelin 2nd ed. New York, Plenum, 1984:97-116.
2. Yakovlev PI, Lecours AR. The myelogenetic cycles of regional maturation of the brain. In: Mankowski A. ed. Regional Development of the Brain in Early Life, Philadelphia: Davis 1967:3-69.
3. Barkovich AJ, Kjos BO, Jackson DE Jr, Norman D. Normal maturation of the neonatal and infant brain: MR imaging at 1.5T. Radiology 1988;166:173-180.
4. Barkovich AJ, Jackson DE Jr. MRI assessment of normal and abnormal brain myelinization. MRI Decisions 1989:19-25.
5. Valk J, van der Knapp MS. Magnetic resonance of myelin, myelination, and myelin disorders. Berlin: Springer-Verlag, 1989.
6. Barkovich AJ. Pediatric Neuroimaging. Raven Press: New York, 1990.
7. Flodmark O., Lupton B, Li D, et al. MR Imaging of periventricular leukomalacia in childhood. AJR 1989;152:583-590.

The Neonatal Brain - Imaging for Prognosis

Olof Flodmark

Department of Neuroradiology, Karolinska Institutet, Stockholm, Sweden

Introduction

Clinical evaluation of the central nervous system is difficult in the neonate. It is particularly difficult to make reliable predictions about outcome in a severely ill newborn with potential for serious disease or damage in several different organ systems. Neuroradiological investigation of the distressed newborn has emerged as a very important adjunct to clinical evaluation of the neonate. Routine imaging has developed in two main directions: Computed Tomography (CT) and later Ultrasonography (US). US has many advantages as the equipment is portable, inexpensive and usually more readily available. The examination can be performed bedside in the incubator but is limited to the first few months of life, and some parts of the brain are poorly visualized. Ultrasonography is very operator dependent and the quality of the study is intimately related to the skill and experience of the sonologist as well as his/her knowledge of the anatomy and pathology of the neonatal brain. US is the imaging method of choice in the immature neonate despite its shortcomings. Although cranial CT scanning may provide additional information in the premature neonate it is rarely used in routine practice. The situation is quite different in assessing the mature neonate suspected of having suffered hypoxic/ischemic damage to the brain. Although ultrasonography may be quite useful, CT should remain the primary mode of imaging in the term neonate. Magnetic Resonance Imaging (MRI), is now more readily available and has been used to study pathology and normal development of the neonatal brain. Technical difficulties limits more general use of this technique during the first few weeks of life [1].

Pathology and pathophysiology

It is important to have some basic knowledge about the pathology and pathophysiology of brain lesions in neonates of varying maturity in order to understand how imaging may assist in predicting the outcome.

The pattern of cerebral injury in the newborn infant depends on the maturity of the brain at the time of insult [2]. This is due to rapid maturation and changing physiology during the third trimester. Rich vascular supply to the basal ganglia and the germinal matrix characterizes the immature brain before 34 weeks of gestation. A thin cortex is supplied by numerous small penetrating branches from leptomeningeal vessels with a watershed area between these two vascular territories in the periventricular white matter. Conversely, the vascular anatomy of the brain after 34 weeks gestation is similar to that of an adult. The evolution of vascular supply to the maturing brain explains why pathology of neonatal hypoxic-ischemic brain injury depends on the maturity of the brain at the time of insult and therefore is different in term and premature newborns. As this process of maturation proceeds whether the baby remains in utero or is born prematurely, an injury caused by an insult in utero may result in a lesion with the characteristics of an injury to the immature brain, e.g. intraventricular hemorrhage or periventricular leukomalacia, despite being seen in a neonate born at term.

Increased cerebral perfusion secondary to damaged cerebral autoregulation is thought to cause *intraventricular hemorrhage* (IVH) [2]. Increased systemic blood pressure will increase cerebral perfusion and cause rupture of the fragile blood vessels in the germinal matrix and hemorrhage. The hemorrhage usually ruptures into the lateral ventricles. The CSF circulation is always compromised when blood is cleared from the ventricular system, but the development of progressive hydrocephalus requiring permanent shunting is much less common than previously thought [3].

In analogy with above, systemic hypotension and subsequent cerebral hypoperfusion may cause brain damage. *Periventricular leukomalacia* (PVL) is caused by such hypoperfusion in the most susceptible watershed area in the periventricular white matter [2]. Lesions occur most commonly close to the trigone and less common adjacent to the frontal horns [4]. Initially coagulation necrosis is found in PVL with subsequent cavitation. These cavities, when small, may collapse and disappear, leading to white matter atrophy and gliosis. Larger cysts may persist and communicate with the lateral ventricles as the ependyma breaks down [5,6]. The lesions in PVL are typically bilateral and more or less symmetrical. PVL is thought to cause spastic diplegia, a specific form of cerebral palsy most commonly seen in prematurely born children [7]. Episodes of both hypo- and hypertension in the distressed neonate may cause PVL complicated by secondary hemorrhage and subsequent extensive brain damage, usually but not always associated with IVH [2].

A third lesion may be seen in the immature brain. This has some of the features of PVL but is typically extensive and unilateral. This lesion is always associated with extensive IVH and is thought to be due to reperfusion following local ischemia in the periventricular white matter caused by the large IVH. Periventricular venous congestion has been suggested. This lesion has been named *hemorrhagic periventricular infarction* and corresponds most closely to the old classification "grade 4 IVH" [8,9].

Intracerebral hemorrhage is uncommon in *term neonates* as the germinal matrix has involuted. If hemorrhage occurs, it is usually due to factors unrelated to asphyxia [10]. Profound and prolonged hypoperfusion with ischemia may lead to cerebral injury in the cortical watershed zones [11]. Diffuse brain injury may occur when the hypoxic-ischemic insult is severe [12]. Cerebral edema is a prominent feature of the pathophysiological process, however its precise role is controversial [13]. Limited damage can cause more focal lesions in the cortex [14-16].

Permanent damage caused by hypoxic-ischemic brain injury in term neonates is seen as cortical necrosis and large portions of cortex may be replaced by cystic spaces [17]. Central gray matter and cerebellum is usually spared due to redistribution of cerebral blood flow during gradual onset of hypoxia. Microcephaly associated with severe mental and motor handicap is common in these infants. Other patterns of brain injury can however involve primarily the basal ganglia showing gliosis and subsequent severe handicap [10].

Neuroradiology of neonatal pathology

The ability to assist the neonatologist in assessing prognosis depends entirely on the ability of the radiologist to detect damage to the neonatal brain and to correctly interpret the findings and predict their consequences. This process has two components. Correct gathering of data at an appropriate time and correct interpretation.

Neurosonography and CT scanning remain the primary imaging tools of suspected pathology in the neonatal brain. Both imaging modalities provide similar results but with different sensitivity and limitations depending on the clinical situation. Although, the maturity of the neonate and suspected pathology should dictate the choice of imaging modality [18], availability of a certain imaging modality is the most important reason to choose a certain mode of investigation. Sonographic equipment of high quality is available in most departments of pediatric radiology. Hence, the radiologists are skilled in the use of this modality. However, accurate interpretation of the study, particularly neurosonography, is possible only if the radiologist has a good understanding of the normal anatomy, patho-physiology and pathology of the neonatal brain. Unless the radiologist is familiar with the limitations of the modality, the results, particularly if negative, are of limited value. The nature of the neurosonographic study is such that a review of the images has limited value, thus the report of the sonologist is extremely important, but also of limited value if the sonologist is less experienced and skilled. Consequently, positive findings are useful, while the method cannot exclude certain types of pathology. This is particularly important in attempting to diagnose cerebral edema in the term newborn. The sensitivity for even severe edema is relatively low and neurosonography should not be relied upon to exclude this pathology. Although CT scanning may not be as readily available as sonography as well as more invasive and cumbersome, the modality has and should maintain an important role in assessing the asphyxiated term newborn. The images are less operator dependent. Accurate interpretation may be as difficult as with neurosonography but the images can be reviewed and reassessed at any time, providing the opportunity for expert evaluation. The role of MRI in the evaluation of the neonatal brain is not yet defined.

The detection of *germinal matrix and intraventricular hemorrhage* is best accomplished by neurosonography, which has an excellent sensitivity and specificity for IVH. However, detection of IVH has no predictive value. Only posthemorrhagic hydrocephalus can be directly attributed to IVH while future handicap is best related to associated parenchymal damage [19]. Bilateral, more or less symmetrical parenchymal hemorrhage is presently thought to represent secondary hemorrhage into an area of *periventricular leukomalacia*. This hemorrhage is thought to be a secondary bleed into an ischemic infarction or may represent an extension from the germinal matrix hemorrhage into the ischemic infarction. Such parenchymal hemorrhage is usually combined with IVH, but the lesion can occur in isolation or in the presence of a very small amount of IVH.

Extensive IVH may create the necessary scenario for an extensive, usually unilateral hemorrhage (*hemorrhagic periventricular infarction*) into the frontal white matter, the most common location for this form of intraparenchymal bleed but a less common location for PVL [8,9]. Although many lesions are extensive and carry a poor prognosis, some may be limited in extent or have a more favorable location indicating a better prognosis. Furthermore, US can not reliably distinguish parenchymal hemorrhage from non-hemorrhagic periventricular infarct (PVL). Hence, the radiologist must carefully describe the sonographic findings to allow a qualified assessment of prognosis by the neonatologist in each individual case (Fig. 1).

Confident diagnosis of *ischemic PVL* is difficult in the newborn. The lesion can readily be found using US when a hemorrhage has complicated the ischemic infarct. PVL without secondary hemorrhage is difficult, unless extensive, to diagnose with US in the neonatal period. Most mild to moderate (70 % and 45 % respectively) lesions escape detection by any imaging modality during the neonatal period [20,21], possibly with the exception of MRI. However, the permanent damage caused by PVL can be detected later during infancy by CT or MRI, as both modalities show a typical pattern of atrophy and white matter damage [22,23]. Such

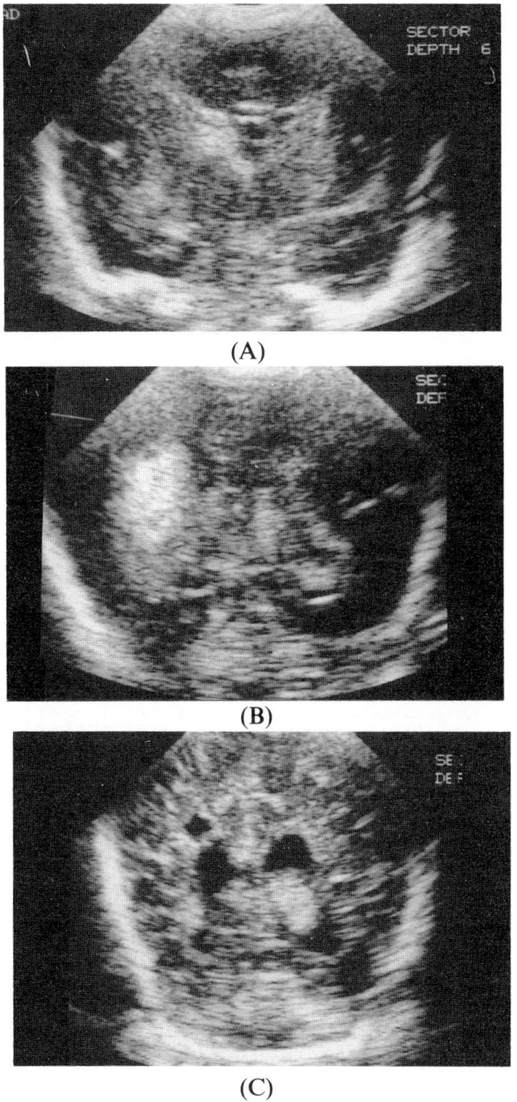

(A)

(B)

(C)

Figure 1. *IVH ASSOCIATED WITH PARENCHYMAL HEMORRHAGE. A one-day-old boy born after 29 weeks gestation. (A) Neurosonographic examination with a coronal view of the region of Foramen Monro shows intraventricular hemorrhage which is more extensive on the right side. (B) A view more posteriorly shows a large parenchymal hemorrhage in the right periventricular white matter. (C) Follow-up examination 10 weeks later shows a cavity having formed in the periventricular white matter. This boy has severe spastic hemiplegia, seizures and is mentally impaired at 4.5 years of age.*

damage can be recognized by the characteristic reduction of periventricular white matter with secondary prominence of the deep portions of the Sylvian fissures. Atrophic ventricular dilatation and in severe cases large cystic spaces adjacent to the ventricles can occur. These findings have been shown in patients with spastic diplegia, the clinical correlate to PVL. Recent experience with MRI confirms these observations and in addition shows evidence of delayed myelination and gliosis in remaining periventricular white matter [23].

It is well documented that CT scanning permits assessment of *hypoxic-ischemic brain injury in term neonates*. Widespread or focal areas of decreased brain tissue attenuation in early CT scans correlate well with adverse neurological outcome [24]. These findings represent cerebral edema developing after hypoxic-ischemic injury with brain tissue attenuation decreasing as the interstitial or intracellular amount of water is increasing. The attenuation of gray matter may approach that of white matter eliminating the distinction between these two tissue-types. The brain appears featureless. The edema peaks 72 hours following the injury, and this is the ideal time of imaging for prognosis (Fig. 2). Even severe edema may have disappeared as early as five days after injury. Gradual onset of hypoxia, common in perinatal asphyxia, results in redistribution of regional cerebral blood flow with preferred perfusion of the basal ganglia and cerebellum. Consequently these structures maintain a more normal attenuation and are clearly visible on the CT image contrasting against the darker background formed by the edematous cerebrum. Neurosonography can detect cerebral edema secondary to hypoxic brain damage as increased echogenicity [25]. However, this finding is only useful if present as it is not possible to confidently exclude cerebral edema using sonography.

Focal areas of brain damage and less severe generalized changes may be difficult to evaluate in CT scans during the first few days of life. Prominent symmetrical areas of low attenuation in the white matter is common and correlates poorly with adverse outcome as long as gray matter can be distinguished from white matter. Errors in interpretation are common with too much significance attached to findings of prominent white matter. Delayed CT scans at 4-7 weeks of age or later may prove most useful in predicting future handicap in these situations.

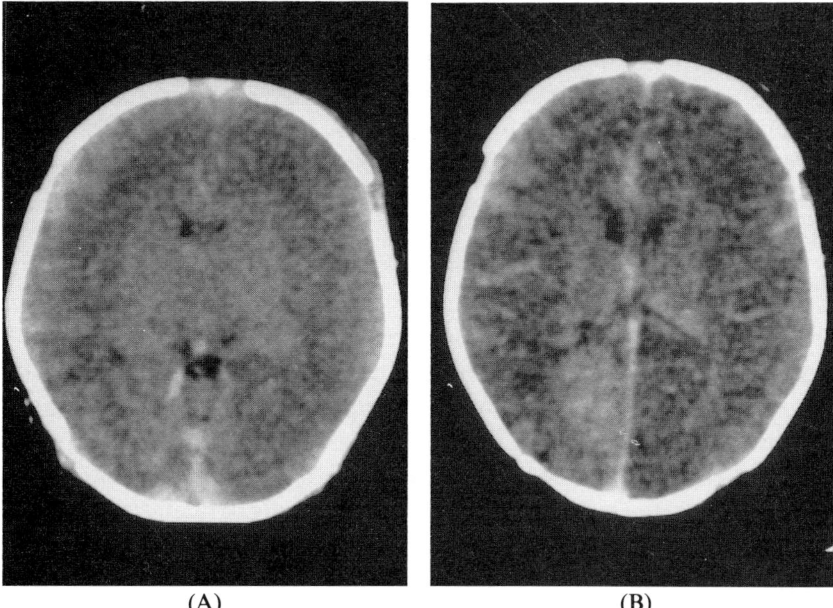

(A)   (B)

Figure 2. *HYPOXIC-ISCHEMIC BRAIN INJURY IN A TERM NEONATE. A one-day-old boy was born at term. He was clinically severely asphyxiated at delivery. (A) The first CT scan was done at 24 hours of age. Note the widespread areas of decreased attenuation and the featureless brain. (B) A second CT scan was performed at 48 hours of age. Radiographic evidence of generalized edema has progressed and the attenuation of brain tissue is still lower. He now has severe psycho-motor delay at six months of age.*

Severe asphyxia in the term neonate may lead to extensive destruction of brain tissue, i.e. "multicystic encephalomalacia" in which cystic spaces replace cortical structures [17]. As atrophy progresses, the ventricles dilate. Bright contrast between the relatively normal tissue attenuation in the basal ganglia and low attenuation throughout the rest of the cerebrum may be mistaken for hemorrhage or even calcifications in the basal ganglia. This very common mistake must be avoided. Confident CT diagnosis of multicystic encephalomalacia depends on careful assessment of brain tissue attenuation [18]. Lesser degrees of atrophy are seen following mild to moderate hypoxic-ischemic brain damage. Loss of brain tissue is diffuse and mainly cortical, although axonal degeneration will cause secondary loss of white matter. Associated microcephaly is commonplace, a piece of information that must be taken into consideration when assessing the degree of atrophy in CT or MRI.

Conclusion

Morphology of a destructive lesion to the brain is more dependent on the stage of maturation at which the injury occurred, than the type of injury. Most important is the difference between the circulatory physiology of the immature brain before and after 34 weeks gestation. This difference in the cerebral vascular supply is thought to explain the occurrence of central atrophy (PVL) in the immature brain, as opposed to predominantly peripheral cortical damage with multicystic encephalomalacia in the mature brain, at or near term. It is extremely important that the neuroradiologist and the neonatalogist both understand the differences between neonates of different maturity when assessing prognosis. The imaging methods have different strengths and weaknesses depending on the maturity of the neonate and correct interpretation depends on intimate knowledge of the limitations in each imaging method.

References

1. McArdle CB, Richardson CJ, Hayden CK, Nicholas DA, Amparo EG. Abnormalities of the neonatal brain: MR Imaging Part II. Hypoxic-ischemic brain injury. Radiology 1987;163:395-403.
2. Pape KE, Wigglesworth JS. Hemorrhage, ischemia and the perinatal brain. Lippincott, Philadelphia 1979
3. Shinnar S, Molteni RA, Gammon K, D'Souza BJ, Altman J, Freeman JM. Intraventricular hemorrhage in the premature infant: a changing outlook. N Engl J Med 1982;306:1464-1468.
4. Shuman RM, Selednik LJ. Periventricular leukomalacia: a one-year autopsy study. Arch Neurol 1980;37:231-235.
5. Banker BQ, Larroche JC. Periventricular leukomalacia of infancy. Arch Neurol 1962;7:386-410.
6. DeReuck J, Chatta AS, Richardson EP Jr. Pathogenesis and evolution of periventricular leukomalacia in infancy. Arch Neurol 1972;27:229-236.
7. Guzzetta F, Shackelford GD, Volpe S, Perlman JM, Volpe JJ. Periventricular intraparenchymal echodensities in the premature newborn: critical determinant of neurologic outcome. Pediatrics 1986;78:995-1006.

8. Volpe JJ. Intraventricular hemorrhage in the premature infant - current concepts. Part I. Ann Neurol 1989;25:3-11.

9. Volpe JJ. Intraventricular hemorrhage in the premature infant - current concepts. Part II. Ann Neurol 1989;25:109-116.

10. Roland EH, Flodmark O, Hill A. Thalamic hemorrhage with intraventricular hemorrhage in the term newborn. Pediatrics 1990;85:737-742.

11. Brann AW, Dykes FD. The effects of intrauterine asphyxia on the full-term neonate. Clin Perinatol 1977;4:149-161.

12. Hill A, Volpe JJ. Pathogenesis and management of hypoxic-ischemic encephalopathy in the term newborn. Neurol Clin 1985;3:31-34.

13. Lupton BA, Hill A, Roland EH, Whitfield MF, Flodmark O. Brain swelling in the asphyxiated term newborn: pathogenesis and outcome. Pediatrics 1988;82:139-146.

14. Roland EH, Hill A, Norman MG, Flodmark O, McNab A. Selective brainstem injury in an asphyxiated newborn. Ann Neurol 1988;23:89-92.

15. Wiklund L-M, Uvebrant P, Flodmark O. Morphology of cerebral lesions in children with congenital hemiplegia: a study with computed tomography. Neuroradiology 1990,32:179-186.

16. Wiklund L-M, Uvebrant P, Flodmark O. Computed tomography as an adjunct in etiological analysis of hemiplegic cerebral palsy. II: Children born at term. Neuropaediatrics (in press).

17. Naidich TP, Chakera TMH. Multicystic encephalomalacia: CT appearance and pathological correlation. J Comp Assist Tomogr 1984;8:631-636.

18. Flodmark O. The neonatal brain. In: Syllabus: A categorical course in diagnostic radiology - neuroradiology. The Radiological Society of North America, Oak Brook, 1987;43-54.

19. Kirks DR, Bowie JD. Cranial ultrasonography of neonatal periventricular/ intraventricular hemorrhage: who, how, why and when? Pediatr Radiol 1986;16:114-119.

20. Flodmark O, Poskitt KJ, Whitfield MF, Roland EH, Hill A. Inability of neurosonography to diagnose periventricular leukomalacia. 27th Annual Meeting of The American Society of Neuroradiology, Orlando, FL, March 19-24, 1989. AJNR 1989;10:891.

21. Hope PL, Gould SJ, Howard S, Hamilton PA, de L. Castello AM, Reynolds EOR. Precision of ultrasound diagnosis of pathologically verified lesions in the brains of very preterm infants. Develop Med Child Neurol 1988;30:457-471.

22. Flodmark O, Roland EH, Hill A, Whitfield MF. periventricular leukomalacia: radiologic diagnosis. Radiology 1987;162:119-124.

23. Flodmark O, Lupton B, Li D, Stimac GK, Roland EH, Hill A, Whitfield MF, Norman MG. Magnetic resonance imaging of periventricular leukomalacia (PVL) in childhood. AJNR 1989;10:111-118.

24. Adsett DB, Fitz CR, Hill A. Hypoxic-ischaemic cerebral injury in the term newborn: correlation of CT findings with neurological outcome. Develop Med Child Neurol 1985;27:155-160.

25. Babcock DS, Ball W Jr. Postasphyxial encephalopathy in full-term infants: ultrasound diagnosis. Radiology 1983;148:417-423.

Congenital Malformations of the Brain

Anne G. Osborn

Department of Radiology, University of Utah, Salt Lake City, Utah, USA

Introduction and General Principles

CNS anomalies are common; over 2000 congenital cerebral malformations have been described and are found in approximately 1% of live births. Seventy-five per cent of fetal deaths have cerebral malformations and one-third of all major anomalies involve the CNS. It is estimated that 10% of intracranial anomalies are due to chromosomal anomalies, 20% to inherited factors, and 10% to adverse intrauterine environment (e.g., infection); 60% have no identifiable causal factor.

A broad spectrum of congenital CNS malformations can be recognized using neuroimaging procedures such as CT, MR, and ultrasound. These malformations are most simply divided into disorders of organogenesis and disorders of histogenesis. Organogenetic abnormalities are further divided into neural tube defects; disorders of diverticulation; disorders of sulcation and migration; disorders of size (microcephaly, macrocephaly); destructive lesions such as hydranencephaly, porencephaly, intrauterine infections. It is appropriate therefore to consider neural tube defects, separate from disorders of histogenesis as represented by the neurocutaneous syndromes.

Disorders of Organogenesis

(Altered brain development, normal histogenesis)

A. Disorders of neural tube closure (myelomeningocele is the most common)
   - Chiari malformations
   - Cephaloceles
   - Agenesis of the corpus callosum
   - Dandy-Walker complex
   - Cranioschisis (meningocele, encephalocele, etc)
B. Disorders of diverticulation or brain cleavage
   - Holoprosencephaly (alobar, semilobar, lobar)
   - Septo-optic dysplasia
C. Disorders of sulcation and cellular migration
   - Agyria (lissencephaly)
   - Schizencephaly
   - Heterotopias
   - Pachygyria, polymicrogyria
D. Disorders of size
   - Microcephaly
   - Macrocephaly
E. Destructive lesions
   - Hydranencephaly
   - Porencephaly
   - Inflammatory diseases (rubella, CMV, toxoplasmosis, herpes simplex)
   - Hypoxia, toxicosis

Disorders of Histogenesis

(Overall brain structure normal but anomalous cells persist and continue to differentiate)

A. Neurocutaneous syndromes
   - Neurofibromatosis
   - Sturge-Weber syndrome
   - Tuberous sclerosis
   - Von Hippel-Lindau disease
B. Vascular lesions
C. Congenital neoplasms

Disorders of Cytogenesis

A. Inborn errors of metabolism
  - Aminoacidurias
  - Mucopolysaccharidoses
  - Lipidoses
B. Leukodystrophies
C. Neuronal degeneration
D. Axonal dystrophies

Disorders of Organogenesis: Disorders of Neural Tube Closure

Disorders of Neural Tube Closure

Disorders of neural tube closure and dorsal induction are the earliest CNS anomalies, occurring within the third and fourth gestational weeks.

A. *Chiari malformations* (I-IV) are a group of unrelated anomalies initially described by Chiari. Originally three types of hindbrain malformations with hydrocephalus were delineated; later severe cerebellar hypoplasia was added as a fourth category. Chiari I and II are relatively common; Chiari III (Chiari II plus encephalocele) is very rare; Chiari IV may not exist as a separate, distinct entity.
  1. Chiari I (Fig. 1)
      a. Tonsillar ectopia (deformed cerebellar tonsils displaced downwards below foramen magnum into upper cervical canal). Not associated with other brain anomalies.
        - tonsillar ectopia of 3-4 mm of uncertain clinical significance; > 5mm often symptomatic.
        - associated syringohydromyelia in 20-25%
        - mild-moderate hydrocephalus 20-25%
        - cranio-vertebral junction anomalies frequent
          - basilar impression 25%
          - C1 to occiput assimilation 10%
          - Klippel-Feil 10%
          - incomplete ossification C1 ring 5%
        - *not* associated with myelomeningocele

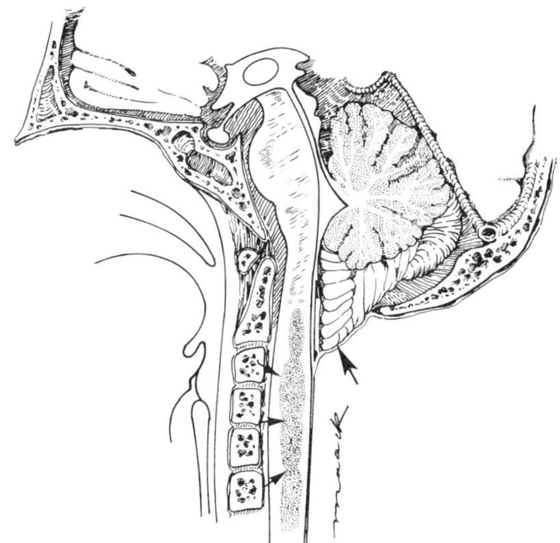

Figure 1. *CHIARI I. Anatomic drawing of Chiari I malformation, lateral view. Note low-lying, pointed cerebellar tonsils (large arrow) and syringohydromyelia of the cervical cord (small arrows).*

2. Chiari II malformation = complex malformation affecting spine, skull, dura, hindbrain. As opposed to Chiari I, Chiari II is almost always associated with some form of spinal dysraphism and meningocele or myelomeningocele and hydrocephalus. There is a high incidence of associated supratentorial anomalies. Abnormalities in Chiari II are numerous and complex; a broad spectrum of radiologic findings may therefore be present in varying degrees or combinations.

   a. Skull and dural abnormalities: (Figs 2, 3)
      - lueckenschaedel: dysplasia of membranous bone resulting in scalloped calvarial thinning. Accompanies and is not caused by the malformation. Rarely prominent after 6 months of age.
      - low-lying torcular and transverse sinuses with small, shallow posterior fossa
      - gaping foramen magnum
      - varying degrees of falx hypoplasia or fenestration with interdigitated gyri give scalloped or serrated appearance to interhemispheric fissure.

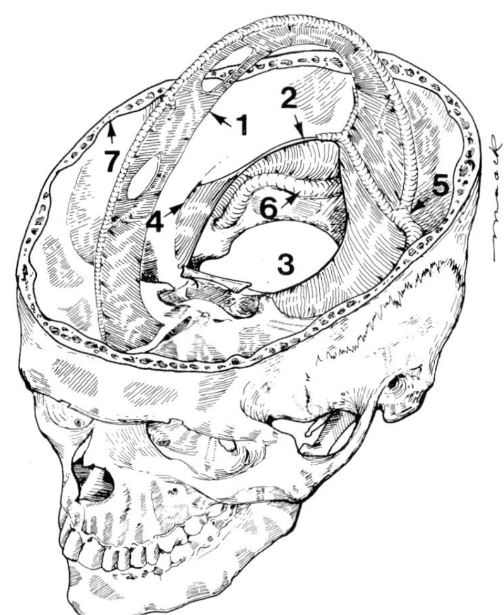

Figure 2. *CHIARI II: SKULL, DURA. Anatomic drawing of the skull and dural abnormalities seen in the Chiari II malformation.* (1) *hypoplastic, fenestrated falx cerebri,* (2) *"heart-shaped" tentorial incisura with towering apex,* (3) *gaping foramen magnum,* (4) *concave petrous ridges,* (5) *low-lying torcular herephili,* (6) *low-lying transverse sinuses,* (7) *residual calvarial thinning (lueckenschaedel)*

- petrous bones, clivus may appear concave posteriorly
- tentorial hypoplasia with wide, broad incisura; vermis and cerebellum bulge upwards through tentorial notch ("cerebellar pseudotumor")

b. Hindbrain and cerebellar abnormalities (Figs 4-6)
  - hindbrain dysgenesis results in downward displacement of medulla and cerebellum
  - medullary kinking (70%)
  - tectal beaking
  - anteromedial growth of cerebellum around sides of brainstem.

c. Ventricles and cisterns (Fig. 4)
  - lateral ventricles vary in size from normal to markedly dilated, are frequently asymmetric with colpocephaly (prominent occipital horns), anterior

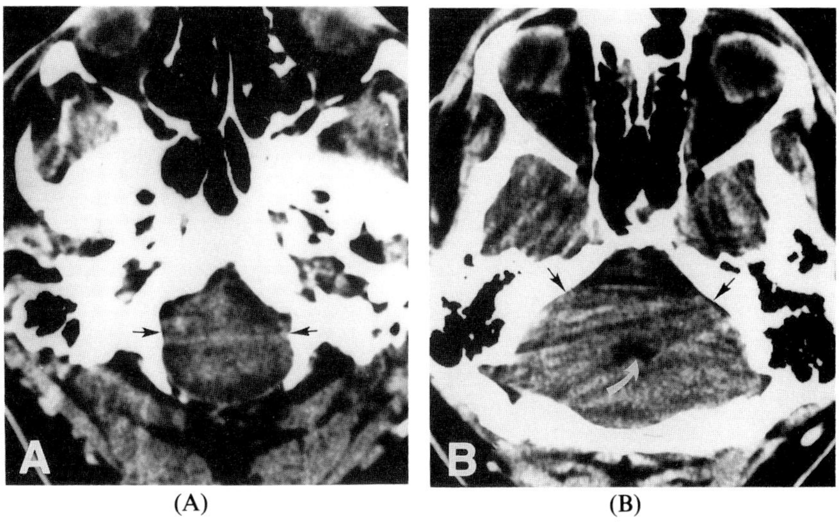

(A)   (B)

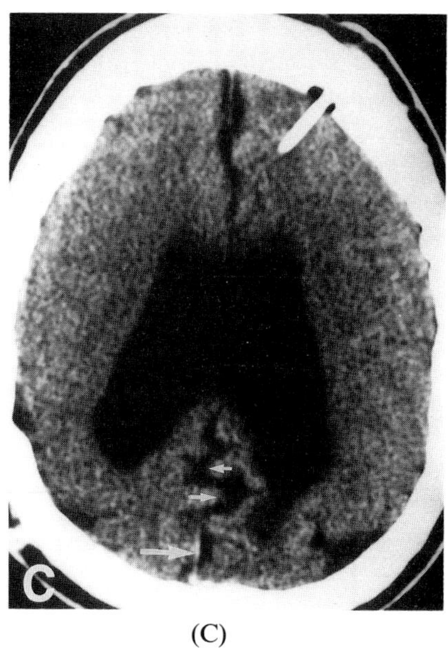

(C)

Figure 3. *CHIARI II. Axial CT scans in a patient with Chiari II malformation show gaping foramen magnum filled with soft tissue (A, arrows), concave temporal bones (B, black arrows) and low-lying deformed fourth ventricle (B, white arrow), hypoplastic falx (C, large white arrow) permits gyri to interdigitate (C, small arrows)*

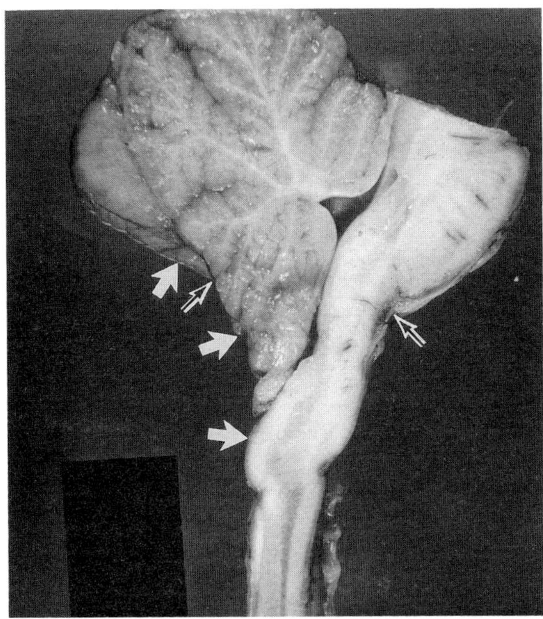

Figure 4. *CHIARI II: HINDBRAIN. Gross pathology of the hindbrain in Chiari II malformation, mid-sagittal section. The fourth ventricle is small, elongated and low-lying. The level of the foramen magnum is indicated by the outlined arrows. The cerebellar tonsils extend inferiorly into the upper cervical canal and, together with the kinked medulla, form a "cascade" of tissues (white arrows) posteriorly along the dorsal surface of the midbrain and spinal cord (specimen courtesy of Dr Lester Alvord).*

and inferior pointing and concavity of frontal horns. Ventricles therefore often have a scalloped appearance.
- third ventricle often enlarged with deformed anterior recesses, enlarged massa intermedia.
- septum pellucidum frequently absent or fenestrated
- fourth ventricle is often elongated and small, displaced caudally
- serrated, often enlarged interhemispheric fissure
- aqueductal stenosis or occlusion may be associated

d. Parenchymal abnormalities
- microgyria/stenogyria
- gray matter heterotopias

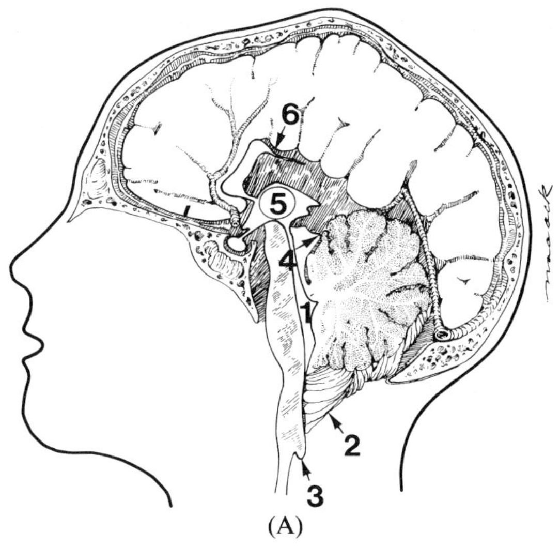

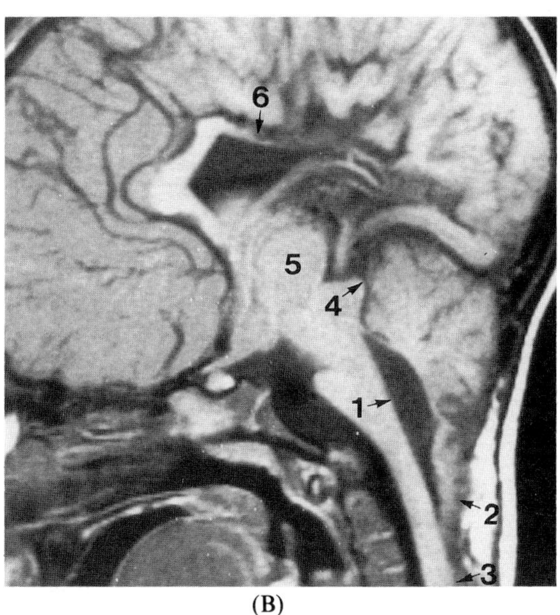

Figure 5. *CHIARI II: HINDBRAIN, VENTRICLES. (A) Anatomic drawing of the Chiari II malformation. (B) Sagittal T1-weighted MR scan of the Chiari II malformation. (1) elongated, low-lying fourth ventricle, (2) pointed, inferiorly displaced tonsils, (3) kinked medulla, (4) beaked tectum, (5) large massa intermedia, (6) partial agenesis of corpus callosum*

    e. Spine and cord. Spinal dysraphism, usually myelomeningocele, virtually always present in some form.
- lumbosacral myelomeningocele in 75%, cervico-thoracic 25%
- syringohydromyelia
- tethered cord usually with lipoma
- diastematomyelia may be associated

    f. Associated anomalies
- corpus callosum anomalies 80-90% (usually partially absent/hypoplastic)

3. Chiari III. Chiari II with low occipital or high cervical encephalocele. Very rare.

4. Chiari IV. Severe cerebellar hypoplasia. Very rare and may not exist as a distinct, separate entity. Findings include absent/hypoplastic cerebellum, small brain stem, large posterior fossa CSF spaces.

B. *Anomalies of the corpus callosum.* The corpus callosum develops during the third and fourth months of fetal life, mostly forming from front to back (exception: rostrum forms last). Agenesis may be complete (Fig. 6) or partial (if partial, genu always present; splenium and/or rostrum absent). Callosal abnormalities are often associated (up to 50%) with other CNS malformations such as gray matter abnormalities (heterotopias, polymicrogyria), Chiari or Dandy-Walker malformations, lipomas, cephaloceles, interhemispheric arachnoid cysts, etc. The classic neuroradiologic findings in corpus callosum agenesis follow (Fig. 7):

1. Lateral ventricles: Frontal horns, bodies widely separated and parallel (not converging). Pointed, sharply angled frontal horns and bodies. Occipital horns frequently disproportionately enlarged ("colpocephaly"). Concave medial borders of lateral ventricles due to protrusion of longitudinal Probst bundles.

2. Third ventricle: Usually somewhat dilated and elevated with varying degree of dorsal extension and interposition between lateral ventricles. Foramen of Monro often elongated.

3. Miscellaneous: Interhemispheric fissure (IHF) appears to be continuous with anterior third ventricle because genu is absent. In coronal views, IHF extends inferiorly between

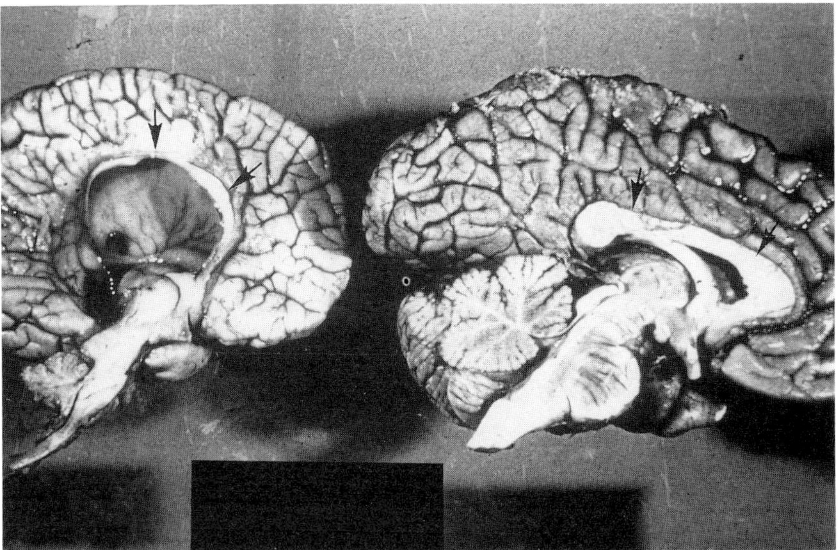

Figure 6. *AGENESIS OF CORPUS CALLOSUM. On the left is a mid-sagittal section of a patient with Chiari II malformation and agenesis of the corpus callosum. The curved paramedian structure indicated by the black arrows is the fornix. Compare with the normal corpus callosum on the right, also indicated by black arrows (from the archives of the Armed Forces Institute of Pathology, Washington, D.C.)*

lateral ventricles to roof of third. In sagittal views, normal cingulate gyrus is absent and the media gyri and sulci have a radial or spoke-like configuration around the third ventricle. Interhemispheric CSF cysts are often seen projecting superiorly between the lateral ventricles. When large, these cysts may assume bizarre configurations, sometimes even obscuring the underlying malformations.

4. Associated anomalies
   - cephaloceles
   - lipoma
     - corpus callosum lipomas = 30% of intracranial lipomas; often associated with callosal anomalies
     - not a true tumor but a brain malformation
     - curvilinear Ca^{++} often present
     - prominent vessels often course through callosal lipoma

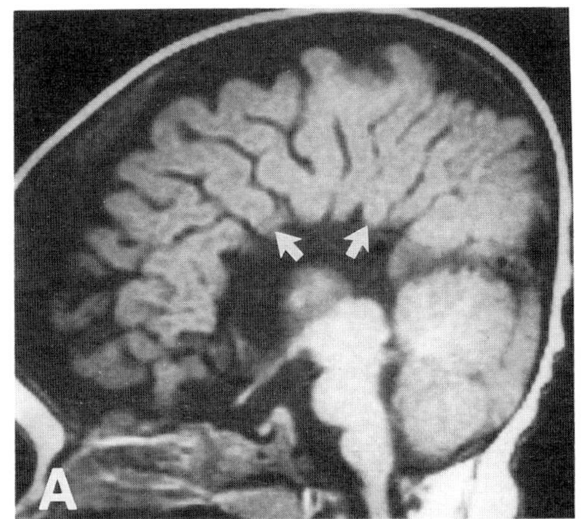

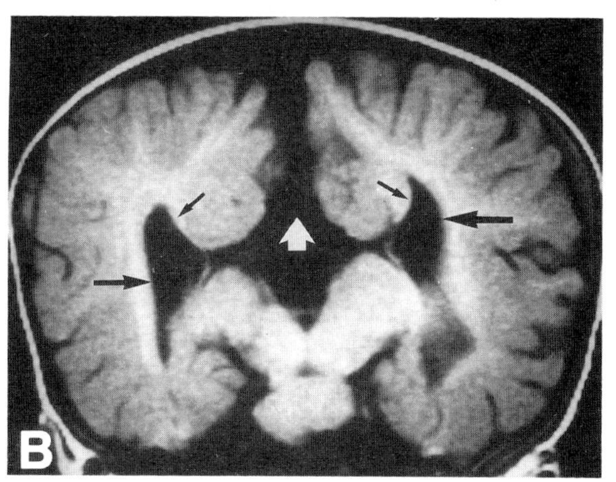

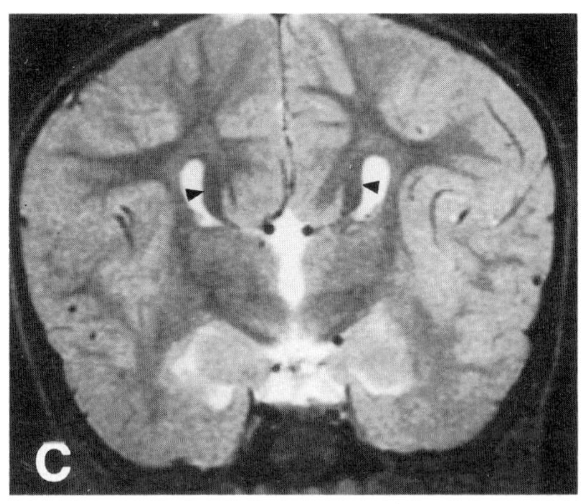

5. Note: An enlarged hippocampal commissure can be seen in some cases of callosal agenesis, mimicking the splenium. A splenium-like bundle of interhemispheric fiber tracts can be seen in some cases of lobar holoprosencephaly. Prognosis varies strikingly (good in former, poor in latter).

C. Dandy-Walker complex (D-W) is a hindbrain congenital malformation characterized by cystic dilatation of the fourth ventricle, associated with varying degrees of vermian aplasia or hypoplasia (Fig. 8). Exact origin of D-W is unknown but theories include failure of development of the anterior medullary velum (embryonic roof of the fourth ventricle), atresia of the outlet foramina, delayed opening of the foramen of Magendie, and insult (of varying severity) to both the developing cerebellar hemispheres and fourth ventricle. The cerebellar hemispheres are usually small. Radiographic features may include some or all of the following (Fig. 9):
1. Large fluid-filled fourth ventricle/cisterna magna complex
2. Large posterior fossa with torcular lying above the lambda (high tentorium)
3. Varying amounts of cerebellar, vermian hypoplasia.
4. Varying degrees of third and lateral ventricular dilatation.
5. Associated abnormalities in > 60% of cases
   * hydrocephalus (75%)
   * corpus callosum dysgenesis (20-25%), with or without interhemispheric cyst
   * polymicrogyria, gray matter heterotopias (5-10%)
   * occipital cephaloceles (< 5%)
   * polydactyly, cardiac anomalies

Figure 7. *AGENESIS OF CORPUS CALLOSUM. (A) Sagittal T1-weighted MR scan in a patient with complete agenesis of the corpus callosum. Note radial or "spoke-like" arrangement of gyri (arrows). (B) Coronal T1-weighted scan in another patient with complete callosal agenesis. The lateral ventricles (large black arrows) are widely spaced and the "high-riding" third ventricle is in continuity superiorly with the interhemispheric fissure (large white arrow). The longitudinally oriented white matter tracts or "Probst bundles" (small black arrows) indent the medial aspects of the lateral ventricles. (C) Coronal T2-weighted scan in still another patient clearly demonstrates the bundles of Probst, seen here as the low signal white matter structures (arrowheads) indenting the lateral ventricles.*

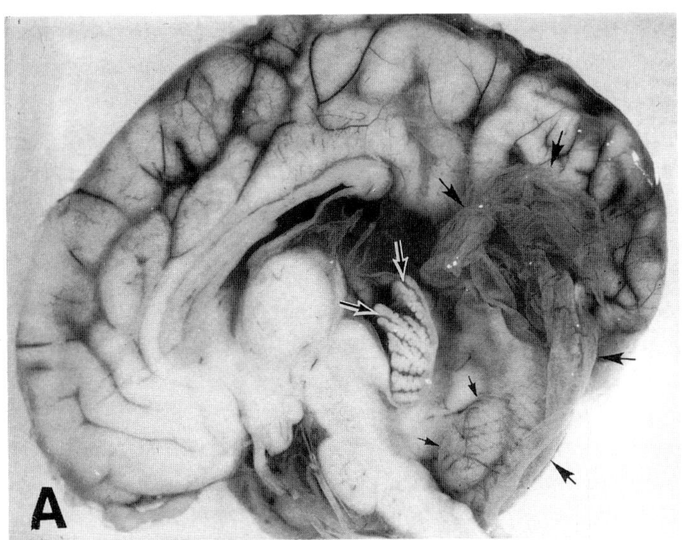

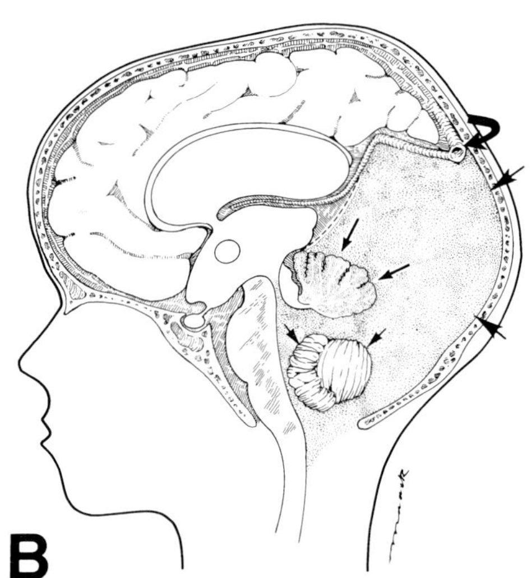

Figure 8. DANDY-WALKER MALFORMATION. Gross specimen (A) and anatomic drawing (B) of Dandy-Walker malformation; mid-sagittal view. A large posterior fossa cyst is indicated by the large black arrows. Only a small part of the anterior vermis is present (outlined arrows); note eversion, elevation and upwards displacement of its few remaining lobules. The cerebellar hemispheres (small black arrows) are hypoplastic and appear to "float" within the cyst. Note elevation of the torcular (B, curved arrow) above the lambda (not shown). (Case courtesy of Dr Lester Alvord).

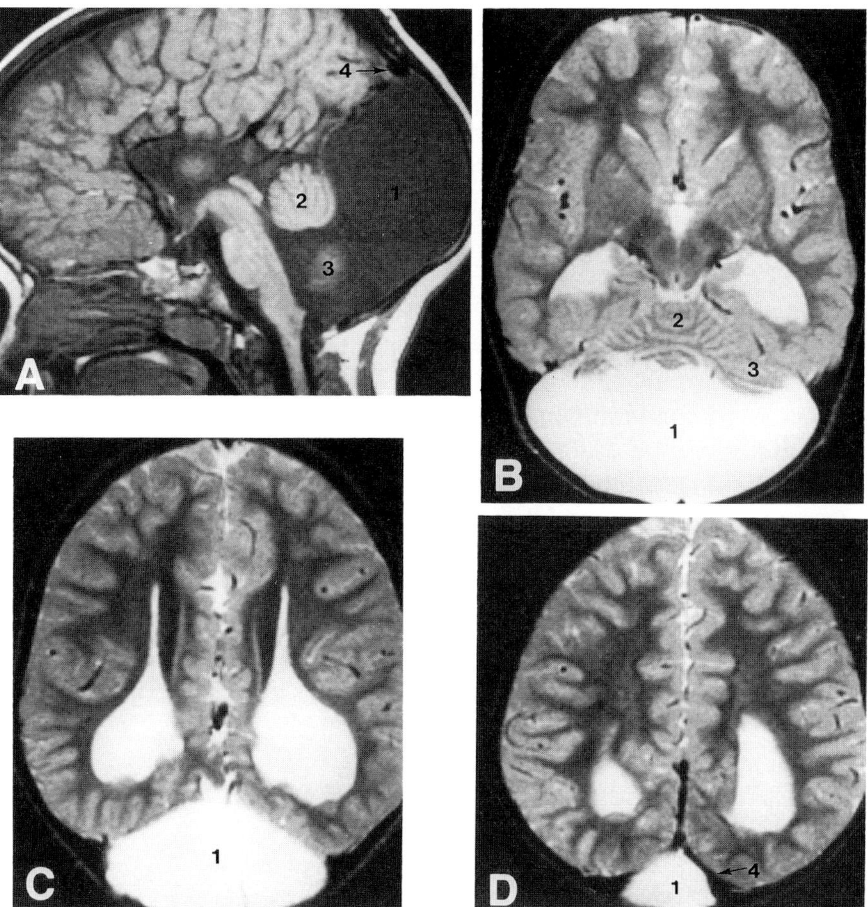

Figure 9. *DANDY-WALKER MALFORMATION. Six-year old girl with Dandy-Walker malformation and co-existing agenesis of the corpus callosum. A = sagittal T1-weighted MR scans; B-D = axial T2-weighted scans. (1) posterior fossa cyst, (2) hypoplastic, everted vermis, (3) small cerebellar hemisphere remnants, (4) high torcular heroptrili.*

6. Differential diagnosis: Retrocerebellar arachnoid cyst (vermis present, displaced but normally formed fourth ventricle). "Mega cisterna magna" (normal positioned torcula Herophili, normal vermis and cerebellum) is probably just a mild variant of the D-W complex. Ventricular or cyst shunting can lead to confusing CT or MR findings so preoperative studies may be necessary for correct diagnosis.

7. To emphasize: the so-called "Dandy-Walker variant" and "mega cistern magna" probably represent points on spectrum of posterior fossa cystic malformation and are not separate entities.

Disorders of Histogenesis: Neurocutaneous Syndromes

Dyshistogenetic disorders include such abnormalities as tuberous sclerosis, neurofibromatosis, von Hippel-Lindau disease and Sturge-Weber syndrome in addition to congenital vascular malformations and possibly congenital neoplasms as well. Only the neurocutaneous syndromes will be discussed here.

The neurocutaneous syndromes are congenital hereditary CNS disorders that affect mainly ectodermal structures and have characteristic associated skin manifestations. Sometimes termed "phakomatoses" (Greek for a lentil-shaped object or spot), they are characterized by the presence of tumor-like malformations with blastomatous tendencies and pigment patches or angiomatoma in tissues of ectodermal origin, particularly the skin and the peripheral and central nervous systems. Included in this interesting disease spectrum are neurofibromatosis (NF), tuberous sclerosis (TS), Sturge-Weber syndrome, and von Hippel-Lindau disease. Miscellaneous less common phakomatoses such as basal cell nevus syndrome and ataxia-telangiectasia also occur. While the manifestations of these disorders are often protean, only the CNS, spine, and skull abnormalities are summarized here.

Neurofibromatosis

At least eight separate forms of neurofibromatosis (NF) (see Table 1) have been described although two types, von Recklinghausen's disease (NF-1) and neurofibromatosis with bilateral acoustic schwannomas (NF-2) are generally agreed upon. The terms "central" and "peripheral" neurofibromatosis should be discarded because they are inaccurate; *both* NF-1 and NF-2 show central nervous system involvement. These neurofibromatosis disorders represent dyshistogenesis of neuroectodermal and mesodermal tissue. Inheritance is autosomal dominant with no sex predilection.

Recently the chromosomal loci for both NF-1 and NF-2 have been pinpointed and the unusual gene responsible for NF-1 isolated.

A. von Recklinghausen's disease (NF-1) seems to be associated with tumors of neurons and astrocytes
  1. Incidence: approximately 1 in 4,000 newborns affected; more than 90% of all NF cases are NF-1
  2. Inheritance:
     - autosomal dominant
     - no sex linkage
     - chromosome 17
     - responsible gene has been isolated
  3. Diagnostic criteria for NF-1 include two or more of these findings:
     - six or more 5 mm or larger cafe-au-lait spots
     - either one plexiform neurofibroma or two or more neurofibromas of any type
     - two or more pigmented iris hamartomas (so-called "Lisch nodules")
     - axillary/inguinal freckling
     - optic nerve glioma
     - first-degree relative with NF-1
     - presence of characteristic bone lesion (e.g., dysplasia of greater sphenoid wing) (Fig. 10)
  4. CNS manifestations in 15-20% of patients with NF-1.
     a. skull lesions (Fig. 10)
        - macrocrania frequent
        - abnormal calcifications
        - hypoplasia of greater sphenoid wing with temporal lobe herniation into orbit, pulsatile exophthalmus (Fig. 10)
        - calvarial defects (e.g., lambdoid suture)
        - can have enlarged internal auditory canals without facial or acoustic nerve masses (from dural ectasia)
     b. optic nerve glioma (ONG) (see Table 1)
        - most common CNS tumor in NF-1 (Fig. 11)
        - lesions can involve one or both optic nerves, chiasm, tracts, lateral geniculate body, optic radiations (Fig. 12)

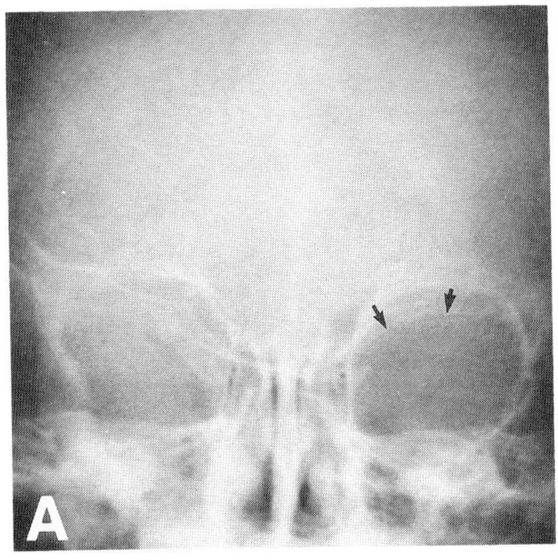

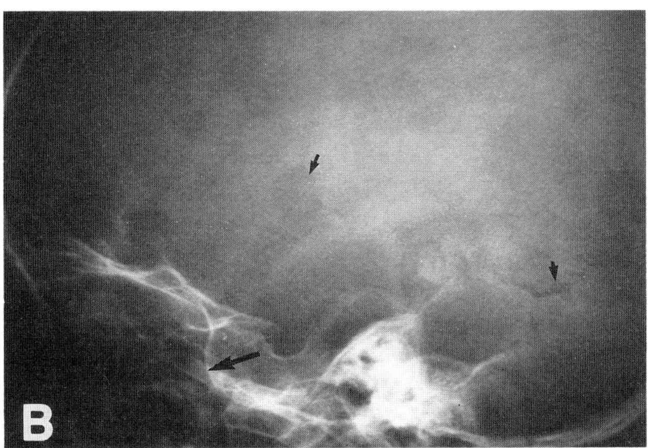

Figure 10. *NEUROFIBROMATOSIS TYPE 1. AP (A) and lateral (B) skull films in a patient with von Recklinghausen's disease (NF-1). Note characteristic bone lesions: absent left greater sphenoid wing (A, arrows) and sutural defects (B, small arrows); on the lateral view only one sphenoid wing is seen (B, large arrow) because the other is absent.*

Table 1. *Neurofibromatosis (NF): comparison between NF-1 and NF-2*

	NF-1		NF-2
1.	von Recklinghausen's disease	1.	Bilateral acoustics schwannomas
2.	1/4000 (represents 90% of NF cases)	2.	1/150,000 (<10% of NF cases)
3.	Chromosome 17	3.	Chromosome 22
4.	Prominent skin manifestations	4.	Minimal skin changes
5.	Associated with tumors of neurons (hamartomas) and astrocytes (gliomas), plexiform neurofibromas, malignant nerve sheath tumors; dual ecstasias	5.	Associated with tumors of meninges (meningiomas) and Schwann cells (cranial nerve schwannomas)
6.	Spinal neurofibromas (usually small, single)	6.	Spinal schwannomas (often large, bilateral, multilevel)
7.	Questionable whether these patients develop spinal gliomas	7.	Spinal ependymomas astrocytomas a prominent feature

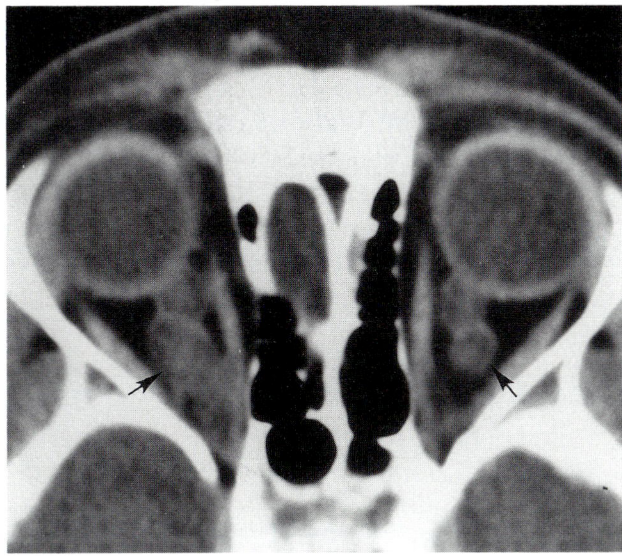

Figure 11. *NEUROFIBROMATOSIS TYPE 1. Axial CT scan in a patient with NF-1, bilateral optic nerve gliomas (arrows)*

- mean age of NF-1 patients with ONG = 5 y; ONG without NF = 12 y
- most are relatively benign histologically (low grade astrocytoma)
- skull films: may show one or both optic canals enlarged
- CT: enlargement of optic nerve sheath complex (Fig. 11)
- MR: lesions are iso/slightly hypointense on T1WI, mildly to strongly hyperintense on T2WI. Often seen on T2WI are other high signal areas without mass effect in basal ganglia, internal capsule, pons, cerebral peduncles, cerebellum, etc. These may be slightly hyperintense on T1WI also and probably represent hamartomas (Fig. 12). Enhancement following contrast administration should raise the suspicion of neoplasm.

   c. nonoptic gliomas: gliomas (most commonly low grade astrocytomas) occur with increased frequency in NF-1; common locations are the tectal and periaquiductal regions, brain stem, etc. Occasionally anaplastic astrocytoma or glioblastoma multiforme may develop (Fig. 13).

   d. nonglial neoplasms: not a feature of NF-1

   e. vascular abnormalities: Dysplastic stenosis of vessels at/near circle of Willis, intra/extracranial aneurysms

   f. cranial nerve tumors: Schwannomas of cranial nerves III-XIII are a feature of NF-2, not NF-1. Optic nerve (CNII) neoplasms are histologically brain neoplasms; CN1 (olfactory) is also anatomically a brain tract, not a nerve and does not give rise to schwannomas.

   g. plexiform neurofibromas: Exocranial origin but often extend intracranially along natural foramina, fissures (e.g., from orbit, pterygopalatine fossa into cavernous sinus) (Figs 14-15)

   h. malignant peripheral nerve sheath tumors 5-10%

5. Spine manifestations

   a. kyphoscoliosis in 1/3-1/2 of patients (Fig. 16)
- probably reflects primary mesodermal dysplasia
- T3-T7 most common

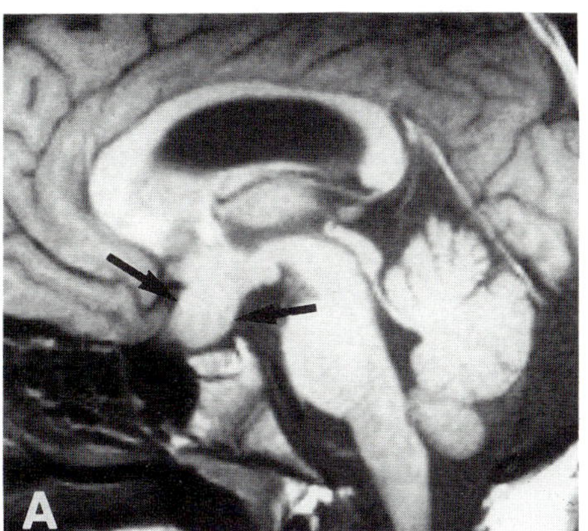
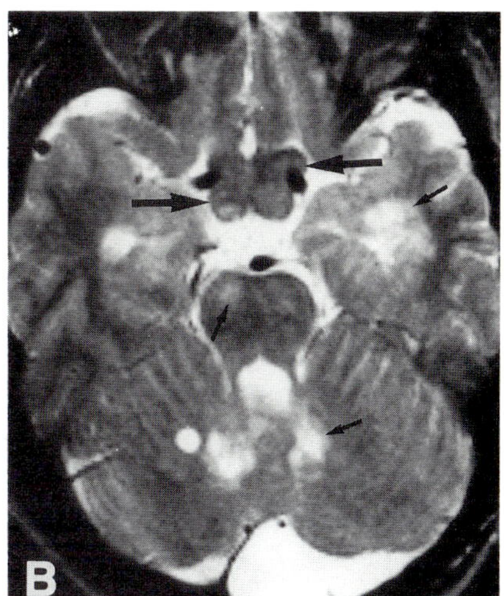
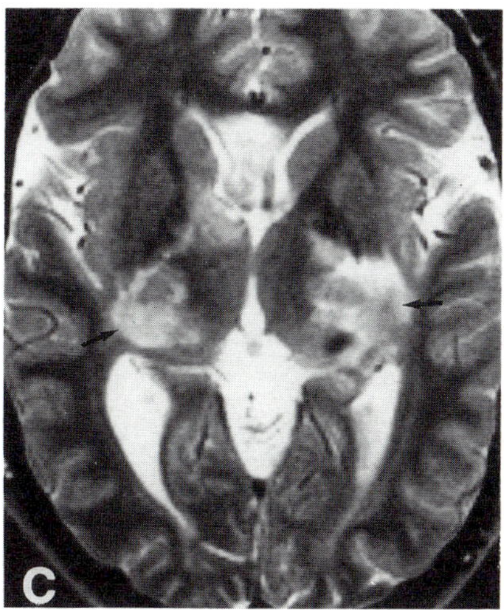

Figure 12. *NEUROFIBROMATOSIS TYPE 1. Five-year-old child with NF-1. Glioma of the optic nerves and chiasm (large arrows) is seen in the sagittal T1 (A) and axial T2-weighted MR scan. Multiple foci of increased signal on T2-weighted images (B, C, small arrows) are often seen in NF-1. Most of these are benign and tend to diminish as the patient ages.*

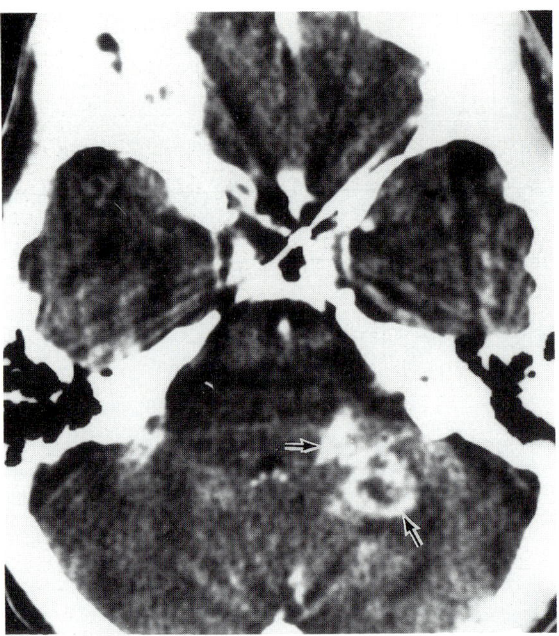

Figure 13. *NEUROFIBROMATOSIS TYPE 1. Axial post-contrast CT scan in a 30-year-old male with NF-1, previous resection of a left optic nerve glioma. Biopsy of the posterior fossa mass (arrows) disclosed glioblastoma multiforme. (Note: gliomas associated with NF-1 are more often low-grade neoplasms.)*

- short segment angular deformities
- usually mild but occasionally can be rapidly progressive, resulting in paraplegia

b. posterior vertebral body scalloping, pedicle erosion (Fig. 16)
  - usually multilevel
  - most often due to dural ectasia
  - "dumbbell" spinal neurofibromas in 13-20%
  - 3% have plexiform neurofibroma causing enlargement

c. lateral meningoceles (Fig. 17)
  - probably caused by weakened, dysplastic meninges that protrude through enlarged intervertebral foramina (pulsion diverticulae)
  - thoracic most common, usually on right side; lumbosacral, cervical occur but are less common

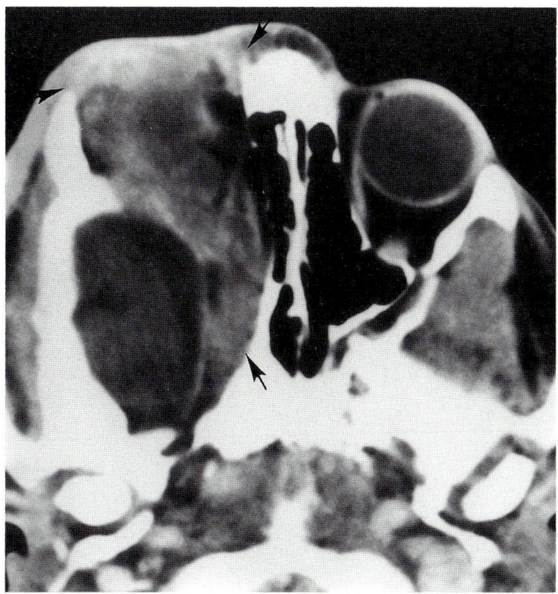

Figure 14. *NEUROFIBROMATOSIS TYPE 1. Axial contrast-enhanced CT scan in a patient with known NF-1. Note hypoplasia of the right greater sphenoid wing. An extensive cutaneous plexiform neurofibroma is present that also involves the orbit and cavernous sinus (arrows).*

- CT: dumbbell-shaped CSF-attenuation lesion protrudes through enlarged neural foramen with adjacent thinned pedicle, scalloped vertebral body
- MR: CSF signal on all sequences

B. Neurofibromatosis with bilateral acoustic neurinomas (NF-2) seems to be associated with tumors of the meninges and schwann cells (Fig. 18)

   1. Incidence: Approximately 1 in 50,000 (much less common than NF-1)

   2. Inheritance
- autosomal dominant
- no sex linkage
- chromosome 22

   3. Diagnostic criteria are one or more of the following:

     a. bilateral eighth nerve masses *or*

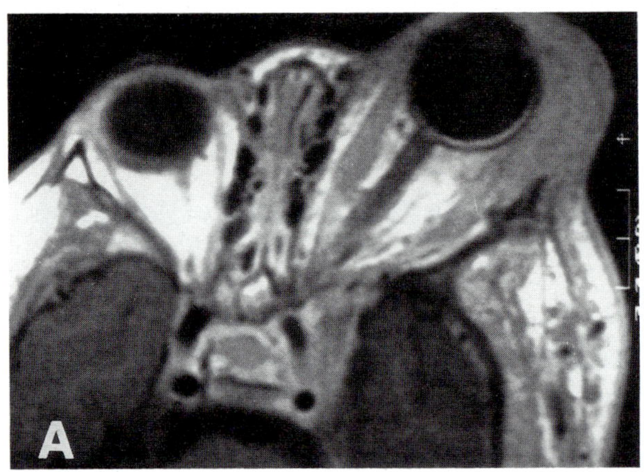

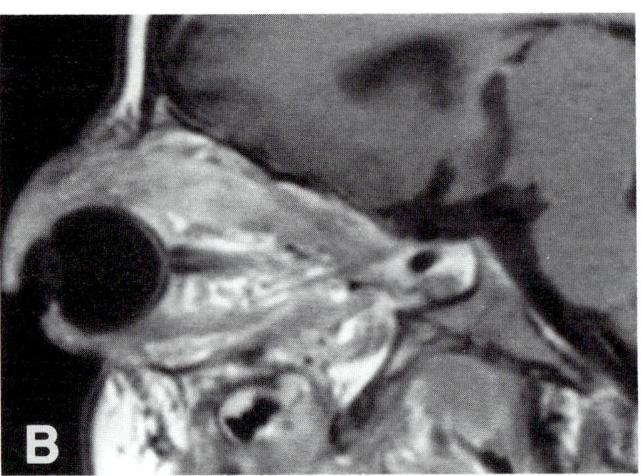

Figure 15. *NEUROFIBROMATOSIS TYPE 1. Axial (A) and sagittal (B) post-contrast T1-weighted scans in a 5-year-old girl with NF-1 and an extensive plexiform neurofibroma that involves the lid and orbit and extends posteriorly through an enlarged orbital fissure into the cavernous sinus (case courtesy of Dr S. Sagon, Bethesda Naval Hospital).*

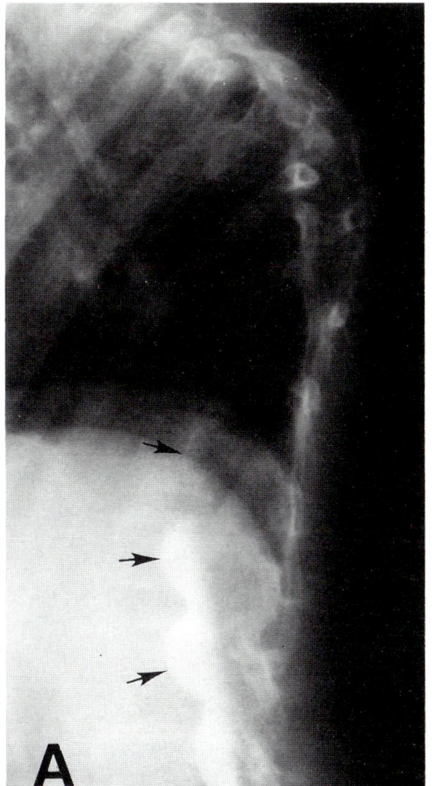
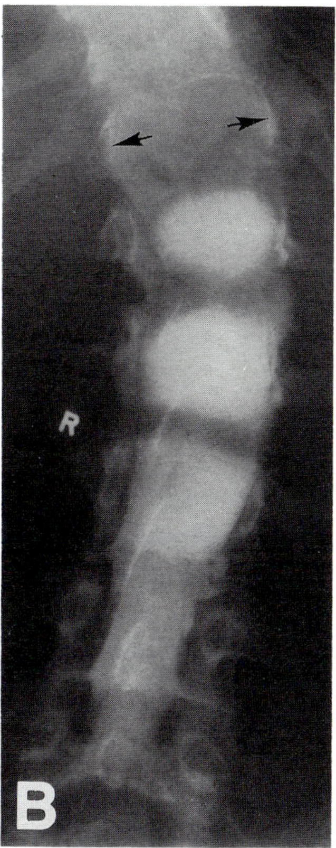

Figure 16. *NEUROFIBROMATOSIS TYPE 1. Lateral (A) and AP (B) views of a lumbar myelogram in a patient with NF-1 and acute kyphoscoliosis. Marked posterior vertebral scalloping and extreme dural ectasia are present (A, arrows). Note thinned pedicles, widened canal (B, arrows). No neurofibromas are identified.*

    b.   first degree relative with NF-2 and either unilateral eight nerve mass or any two of the following: neurofibroma, meningioma, glioma, schwannoma, or juvenile posterior subcapsular lenticular opacity

4. Cutaneous manifestations much less common than with NF-1, therefore NF-2 patients often older when initially diagnosed.
   - few/small pale cafe-au-lait spots
   - minimal/absent cutaneous neurofibromas
   - no lisch nodules

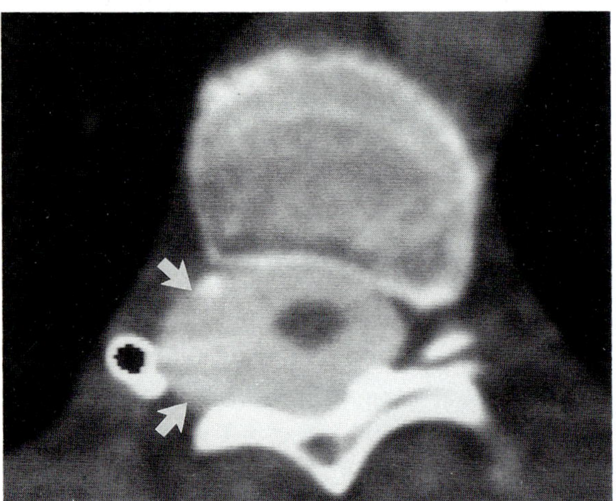

Figure 17. *NEUROFIBROMATOSIS TYPE 1. Post-contrast CT scan in a patient with NF-1 shows a small lateral thoracic meningocele (arrows).*

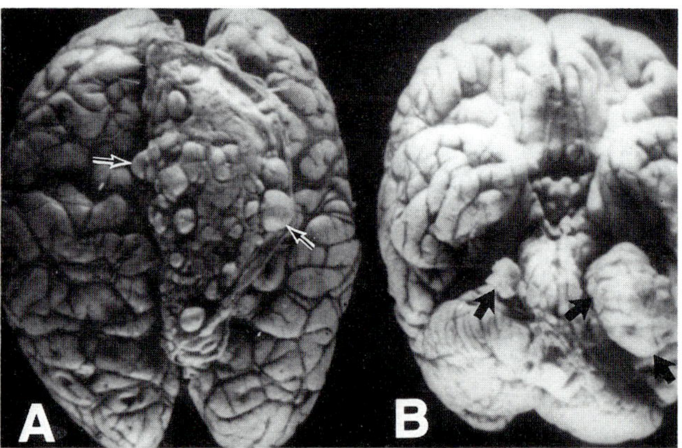

Figure 18. *NEUROFIBROMATOSIS TYPE 2. Gross specimen from a patient with Type 2 neuro- fibromatosis (NF-2). (A) Viewed superiorly. Note multiple convexity and falx meningiomas (outlined arrows). (B) Viewed from below. Note bilateral acoustic neuromas (black arrows) (from the archives of the Armed Forces Institute of Pathology, Washington, D.C.).*

5. CNS manifestations (Fig. 19)
   a. vestibulocochlear schwannomas (N.B. - dural ectasia without acoustic neurinomas can widen the internal auditory canals in these patients)
   b. schwannomas of other cranial nerves (III-XII)
   c. solitary/multiple meningiomas (both spinal, intracranial)
   d. other tumors
      * questionable whether patients with NF-2 develop intracranial gliomas
      * astrocytomas of cord
      * ependymomas of cord (most common intrinsic cord neoplasm in NF-2)
   e. multiple paraspinal schwannomas (often large, bilateral multilevel) (Figs. 20, 21)

Sturge-Weber Syndrome (SWS)

(Also known as encephalotrigeminal angiomatosis). "Sporadic, port-wine" vascular nevus flammeus in CNV distribution (part or all of face, may involve sclera), leptomeningeal venous angiomatosis, seizures, dementia, mental retardation, hemiparesis, hemianopsia, congenital glaucoma and buphthalmos ("cow-eye") and visceral angiomas can all be features of this disease.

A. General (Fig. 22)
   1. Pathology: May be due to faulty development of venous drainage with resulting venous angioma confined to pial layer of leptomeninges; ipsilateral choroid plexus of lateral ventricle often also involved; 30% have ocular choroidal angioma, glaucoma; 15% have buphthalmos
   2. Intracranial lesions typically unilateral, ipsilateral to facial nerve but can be bilateral, occasionally even contralateral
B. Imaging findings: It is typically the sequelae of the angiomatous malformations, not the malformation itself, that are visualized
   1. Skull films (Fig. 23)
      a. curvilinear/gyriform calcifications, most often parieto-occipital area
      b. ipsilateral calvarial thickening, enlarged sinuses and elevated petions ridge if affected hemisphere is severely atrophic

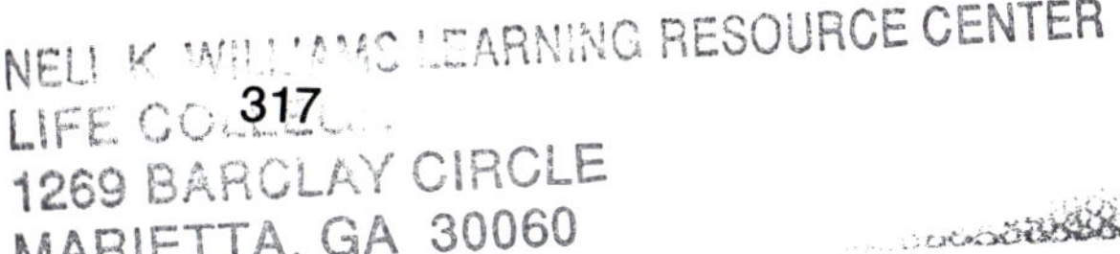

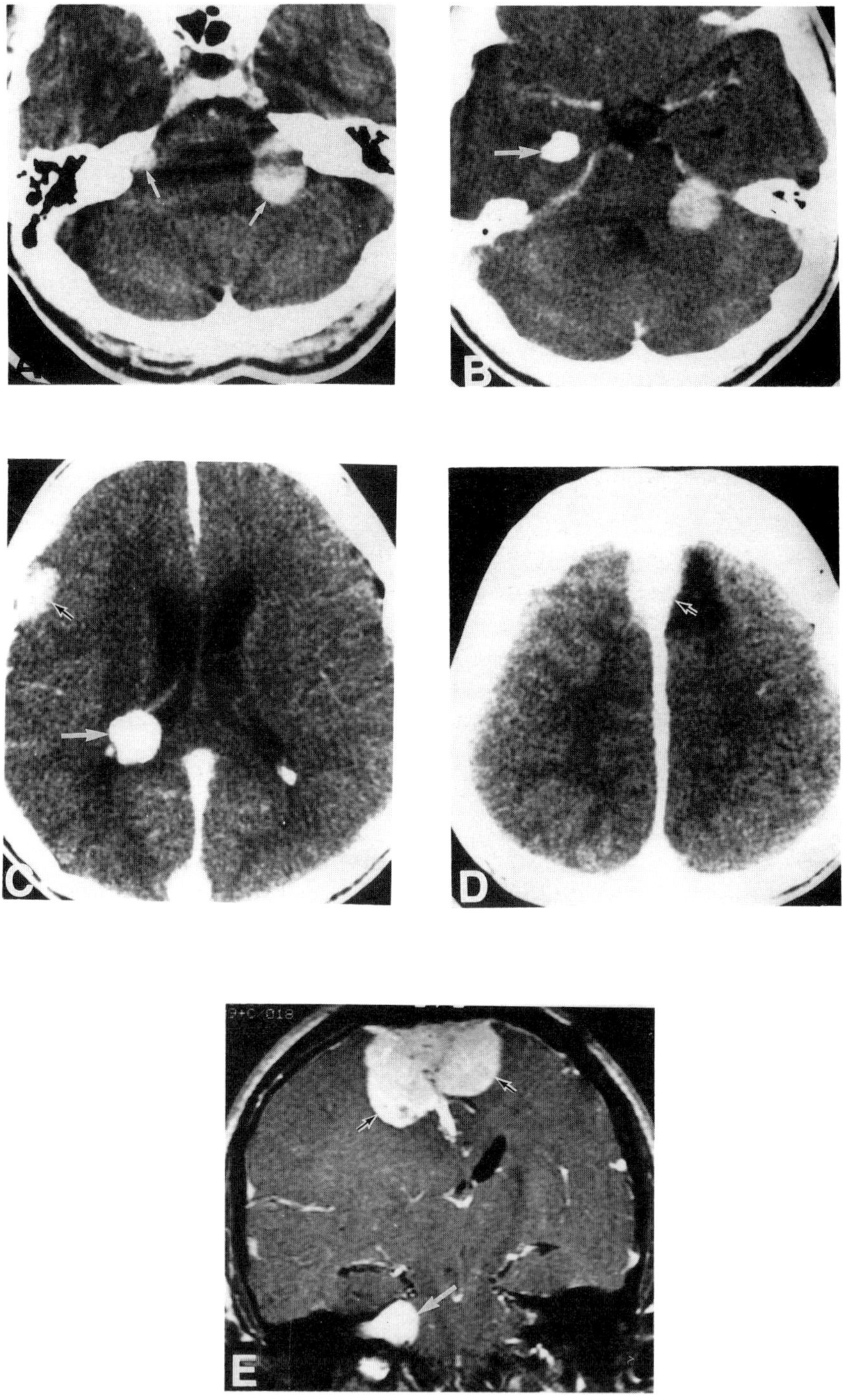

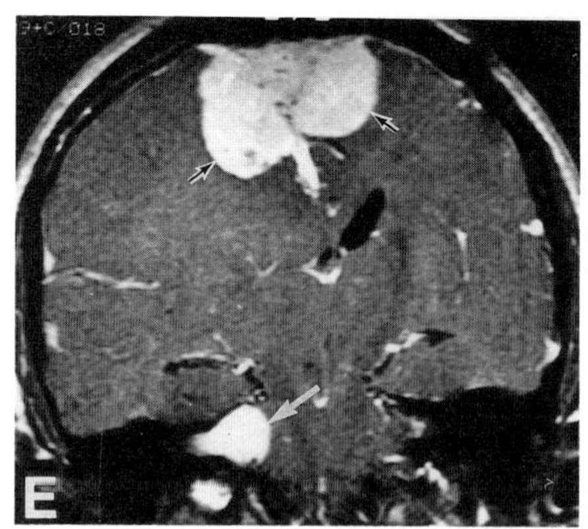

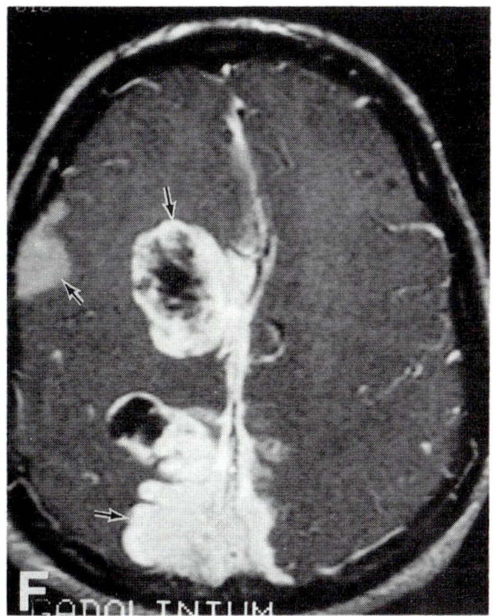
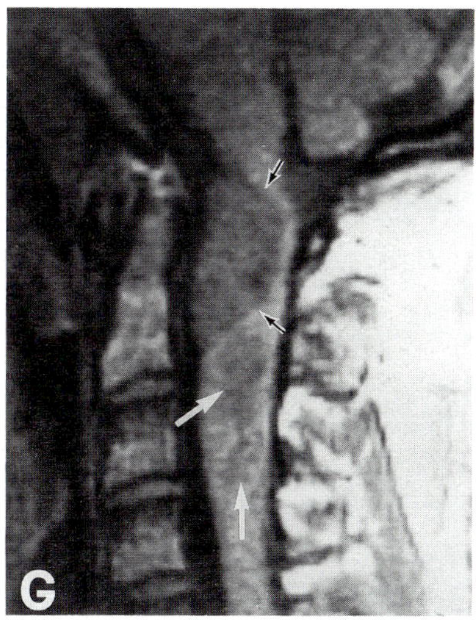

Figure 19. *NEUROFIBROMATOSIS TYPE 2. Nineteen-year-old male with NF-2. Contrast-enhanced CT scans show bilateral acoustic neuromas (A, small arrows), calcified choroid plexus (B, C solid arrows) and multiple meningiomas (C, D outlined arrows). MR scans were performed 4 years later after the left-sided acoustic neuromona was removed. Coronal (E) and axial (F) post-contrast T1-weighted MR scans show the right-sided acoustic neurinoma (solid arrow) and multiple meningiomas (outlined arrows) are more numerous and larger. Scan of the cervical spinal cord shows a meningioma (G, outlined arrows) and astrocytoma (G, solid arrows).*

2. CT
   a. calcification = most frequent findings in SWS
      - curvilinear calcifications following cerebral gyri
      - rarely seen before age 2
      - usually starts in occipital lobe
      - progresses anteriorly
      - located in dystrophic cerebral cortex underlying the pial angioma (possibly related to chronic hypoxia and/or venous infarctions), typically at the second/third cortical layers
      - bilateral in up to 20%, occasionally contralateral to facial lesion
   b. cerebral atrophy
      - usually unilateral, ipsilateral to facial nervus
      - typically occipital but can involve entire hemisphere

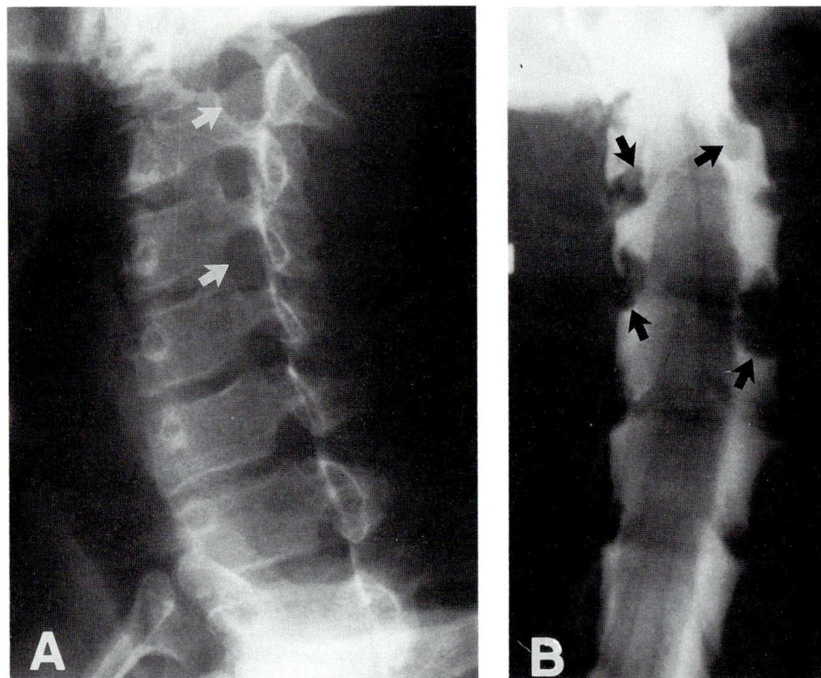

Figure 20. *NEUROFIBROMATOSIS TYPE 2. (A) Oblique plain film cervical spine radiograph in a twenty-three-year-old male with neurofibromatosis. Note multiple enlarged neural foramina (arrows). (B) Myelogram shows multiple extramedullary intradural filling defects (arrows). Presumed schwannomas, NF-2.*

    c.   gyral enhancement following contrast
    d.   enlarged, intensely enhancing ipsilateral choroid plexus in 75% (often hyperplasia although frank plexal angiomas have also been reported)
3. MR (Fig. 24):
    a.   hypointensity on T2WI in areas of cortical calcification can be seen
    b.   cerebral atrophy, miscellaneous parenchymal abnormalities
        • thickened diploe in overlying calvarium
        • widened sulci
        • some focal hyperintensities on T2WI may represent reactive gliosis of underlying white matter

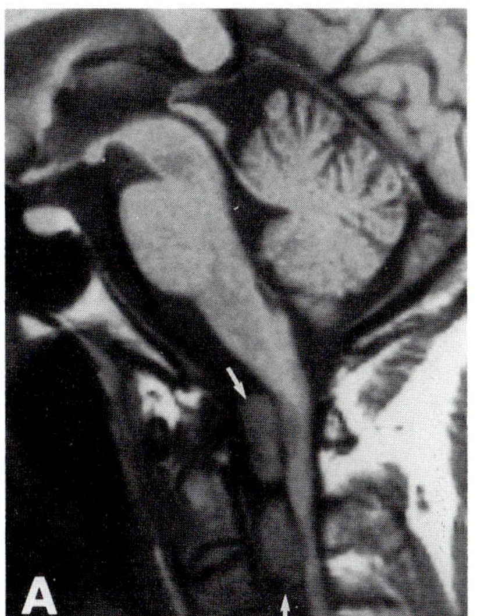
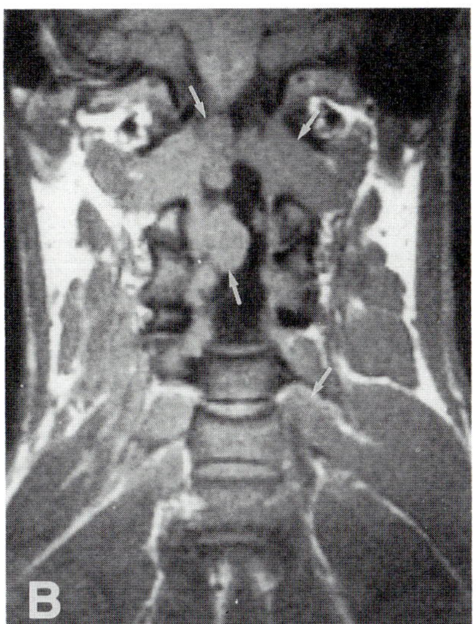
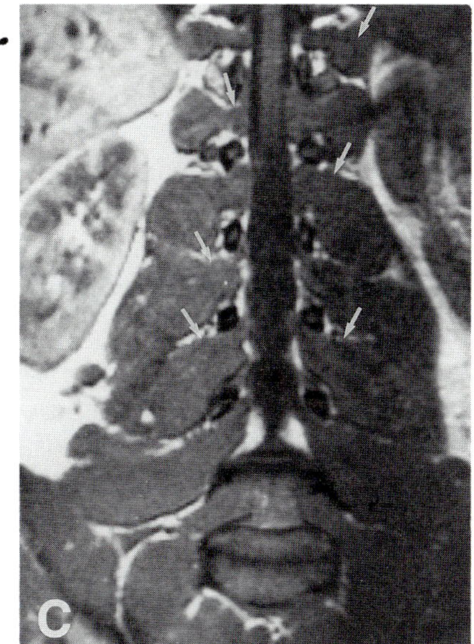

Figure 21. *NEUROFIBROMATOSIS TYPE 2. Twenty-year-old male with NF-2, multiple spinal nerve root schwannomas. Sagittal (A) and coronal cervical (B) and lumbar (C) MR scans show the lesions (a few are indicated by the arrows).*

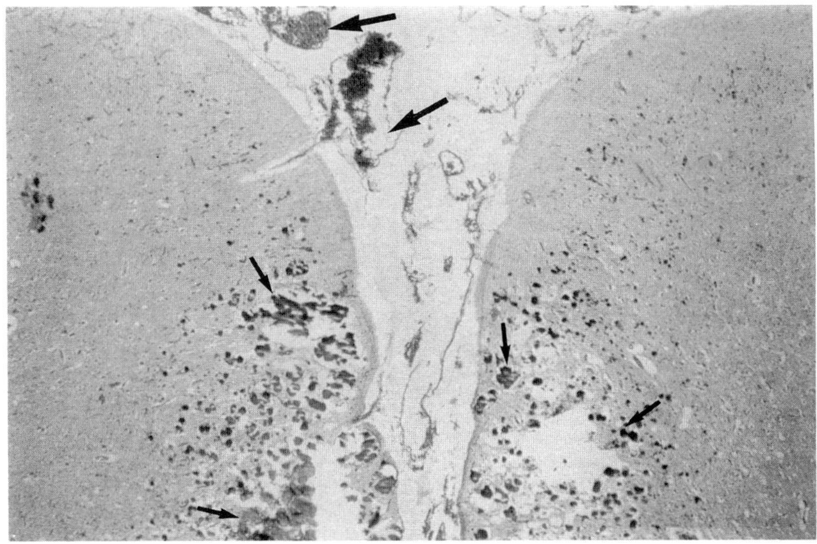

Figure 22. *STURGE-WEBER SYNDROME. Low-power Photomicrograph of Sturge-Weber Syndrome. The pial (leptomeningial) angioma (large black arrows) lies over the gyri in the subrachnoid space. The underlying cortex shows atrophy, encephalomalacic changes and dystrophic calcification (small black arrows).*

- calcifications may be effectively demonstrated with gradient echo scans
- c. enlarged enhancing choroid plexus in 75%
- d. gyral enhancement following contrast frequent, may be faint or striking
- e. collateral venous drainage may be manifested by enlarged tortuous medullary, subependymal veins
- f. accelerated myelination in some infants with SWS
4. Angiography
    - a. arterial phase normal
    - b. diffuse homogeneous capillary blush may be present; this is *not* the angioma itself but probably represents vascular stasis and delayed venous wash-out due to abnormal cortical venous drainage
    - c. paucity of superficial cortical draining veins, and are often dysplastic, sparse, bilateral and irregular
    - d. medullary (deep white matter) and subependymal veins enlarge to provide collateral pathways for venous drainage

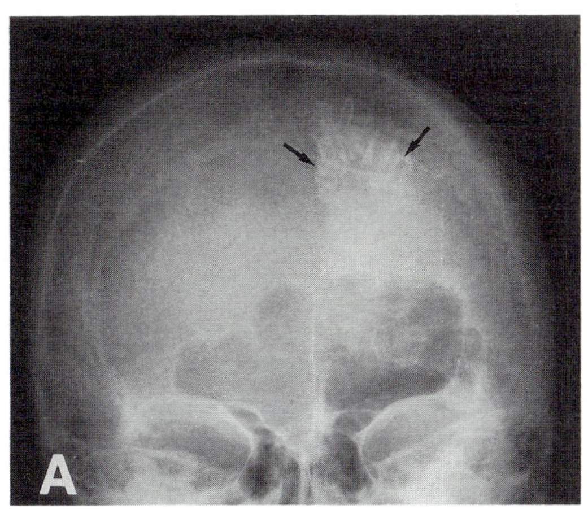

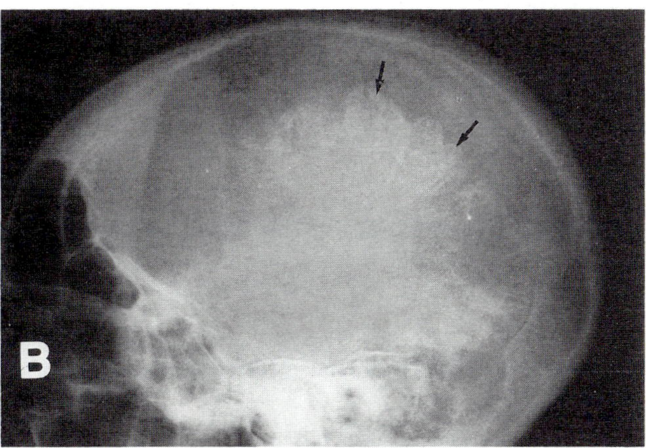

Figure 23. *STURGE-WEBER SYNDROME. AP (A) and lateral skull radiograph in a 5-year-old male with Sturge-Weber syndrome. Note curvilinear calcifications in the parieto-occipital area (arrows). Also note enlargement of the left frontal sinus and thickening of the ipsilateral calvarium secondary to atrophy of the affected hemisphere.*

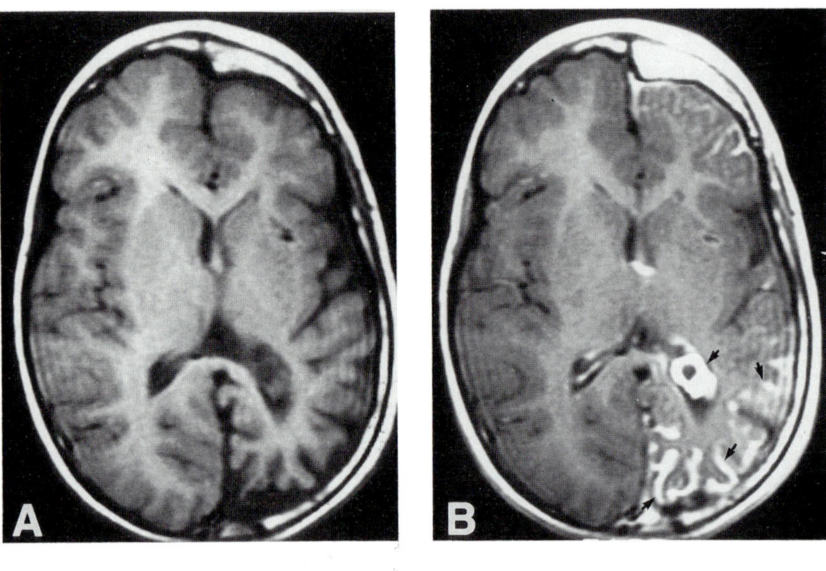

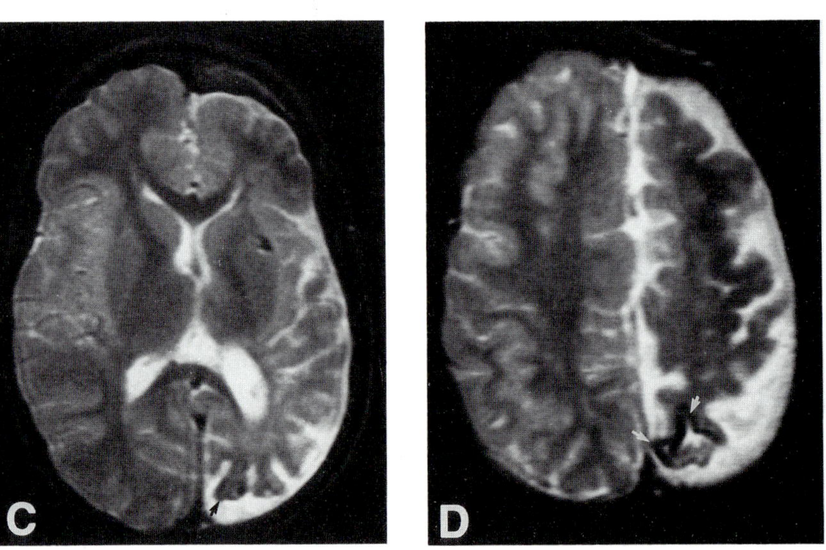

Figure 24. *STURGE-WEBER SYNDROME. Pre- (A) and post-contrast (B) axial T1 weighted MR scans in patient with a left-sided port wine stain. Leptomeningeal and choroidal enhancement (B, arrows) is striking. Note evidence for cortical atrophy and calcification seen on the T2-weighted studies (C, D, arrows). The overlying calvarium is thickened compared to the normal opposite side.*

Tuberous Sclerosis (TS)

(Also known as Bourneville's disease). TS is an hereditary disorder with a widespread potential for hamartomatous growths in multiple organ systems

A. General
  1. Incidence: 1:10,000-50,000 patients
  2. Inheritance
      a. autosomal dominant, low penetrance
      b. no sexual, racial predilection
  3. Clinical
      a. classic triad (not always present)
        ● adenoma sebaceum (90%); ash leaf spots on slit-lamp
        ● seizures (80-90%)
        ● mental retardation (50-80%)
  4. Pathology (Fig. 25)
      a. subependymal hamartomas, giant cell astrocytomas
      b. cortical hamartomas (as opposed to subependymal hamartomas, these rarely if ever undergo neoplastic degeneration)

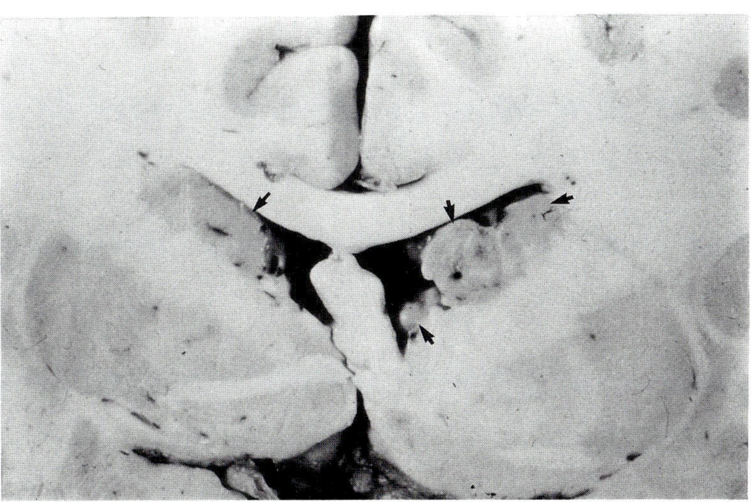

Figure 25. *TUBEROUS SCLEROSIS. Gross pathology specimen, coronal section through the lateral ventricles in a patient with tuberous sclerosis. Note multiple subependymal nodules (arrows).*

    c.   ocular hamartomas ("giant drusen"): 50% have retinal hamartomas; seen as calcifications at/near optic nerve head

    d.   other lesions
- renal: angiomyolipomas 40-80%
- cardiac: rhabdomyomas (50% of patients with cardiac myomas have TS)
- lung: cystic lymphangiomyomas, chronic fibrosis
- liver: leiomyomas, adenomas
- spleen, pancreas: adenomas
- extremities: cystic bone changes, subungual fibromas
- skull: multiple bone islands in diploic space
- vascular: a rare cause of nonatheromatous stenosis

5. Imaging
    a.   skull films (Fig. 26): periventricular calcifications
    b.   CT:
- intracranial abnormalities in up to 90%
- calcifications. Increase with age (rare before age 1), seen in up to 50% of all patients with TS

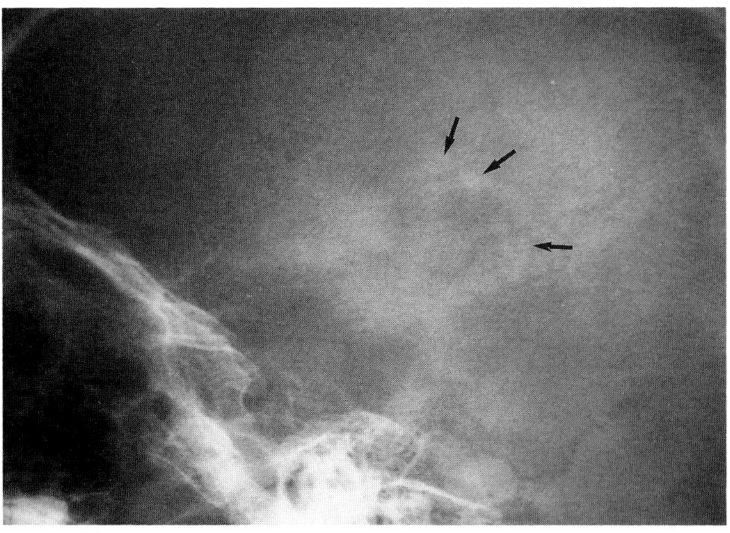

Figure 26. *TUBEROUS SCLEROSIS. Lateral skull radiograph in a 5-year-old male with mental retardation and onset of seizures at age 3 months. At two years of age he developed a papular "rash" on his jaw and forehead. Note nodular calcific foci (arrows) in the periventricular area.*

- 10-15% of patients with TS develop malignant degeneration (giant cell astrocytoma)
- enhancement following contrast should be considered indicative of neoplastic transformation
- typical neoplasm = subependymal giant cell astrocytoma; most common near foramen of Monro
- 10-15% have parenchymal hamartomas demonstrable on CT
- ventricular dilatation (either dysplastic or secondary to foramen of Monro obstruction by giant cell astrocytoma)

c. MR (Fig. 27):
- subependymal nodules (signal intensity similar to white matter)
- cortical tubers (lesions with somewhat indistinct borders that are typically iso/hypointense on T1WI, hyperintense on T2WI, possibly because of fibrillary gliosis or demyelination. Don't enhance.

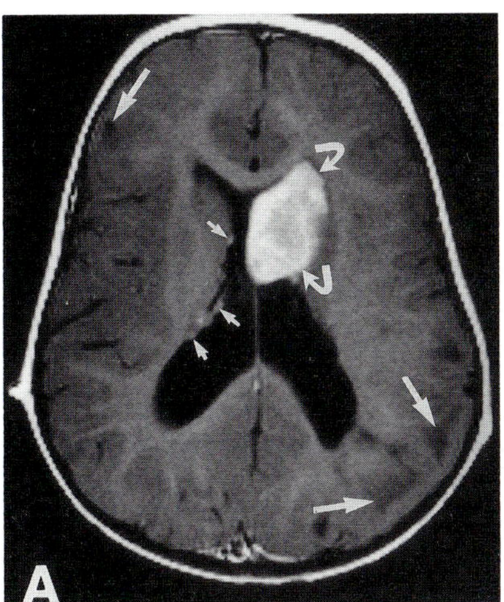
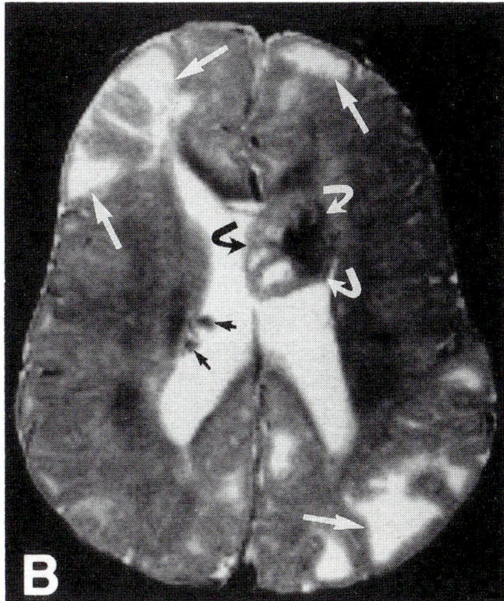

Figure 27. *TUBEROUS SCLEROSIS WITH GIANT CELL ASTROCYTOMA. Axial post-contrast T1 (A) and T2-weighted MR scans in a 14-month-old girl with seizures, no skin stigmata. Note subependymal nodules (small arrows), extensive subcortical white matter abnormalities (large arrows) and contrast-enhancing intraventricular mass at the foramen of Monro (curved arrows). The mass was resected and found to be a giant cell astrocytoma.*

- white matter heterotopias/gliosis (signal similar to cortical tubers)
- giant cell astrocytoma: enhancing mass near foramen of Monro. If subependymal nodules elsewhere enhance they should probably be considered malignant or at least histologically active lesions with the potential to evolve.

References

1. Harwood-Nash DC, Fitz CR. Neuroradiology in infants and children. St. Louis, CV Mosby 1976;1000-1014.
2. Boyer RS. MR in brain formation and malformation. Sem US, CT, MR 1988;9:183-185.
3. van der Knaap MS, Valk J. Classification of congenital abnormalities of the CNS. AJNR 1988;9:315-326.
4. Poe LB, Coleman LL, Mahwad F. Congenital central nervous system anomalies. RadioGraphics 1989;9:801-826
5. Naidich TP, Pudlowski RM, Naidich JB, Gornish M, Rodriguez FJ. Computed tomographic signs of the Chiari II malformation. Part I: skull and partitions. Radiology 1980;134:65-67.
6. Naidich TP, Pudlowski RM, Naidich JB. Computed tomographic signs of the Chiari II malformation. Part II: midbrain and cerebellum. Radiology 1980;134:391-398
7. Naidich TP, Pudlowski RM, Naidich JB. Computed tomographic signs of the Chiari II malformation. Part III: ventricles and cisterns. Radiology 1980;134:657-663.
8. Naidich TP, McLone DG, Fulling KH. The Chiari II malformation. Part IV: the hindbrain deformity. Neuroradiol 1983;25:179-197.
9. Barkovich AJ, Kjos BO, Norman D, Edwards MS. Revised classification of posterior fossa cysts and cystlike malformations based on the results of multiplanar MR imaging. AJNR 1989;10:977-988.
10. Barkovich AJ. Congenital malformations of the brain. In: Pediatric Neuroimaging, New York, Raven Press 1990;77-121.
11. Altman NR, Purser RK, Post MJD. Tuberous sclerosis: characteristics at CT and MR imaging. Radiology 1988;167:527-532.
12. Crawford SC, Boyer RS, Harnsberger HR, et al. Disorders of histogenesis: the neurocutaneous syndromes. Sem US, CT, MR 1988;9:247-267.
13. Aoki S, Barkovich AJ, Nishimura K, et al. Neurofibromatosis types 1 and 2: cranial MR findings. Radiology 1989;172:527-534.
14. Barkovich AJ. Phakomatoses. In: Pediatric Neuroimaging, New York, Raven Press 1990;123-137
15. Wasenko JJ, Rosembloom SA, Duchesneau PM, et al. The Sturge-Weber syndrome: comparison of MR and CT characteristics. AJNR 1990:11:131-134.
16. Elster AD, Chen MYM. MR imaging of Sturge-Weber syndrome. AJNR 1990;11:625-689.
17. Braffman BH, Bilaniuk LT, Zimmerman RA. MR of central nervous system neoplasia of the phakomatoses. Sem Roentgenol 1990;25:198-217.

Hydrocephalus

Olof Flodmark

Department of Neuroradiology, Karolinska Institutet, Stockholm, Sweden

Introduction

The terminology and classification of hydrocephalus is confusing and many older terminologies, often influenced by the way the condition was investigated, should be eliminated. The strict definition of the word hydrocephalus is increased amount of fluid in the cranial cavity without any reference to the cause. This definition would also include cases in which decreased amounts of brain tissue has been replaced by increased amount of CSF. Hydrocephalus should in modern neuroradiology be considered a dynamic process in which there is an imbalance between the production and reabsorption of CSF causing pressure buildup within all or parts of the ventricular system. Hydrocephalus is not a disease by itself but rather a condition with many different expressions. From a diagnostic and therapeutic point it is practical to classify patients with hydrocephalus in those who have a block to CSF flow in the ventricular system as having obstructive or non-communicating hydrocephalus, and those who have the block outside the ventricular system, communicating hydrocephalus.

Hydrocephalus is commonly associated with increased ventricular size, ventriculomegaly. However, all patients with ventriculomegaly do not have hydrocephalus. Ventriculomegaly, even progressive, may be secondary to a static or progressive form of brain tissue loss. On the other hand, ventriculomegaly due to abnormal CSF circulation can be stable as compensation has occurred and the production and reabsorption of CSF has balanced. Finally, a destructive process causing loss of brain tissue may coexist with abnormal CSF circulation and hydrocephalus. This situation may be very difficult to evaluate, both clinically and using neuroradiology [1].

Diagnosis of Hydrocephalus

The clinical symptoms of hydrocephalus relates to raised intracranial pressure. The symptoms vary with the age of the patient at onset and the severity of the abnormality. The growth of the skull in a young infant depends on the growth of the intracranial content. Increased ventricular size due to CSF build-up under pressure will increase the size of the intracranial content and the head circumference will increase more rapidly than normal. Accelerated head growth is commonly the first symptom of hydrocephalus in an infant. As the sutures of the skull in the older child are more resistent to widening, other symptoms of raised intracranial pressure will be seen before or at the same time as splitting of the sutures. Headaches, nausea and vomiting are symptoms seen in older children and adults as the skull gradually looses its ability to accommodate a larger intracranial volume. A gradual build up of pressure will delay onset of symptoms in the child as the sutures can accommodate the increased pressure. However, only a very small infant can accommodate a rapid increase in intracranial pressure by means of widening of the sutures [1].

Radiographic Diagnosis

The first responsibility of the neuroradiologist is to confirm the presence of abnormal CSF circulation. In most situations this is easy but may in others be extremely difficult. Just as every patient with wide cortical sulci does not have atrophy, the neuroradiologist must not assume that every patient with ventriculomegaly has hydrocephalus. This is particularly difficult in the assessment of children and neither the diagnosis of hydrocephalus, nor atrophy can be made with confidence without clinical support for the diagnosis. Having confirmed abnormal CSF circulation, the neuroradiologist must evaluate the etiology of the hydrocephalus. No efforts can be spared in this endeavor as hydrocephalus is secondary to a pathological process which should be possible to establish in most cases. Finally the neuroradiologist should be able to address the state of progression associated with the diagnosis of hydrocephalus [2].

Imaging of the brain using CT scanning or lately MRI, is the primary investigation when hydrocephalus is suspected, as the brain and CSF-containing spaces can be assessed without interfering with the CSF dynamics. Intravenous injection of contrast material is only necessary when investigating the etiology of the hydrocephalus. Diagnosis of hydrocephalus rests primarily on assessment of the lateral ventricles. Dilatation of the lateral ventricles is usually symmetrical with increased roundness of the anterior horns. The temporal horns typically dilate and the size of these is a sensitive indicator of raised intraventricular pressure (Fig. 1). The occipital horns dilate out of proportion in the neonate with hydrocephalus. The reason for this is not understood. A particular type of ventricular dilatation may be seen in infants, where the medial aspect of trigonum is weak and a diverticulum may develop as the ventricle dilates. This diverticulum will expand medially and into the posterior fossa and will act as a mass. It is important to recognize this condition as the posterior fossa mass may simulate a cyst and be mistaken as the cause of hydrocephalus rather than a secondary feature (Fig. 2). Decompression of the lateral ventricle will eliminate the mass in the posterior fossa [3]. Periventricular edema may be seen in increased intraventricular pressure, particularly with the first occasion of raised pressure (Fig. 1b). This finding is useful only if present, as edema may be absent even if the pressure is high, particularly in cases of shunt failure. Ventricular dilatation may be quite irregular when associated with brain damage and loss of brain tissue.

The third ventricle is surrounded by dense brain structures. Hence, dilatation of this part of the ventricular system is relatively late. It is also the part of the ventricular system that is first to resume normal size following normalization of the ventricular pressure. A third ventricle dilated due to high pressure has a round shape in the transaxial plane while a square shape is seen if the ventricle is dilated due to atrophy.

The size of the ventricular system has to be related to the size of the skull. This is particularly important in a child found to have

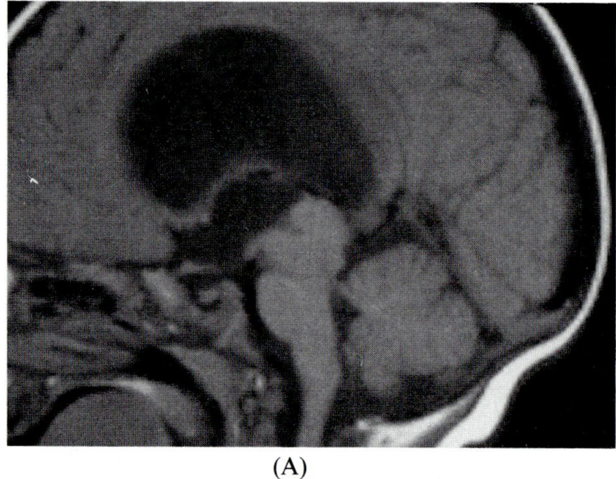

(A)

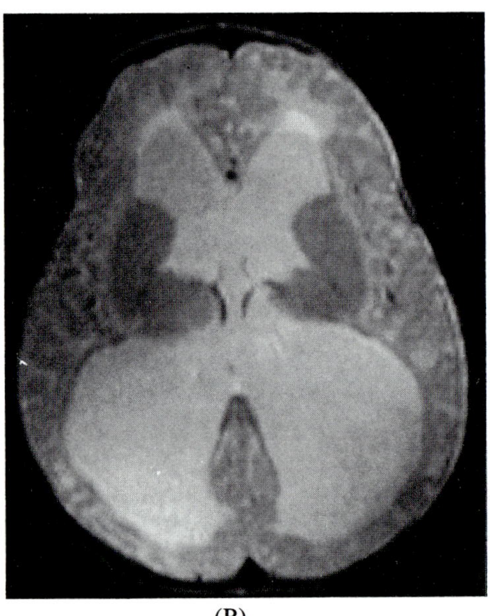

(B)

Figure 1. *OBSTRUCTIVE HYDROCEPHALUS. This girl presented at 10 months of age with a large head and clinical evidence of raised ICP. (A) MRI (T1 weighted sagittal image) confirmed the presence of hydrocephalus. The aqueduct was compressed by a mass in the quadrigeminal plate. Stereotaxic biopsy showed an astrocytoma grade II. (B) Axial T2 weighted image shows marked ventriculomegaly with predominance for the occipital horns. High signal along the frontal horns indicates periventricular edema, confirming the presence of abnormal CSF circulation.*

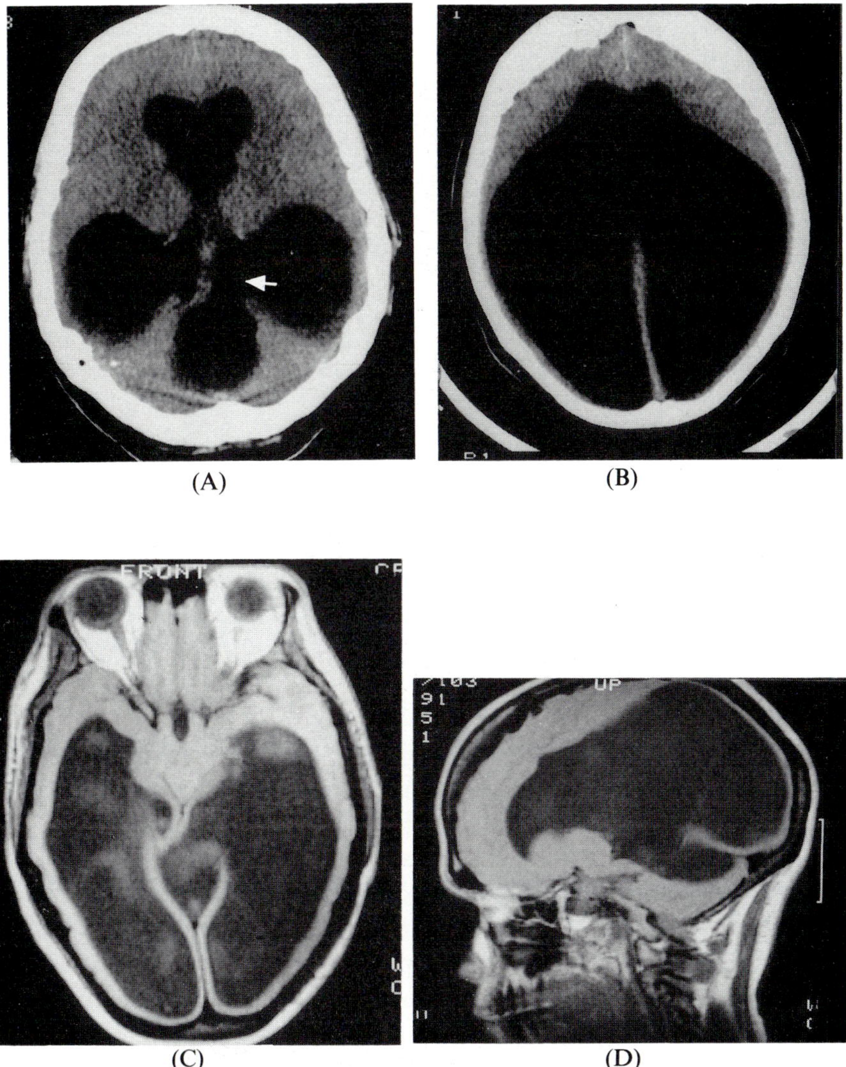

Figure 2. *ARRESTED HYDROCEPHALUS. A 53-year-old female, previously well and of normal intelligence, presented to the emergency room with painful neck and torticollis following minor trauma. The head was large. (A+B) The initial CT scan showed marked ventriculomegaly with very thin cortex in the parietal and occipital regions. The lower cut shows a cystic structure in the posterior fossa communicating with the left lateral ventricle (arrow). (C+D) T1 weighted images from a subsequent MR scan confirmed the communication between the posterior fossa cyst and the lateral ventricle. The cystic structure in the posterior fossa represents an atrial diverticulum. This patient has arrested hydrocephalus likely since childhood.*

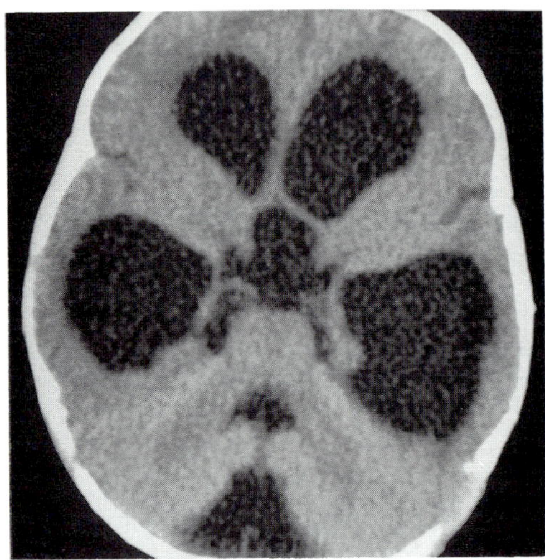

Figure 3. *COMMUNICATING HYDROCEPHALUS. Initial CT scan shows marked dilatation of the lateral ventricles and the third ventricle. The fourth ventricle appears relatively smaller. This constellation would indicate obstruction at the level of the aqueduct. However, contrast injection through a shunt that was inserted showed immediate opacification of all ventricles and the basal cisterns.*

slightly increased size of all ventricles. The subarachnoid spaces over the hemispheres are often generous. This constellation of findings may represent abnormal CSF dynamics with raised pressure, a normal variant with normal pressure or generalized loss of brain tissue, atrophy. It is usually not possible to differentiate between these three conditions using only neuroradiological criteria. Knowledge about the clinical symptoms and particularly information about head size and head growth is essential for the interpretation and hence diagnosis [2,4]. It is unlikely that a patient with large ventricles suffers from raised intracranial pressure should the head size be small and growing at a normal or slower pace. Similarly, it is quite unlikely that a patient with a larger than normal head growing at a normal pace should have atrophy. Yet misinterpretation of this situation is most common, even among neuroradiologists. A similar assessment should be done in an adult found to have large ventricles but little evidence of raised intracranial pressure. Should the patient have a large head, this may represent a since long arrested hydrocephalus (Fig. 2).

Although it may be very easy to confirm the presence of abnormal CSF dynamics using CT scanning, MRI or neurosonography, the diagnosis may in some cases be impossible. Invasive monitoring of the intraventricular pressure over 24 hours may then be the only way to prove the intraventricular pressure to be elevated [5].

It is generally accepted that ventricular dilatation due to raised pressure will compress brain tissue. It is assumed that this process may harm the brain. This appears true in adults as even limited ventricular dilatation will cause severe symptoms. However, neonates may have had longstanding ventriculomegaly during fetal life and yet very little symptoms. Assessing intelligence in children with hydrocephalus has shown poor correlation between ventricular size and intelligence but strong correlation between the etiology of hydrocephalus and mental capacity [6]. These results appear to contradict the surgical dogma that large ventricles always are bad for the brain. It is more likely raised pressure that can cause damage to the brain. Although ventriculomegaly is secondary to raised pressure, the size of the ventricles is a poor indicator of the intraventricular pressure, particularly in children (Fig. 2).

Etiology of Hydrocephalus

The cause of hydrocephalus is in most situations clear. A tumor in the posterior fossa may obstruct the CSF pathways and cause hydrocephalus. Ventriculomegaly following subarachnoid hemorrhage can safely be assumed secondary to the bleed while ventriculomegaly following meningitis may be due either to hydrocephalus or atrophy or a combination of both. Although congenital malformations may be associated with abnormal CSF dynamics, it is not safe to assume that hydrocephalus in a neonate is of congenital origin unless other reasons have been ruled out. No efforts should be spared in evaluating the etiology of hydrocephalus [2].

Assessing the size of each individual part of the ventricular system may give some indication of the location of an obstruction to CSF flow. But this evaluation is not as reliable as usually thought (Fig. 3). Although the appearance may be that of an aqueduct stenosis, the neuroradiologist must be prepared to reassess the cause of hydrocephalus when the aqueduct is seen to be patent and with flow on MR. The evaluation of etiology may be deferred until the ventricles have been decompressed and intraventricular pressure normalized. However, it must not be omitted or forgotten. The work-up should as a minimum include a CT scan performed with contrast enhancement. The site of obstruction can also be determined by puncture of the shunt system and retrograde injection of contrast followed by CT. MR imaging is very powerful in the assessment of etiology. Increased sensitivity may detect small mass lesions in critical locations such as in the quadrigeminal plate in patients thought to have aqueduct stenosis of congenital type [7] (Fig. 1). Its sensitivity for the composition of fluids allows detection of cysts within the ventricular system not shown by CT scanning. In addition MRI has the potential of showing CSF flow in various parts of the ventricular system and subarachnoid space and thus may increase our knowledge and understanding of hydrocephalus [8-9].

Mass lesions may obstruct CSF flow at any point in the system of CSF pathways. Tumors rarely pose any major diagnostic challenge while mass lesions other than tumors may be more difficult to detect, such as intraventricular cysts of ependymal or arachnoid origin. Ependymal cysts may vary in size and cause intermittent hydrocephalus (Fig. 4). Arachnoid cysts in the suprasellar region are not uncommon and have a tendency to invaginate into the third ventricle, thus simulating a dilated third ventricle [2]. Congenital aqueductal stenosis is a diagnosis by exclusion and with the visualization of a stenotic aqueduct on MRI. Tumors in the cerebellar hemispheres or vermis commonly present with clinical symptoms of raised intracranial pressure while hydrocephalus is a late symptom of a mass in the brain stem or pons.

The obstruction to CSF flow is quite commonly found outside the ventricular system. Intraventricular hemorrhage in the prematurely born neonate is a less common cause of hydrocephalus, most often due to obstruction of CSF pathways in the posterior fossa. On the other hand, neonates born at term who suffer significant hemorrhage into the ventricular system commonly develop hydrocephalus. The reason for this discrepancy is not known. Posthemorrhagic hydrocephalus is not an uncommon sequelae after subarachnoid hemorrhage in an adult. Meningitis may cause obstruction over the hemispheres with adhesions in CSF pathways, while an unknown process with similar results operates in older patients who develop abnormal CSF dynamics better known under the name of "Normal pressure hydrocephalus." The transportation of CSF over the arachnoid villae to the intracranial venous sinuses is passive and driven by a pressure gradient. Hence increased intracranial venous pressure will raise the intracranial pressure as the reabsorption of CSF is decreased. This mechanism has been proven to operate in children with achondroplasia [10] and high flow intracerebral arterio-venous malformations. Slightly elevated venous pressure will decrease CSF reabsorption and subsequently raise the intracranial pressure slightly but enough to increase the size of the head in a neonate. Hence pathological processes with raised venous pressure will only cause hydrocephalus while operating early in life when the sutures still are open. Later in life, similar pathology with thrombosis of the intracranial veins will cause raised intracranial pressure but without hydrocephalus. The pathophysiology of benign intracranial hypertension may also be similar.

"Normal Pressure Hydrocephalus"

The clinical triad of dementia, incontinence and abnormal gait was described by Hakim and Adams. It has later been found to be associated with ventriculomegaly but normal CSF pressure. The term normal pressure hydrocephalus (NPH) was applied and used to describe the radiological findings of ventriculomegaly without general prominence of the cortical sulci [11,12]. However, only few patients with this radiological picture have the clinical triad of Hakim and Adams. Furthermore, the use of the term NPH to describe the radiological findings has generated much confusion. Surgical decompression of ventriculomegaly in patients with "NPH" has showed depressing results but have been most successful in patients with Hakim-Adams syndrome. The most sensible approach appears to be clinical diagnosis of Hakim-Adams triad and then surgically decompression only in those patients who have the radiological picture of abnormal CSF dynamics [13]. Radiological criteria of abnormal CSF circulation includes enlargement of the lateral ventricles and third ventricle associated with focal dilatation of the Sylvian fissures and one or two cortical sulci over the hemispheres. Other cortical sulci should be small and probably compressed. MR imaging of these patients have shown increased

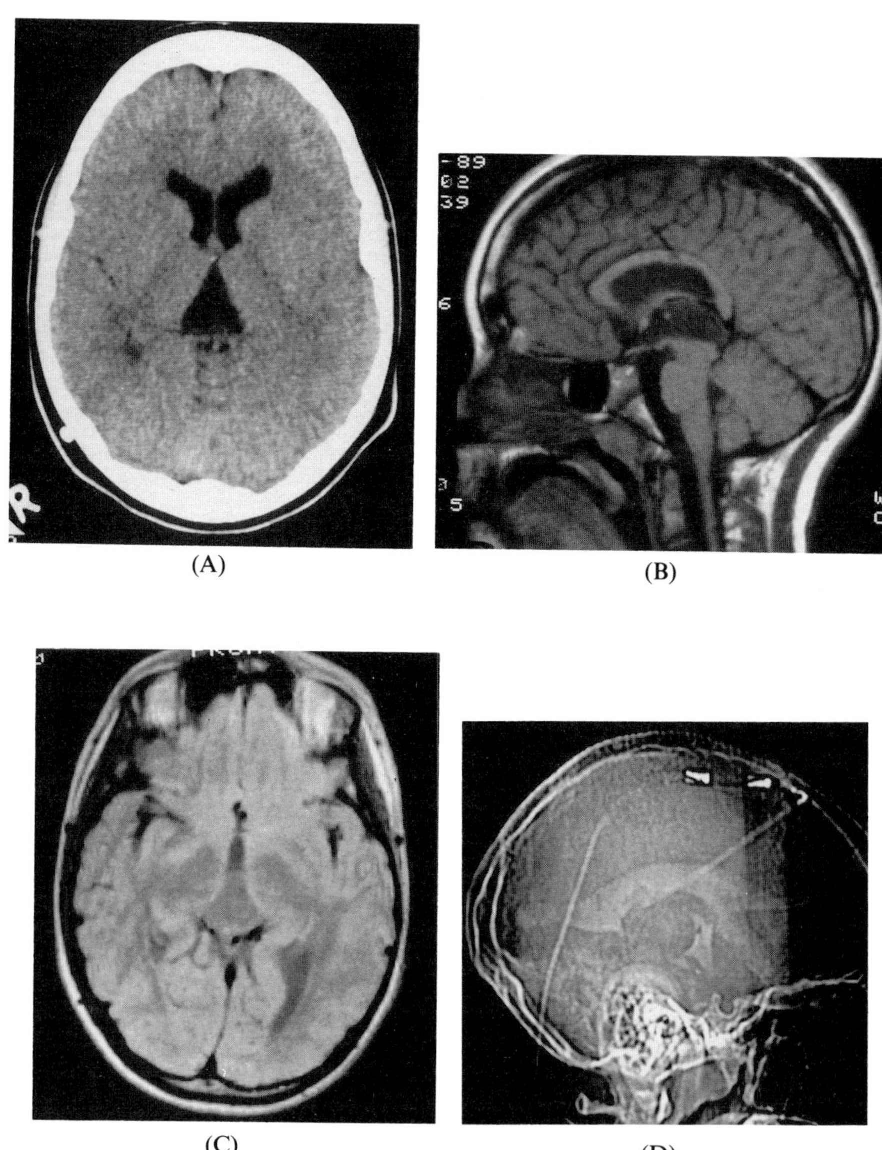

(A)

(B)

(C)

(D)

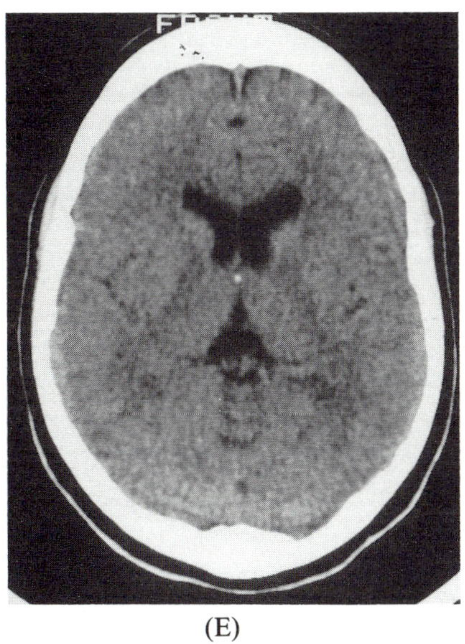

(E)

Figure 4. *INTERMITTENT OBSTRUCTIVE HYDROCEPHALUS. A 14-years-old female had had three episodes during the last four years of clinical evidence of raised ICP with only minimal transient increase in ventricular size. Treated with ventriculo-peritoneal shunting with good results. (A) A CT scan shows a triangular fluid filled space which separates the thalami and flattens the medial aspect of these structures. (B) Sagittal MR (T1 weighted image) scan shows compression of mesencephalon from above as from a mass in the posterior aspect of the third ventricle. (C) Axial MR image (proton weighted image) shows different signal intensities in the anterior and posterior parts of the third ventricle. (D) Digital radiograph (Scoutview) in lateral projection following contrast injection through the shunt system demonstrates a mass in the third ventricle. Stereotaxic biopsy of the mass showed an ependymal cyst which was opened and evacuated. (E) Repeat CT scan obtained following removal of the shunt system shows no residual mass. The thalami have returned to normal shape, and the patient is clinically free of symptoms.*

signal void in a dilated aqueduct of Sylvius suggesting increased pulsatile flow in patients with abnormal CSF dynamics [9]. Careful selection of patients suitable for surgery is very important as the complication rate is high [11].

Congenital Malformations with Hydrocephalus

Congenital malformations of the brain may be associated with hydrocephalus. The component of hydrocephalus is commonly so prominent that it may be difficult to recognize the primary malformation, let alone to establish the type of malformation. As the results of decompression depend more on the etiology of hydrocephalus than the degree of ventriculomegaly, it is extremely important to correctly diagnose the malformation in order to best assess prognosis for the child. In no other situation is this as important as in the discussion about intervention during fetal life when ventriculomegaly has been detected by obstetrical ultrasound [14].

The Chiari malformation type II is a constant finding in patients with open spinal dysraphism. It is associated with, usually rapidly progressing, hydrocephalus in 95%. The site of obstruction has been shown to vary but standard treatment includes ventriculo-peritoneal shunting. More severe dysplasia of the brain can also be associated with hydrocephalus. Extensive abnormalities of neuronal migration are found in this group as is holoprosen-cephaly. Complete absence of corpus callosum is most commonly secondary to abnormal migration in one or both of the cerebral hemispheres. A cyst located in the interhemispheric fissure is a common feature of this malformation. The cyst can be very large and occupy a large portion of the cranial cavity. The ventricles are compressed by the cyst but the cyst can simulate marked dilated ventricles. Recognition of this malformation is important as proper treatment is decompression of the cyst and not the ventricular system. Hydra-nencephaly, thought to be of destructive etiology during late fetal life, is another malformation which may simulate the radiographic picture of massive hydrocephalus. Although hydranencephaly may be associated with some disturbance of CSF circulation, decompression will be of importance to the care givers. The Dandy-Walker malformation of the posterior fossa is typically associated with hydrocephalus. Primary decompression of the posterior fossa cyst may also but not always decompress the supratentorial ventricles [2].

Neuroradiology in Indications for Treating Hydrocephalus

Treatment of hydrocephalus is today limited to implantation of devices which temporarily or permanently divert CSF usually to the peritoneal cavity. This procedure is not without complications and neuroradiology plays an important role in assessing the results of shunting and possible complications.

The treatment of hydrocephalus has the single objective to normalize the intraventricular pressure. Decreasing ventricular size is commonly the effect of successful reduction of intraventricular pressure. Monitoring of ventricular pressure would ideally be the way to secure the indications for shunting and to assess the success of this procedure. However, no such method exists that is both reliable and non-invasive. The indications for treatment and assessment of successful decompression must therefore depend on clinical assessment of intracranial pressure supported by radiographic visualization of ventricular size.

Ventriculomegaly and clinically raised ICP represent clear indication of surgical decompression [1]. The situation may be much more difficult in patients in whom one of these components is less obvious or even missing. Raised ICP with normal ventricular size is seen in cases of benign intracranial hypertension and in some patients with block to CSF flow outside the ventricular system. Neuroradiological investigations are of little help in this situation and other methods are necessary to confirm the presence of raised ICP. The other side of this problem is represented by patients with ventriculomegaly but without obvious signs of raised pressure. These patients are usually thought to have arrested hydrocephalus. CT scanning and even MRI offer little assistance in these very difficult treatment decisions. The insertion of a permanent shunt has far reaching consequences for the patient, particularly children, and should not be done unless necessary. Neonates with intraventricular hemorrhage can illustrate this dilemma. Every neonate with intraventricular hemorrhage will develop abnormal CSF dynamics and ventriculomegaly. Conservative treatment will reduce the group needing a permanent shunt to less than 20%. Conversely, aggressive shunting early in the process will transform an incomplete or transient obstruction to a permanent, complete block and make a much larger number of children dependent for life on a working shunt.

Neuroradiological Assessment of Shunting

Neuroradiology can, as explained above, assess only the secondary effects to reduce ventricular pressure. MRI can assess the periventricular edema and confirm its reduction while both MRI and CT can assess ventricular size, in practice the way we evaluate the success of surgical decompression. The reduction in ventricular size depends on many factors such as age, type of shunt and previous shunting procedures. Much of the reduction is generally achieved soon after shunting while it will take several weeks before final balance is reached. Ventricular size may in children change over a longer perspective as brain growth will occur. The lateral ventricle with the shunt catheter is always smaller than the contralateral ventricle.

The placement of a permanent shunt is affiliated with complications, some severe. Excessive drainage may create clinical symptoms similar to those of shunt failure, however, CT or MRI will usually differentiate. Excessive drainage, particularly of long standing large ventricles may also precipitate extracerebral hemorrhage. Complete collapse of the ventricular system is not desired, particularly in children as the sutures may fuse prematurely resulting in a small head. Small ventricles per se are not harmful in older children as the ability to dilate in response to raised pressure is preserved. The specific term "slit ventricle syndrome" should be reserved for those few patients who have lost their ability to dilate the ventricles in response to raised pressure. This is a severe complication to shunting as shunt revision is difficult in the presence of small ventricles [2].

Neuroradiological assessment of ventricular size is important as a preoperative procedure in patients with suspected shunt failure. However, proper assessment is only possible with access to a base line study when the shunt is presumed to work properly and the patient is free of symptoms. Routine imaging at regular intervals of patients with a shunt is of no value and should be avoided to minimize radiation exposure. Furthermore, shunt revision should not be undertaken based on radiographic evidence of increased ventricular size alone.

References

1. McCullough DC. Hydrocephalus: etiology, pathological effects, diagnosis and natural history. In: McLaurin RL, Venes JL, Schut L, Epstein F, eds. Pediatric neurosurgery. W.B. Saunders, Philadelphia, 1989:180-190.
2. Flodmark O, Hydrocephalus. In: Putman CE, Ravin CE, eds. Textbook of diagnostic imaging. W.B. Saunders, Philadelphia, 1988:153-166.
3. Naidich TP, McLone DG, Hahn YS, Hanaway J. Atrial Diverticula in severe hydrocephalus. AJNR 1982;3:257-266.
4. Maytal J, Alvarez LA, Elkin CM, Shinnar S. External hydrocephalus: radiologic spectrum and differentiation from cerebral atrophy. AJR 1987;148:1223-1230.
5. Whittle IR, Johnston IH, Besser M. Intracranial pressuer changes in arrested hydrocephalus. J Neurosurg 1985;62;77-82.
6. Dennis M, Fitz CR, Netley CT, Sugar J, Harewood-Nash DCF, Hendrick EB, Hoffman HJ, Humphreys RP. The intelligence of hydrocephalic children. Arch Neurol 1981;38:607-615.
7. Britton J, Marsh H, Kendall B, Kingsley D. MRI and hydrocephalus in childhood. Neuroradiology. 1988;30:310-314.
8. Citrin CM, Sheman JL, Gangarosa RE, Scanlon D. Physiology of the CSF void sign: modification by cardiac gating. AJR 1987;148:205-208.
9. Sherman IL, Citrin CM, Gangarosa RE, Bowen BJ. The MR appearance of CSF flow in patients with ventriculomegaly. AJR 1987;148:193-199.
10. Steinbok P, Hall J, Flodmark O. Hydrocephalus in achondroplacia: the possible role of intracranial venous hypertension. J Neurosurg 1989;71:42-48.
11. Wikkelsö C, Andersson H, Blomstrand C, Matousek M, Svendsen P. Computed tomography of the brain in the diagnosis and prognosis in normal pressure hydrocephalus. Neuroradiology 1989;31:160-165.
12. Clifford RJ, Mokri B, Laws ER, Houser OW, Baker HL, Petersen RC. MR findings in normal-pressure hydrocephalus: significance and comparison with other forms of dementia. JCAT 1987;11:923-931.
13. Huckman MS. Normal pressure hydrocephalus: evaluation of diagnostic and prognostic tests. AJNR 1981;2:385-395.
14. Nyberg DA, Mack LA, Hirsch J, Pagon RO, Shepard TH. Fetal hydrocephalus: sonographic detection and clinical significance of associated anomalies. Radiology 1987;163:187-191.
15. Flodmark O, Scotti G, Harwood-Nash DC. The clinical significance of ventriculomegaly in children who suffered perinatal asphyxia with or without intracranial hemmorhage: an 18 month follow-up study. JCAT 1981;5:663-673.

Cerebral Vascular Malformations in Children

Francis Brunelle

Department of Radiology, Hôpital des Enfants Malades, Paris, France

Cerebral vascular malformations form an heterogeneous group and include various abnormalities such as true arteriovenous malformations either parenchymal or meningeal, cavernous angioma, and venous malformations. Neurocutaneous syndromes may be associated with vascular abnormalities such as arterial aneurysms in neurofibromatosis and meningeal angioma in Sturge-Weber syndrome.

Classification

The classification of arteriovenous malformations is histologic [1,2].

A. Arteriovenous malformations sensu strictu are made of large arteries and veins intermingled with brain tissue. There is a high flow in this malformation responsible for hemodynamic steal from the normal territories. The vascular walls are abnormal and may show hyalinization, fibrosis and ectasia. Calcifications and thrombosis may occur within the malformation.

B. Cavernous angiomas are made of vascular spaces separated by fibrous walls. They very frequently calcify. The circulation of blood is very slow in this type of malformation.

C. Telangiectasias : they are masses of capillary channels lacking of normal muscle fibers in their walls.

D. Venous malformations consist of dilated tortuous veins without arteriovenous shunt.

Clinical Findings and Radiological Features

Arteriovenous Malformations

They are the most frequent vascular malformations in children. Mean age at time of diagnosis is 10 years [3] (Figs. 1, 2).

Revealing symptoms include intracranial hemorrhage, epilepsy and motor deficits. Plain skull films may show calcifications and vascular grooves on the vault especially in malformations with dural drainage.

On CT, AVM are seen as an area of heterogeneous high intensity mass. Focal atrophy adjacent to the AVM is frequently seen.

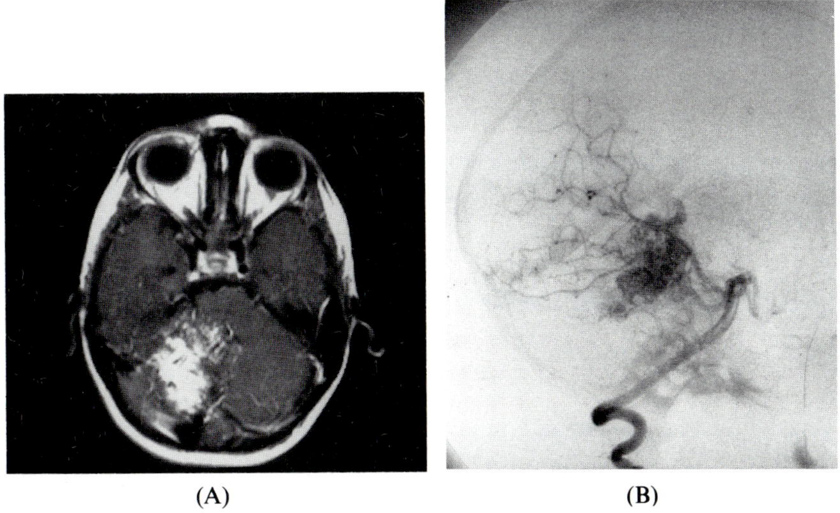

(A)   (B)

Figure 1. *POSTERIOR FOSSA AVM. Seven-year-old boy with subarachnoid hemorrhage. (A) Axial T1 weighted MRI with Gadolinium shows a posterior fossa malformation. (B) Lateral vertebral angiogram. The malformation is well demonstrated but its exact relationship to the brain is only shown by MRI.*

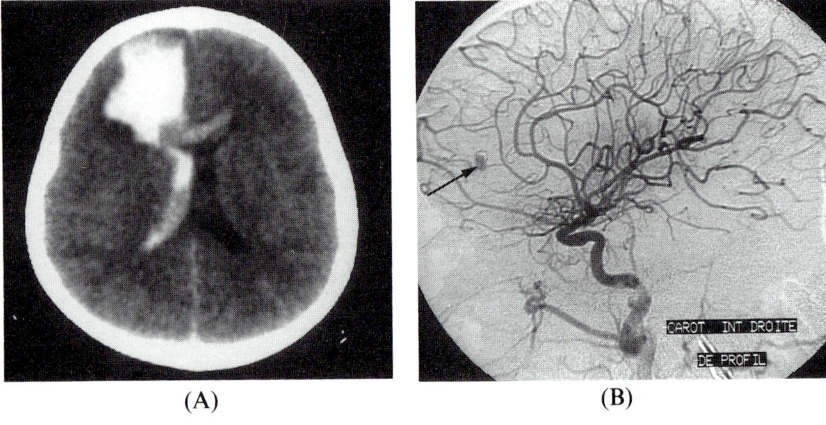

(A)   (B)

Figure 2. *AVM PLUS HEMATOMA. Fourteen-year-old boy with sudden onset of headaches. (A) CT. A large hematoma is seen in the right frontal lobe as well as intraventricular hemorrhage. (B) Right carotid angiogram. A small arteriovenous malformation is seen in the frontal lobe (→).*

After contrast injection, the AVM enhances and abnormal arteries and veins are opacified. A spontaneous dense mass on CT can be seen in case of hematoma complicating the AVM.

Angiography gives information about the feeding vessels and draining veins. It is the first step before treatment is started either surgical or by embolization. Stereotaxic radiotherapy may cure small AVMs.

A peculiar form of AVMs is spontaneous hematomas. CT and angiography fail to demonstrate any abnormal vessel. Compression or thrombosis of the AVM by the hematoma may explain this peculiar clinico-radiological presentation.

Cavernous Hemangiomas

Classically seen in adults, it is more and more often diagnosed in children. Epilepsy is the most frequent clinical manifestation. Plain skull films are usually normal. Calcifications are very rarely seen [4,5] (Figs. 3, 4).

On CT cavernous hemangiomas present usually as a small dense lesion cortical in location. After contrast, the spontaneous high density of the lesion usually does not show enhancement.

MRI is virtually diagnostic in showing an hyperintense lesion on

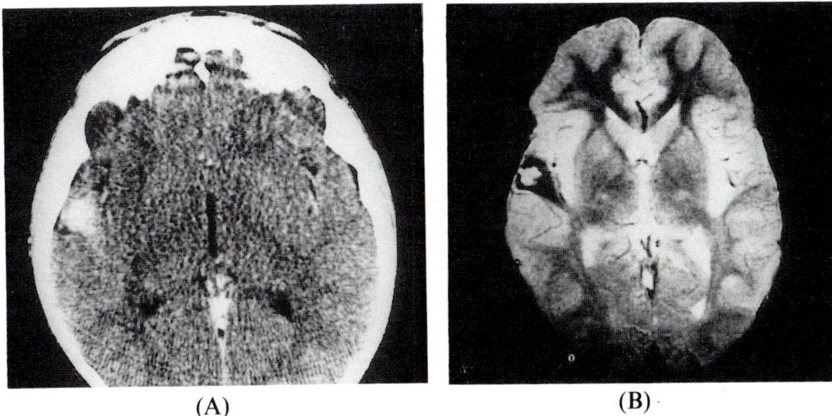

(A)   (B)

Figure 3. *CAVERNOUS ANGIOMA. Eleven-year-old boy with seizures. (A) CT scan after injection shows a dense right parietal lesion. (B) MRI shows on T2 weighted sequence an hyperintense lesion with an hypointense rim.*

T2 with an hypointense rim due to the presence of hemosiderin due to chronic bleed. On T1 sequences the lesion may be isointense to the brain, then not visible.

Angiography is usually normal as the flow in this cavernous hemangioma is low.

Venous Malformations

They may be revealed by migraine-like headaches or spontaneous hemorrhage, but the discovering may be fortuitous [6] (Fig. 5).

CT is normal before contrast. After contrast an abnormal vein tracing from the white matter to the cortex is seen.

On angiography arterial phase is normal. On the venous phase an umbrella like group of veins draining into a large single vein to the cortex is seen. They correspond to dilated deep medullary veins. They can be seen in the cerebral hemispheres as well as in the cerebellum.

Vein of Galien Varix

Vein of Galien varix is due to secondary dilatation of the vein of Galien due to arteriovenous malformation of the meninges of the roof of the third ventricle [7] (Fig. 6).

Clinical findings depend on the age of presentation.

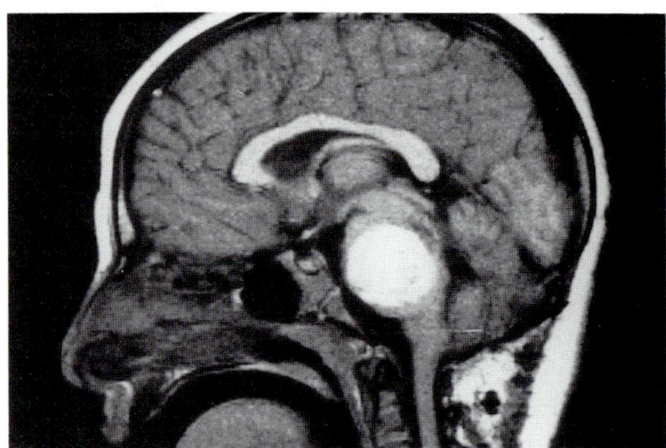

Figure 4. *CAVERNOUS HEMANGIOMA AND BLOOD CLOT. Eleven-year-old girl with increased intracranial pressure, left hemiparesis. (A) MRI sagittal midline T1 weighted. A spontaneously hyperintense lesion is occupying the pons.*

Neonatal Form

Cardiac failure is the most common clinical presentation. The diagnosis may be suspected in utero. The head circumference is enlarged and dilated facial veins are seen. Cardiomegaly is present on chest films.

Ultrasound, doppler and color doppler make the diagnosis thanks to a transfontanellar approach.

CT shows the arteriovenous malformation and the dilatation of the vein of Galen. After contrast injection multiple arterial feeders and enhancement of the vein is seen.

Variable ventricular dilatation is present. Cerebral atrophy may be extreme due to chronic ischemia of the brain.

Prognosis is poor and most patients die within days or weeks from cardiac failure.

Infantile Form

Usually revealed by progressive increased head circumference due to hydrocephalus during the first year of life.

Associated dilated facial veins and intracranial bruit are present.

Variable neurologic signs such as moderate mental retardation may be present.

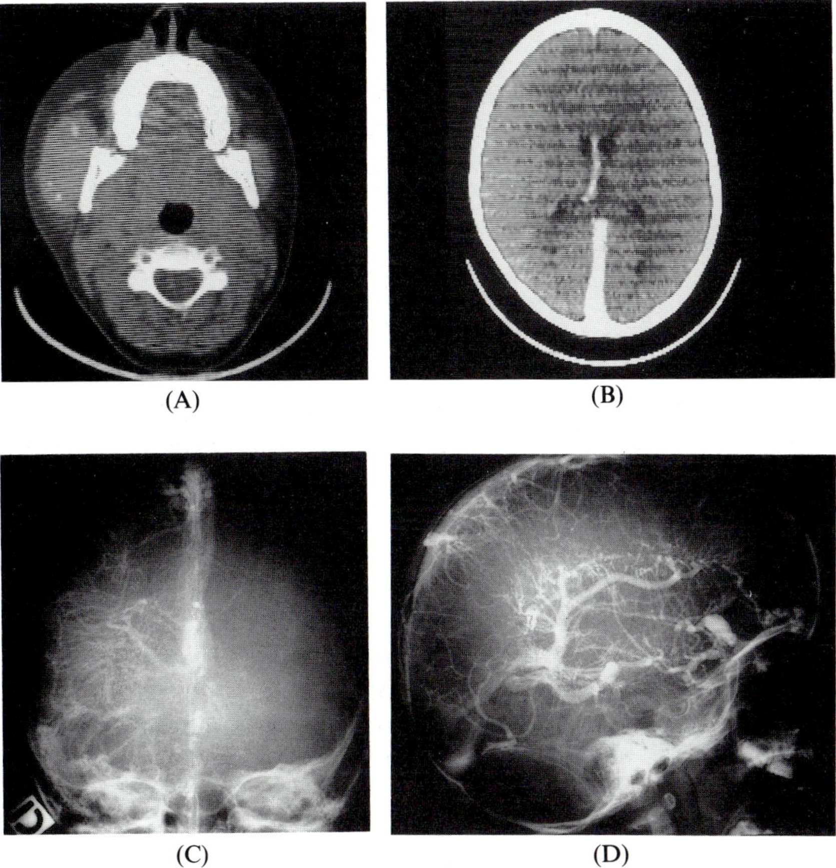

Figure 5. *VENOUS MALFORMATION. Sixteen-year-old girl with Bonnet Blanc Dechaume syndrome associating a venous angioma on the right side of the body involving the two limbs, the face and the brain. (A) CT shows the venous angioma of the cheek with phleboliths. (B) Brain CT shows the dilated abnormal vein. (C) AP view of the venous phase of a carotid angiogram showing the multiple dilated veins. (D) Same patient lateral view.*

CT shows the same findings but may reveal white matter calcifications due to chronic ischemia of the brain.

MRI should be performed as a pretherapeutic tool to evaluate the extension of the malformation.

Arterial embolization during or after a complete angiographic work-up aims to occlude most of the arterial feeders.

Spontaneous thrombosis of the malformation may occur.

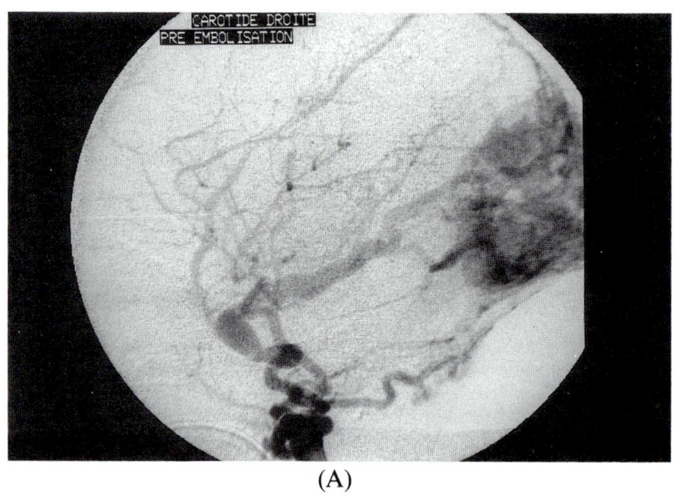

(A)

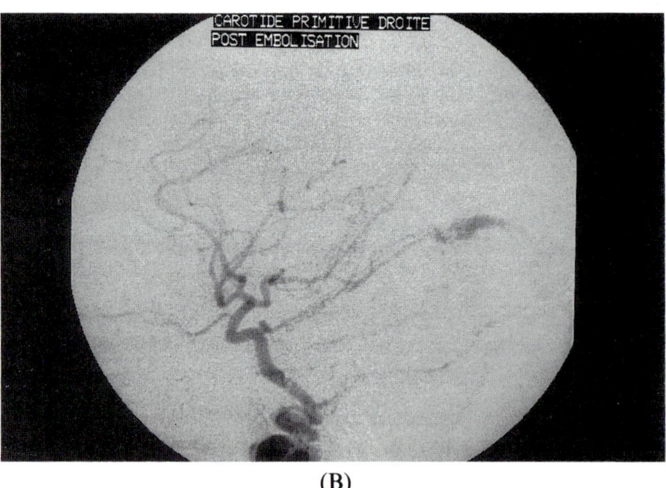

(B)

Figure 6. *DURAL ARTERIOVENOUS MALFORMATION. One-month-old boy with cardiac insufficiency and intracranial bruit. (A) Right common carotid artery injection. The middle meningeal artery is dilated and drains into a huge venous sinus. (B) Same injection after embolization of the meningeal artery.*

Calcifications of the walls of the vein of Galen can be seen as well.

Dural Arteriovenous Malformation

Dural AVMs are extremely rare in children. They are usually revealed by cardiac insufficiency or hydrocephalus.

CT will show only dilated draining sinuses. After contrast arterial feeders and dilated sinuses are seen.

Angiography will show extreme dilatation of meningeal arteries taking off from the external carotid artery. But accessory meningeal branches from the internal carotid and the vertebral arteries may participate as well to the malformation.

In conclusion recent advances in the knowledge of vascular malformations in children has come from MRI and development of interventional radiology techniques.

References

1. McCormick WF. The pathology of vascular (arterio-venous) malformations. J. Neurosurg 1966;24:807-816.
2. Brunelle FO, Harwood-Nash DC, Fitz CR, et al. Intracranial vascular malformations in children : computed tomographic and angiographic evaluation. Radiology 1983; 149:455-461.
3. Celli P, Ferrante L, Palura L, et al. Cerebral arterio-venous malformations in children. Surg neurol 1984;22:43-49.
4. Savoiardo M, Strada L, Passerini A. Intracranial cavernous hemangioma. Neuroradiological review of 36 operated cases. AJNR 1983;4:945-950.
5. Lee BCP, Herberg L, Zimmerman RD, et al. MR imaging of cerebral vascular malformations. AJNR 1986;6:863-870.
6. Olson E, Gilmor RC, Richmond B. Cerebral venous angiomas. Radiology 1984;151:97-104.
7. Seidenwurm D, Berenstein A, Hyman A, et al. Vein of Galen malformation : correlation of clinical presentation, arteriography and MRI. AJNR 1991;12:347-354.

Introduction to the NICER Lecturer

Derek C. Harwood-Nash
The Hospital for Sick Children, Toronto, Ontario, Canada

Mummification as practiced by the ancient Egyptians and as described in great detail by Herodotus has provided the medical fraternity with a mother lode of actual and potential subjects of great antiquity on whom a large variety of imaging techniques may be employed with revelations of considerable interest and excitement.

The first computed tomogram in 1978 of a whole mummy [1] - Djemaetesankh of the twenty-second Dynasty (9th century BC) and of a desiccated brain of a 14-year-old boy weaver Nakht, who died in approximately 1400 BC, did not reveal any paleopathological peculiarities or scientific breakthroughs! They were simply remarkable images both to the experienced Egyptologist and to the neophyte "Egyptoradiologist."

Others followed, but exceptionally did the Manchester Museum Mummy Project - publish their findings simply, exhaustively, and most interestingly in 1979 [2]. Prominent amongst the investigators was Professor Ian Isherwood, Head of the University of Manchester, Department of Radiology, who described so expertly the radiography of the studied mummy. His interest and investigations have continued with great effect to the present.

References

1. Harwood-Nash DC. Computed tomography of ancient Egyptian mummies. J Comp Ass Tomogr 1979;3:768.
2. Isherwood I, Jarvis H, Fawcitt RA. Radiology of the Manchester mummies. In: David AR, ed. The Manchester Museum mummy project. Manchester. Manchester Museum 1979;25-64.

NICER Lecture:
Science in Egyptology

Ian Isherwood
Department of Diagnostic Radiology, University of Manchester,
Manchester, England

One of the earliest retrospective surveys of ancient Egyptian remains is that of Herodotus, the Greek traveller, who, writing in the Vth century B.C., described in detail the process of mummification.

There are two main areas of interest in the scientific investigation of human and animal remains, one concerned with the archaeology of the specimen and its relationship to contemporary living conditions and the time scale of cultural development, and the other with the study of diseases, injury and causes of death in ancient civilizations.

Knowledge of disease in Ancient Egypt has been gained in the past from studies of the medical papyri and from examination of works of art such as drawings and statues showing malformed persons. The term palaeopathology was devised by Ruffer in 1913 to describe "the science of the diseases which can be demonstrated in human and animal remains of ancient tissues".

One of the earliest scientific investigations of Egyptian mummies was carried out by Dr Margaret Murray, Egyptologist at the Manchester Museum together with a multidisciplinary team in 1907. It consisted mainly of an unwrapping and a dissection of Two Brothers in the Manchester collection. A great variety of scientific techniques have since been applied to the investigation of Egyptian mummified remains of humans, animals and birds. The approaches have included radiology, histopathology, electron microscopy, endoscopy, fingerprinting, carbon dating, spectroscopy, blood grouping, and an analysis of DNA. Studies of ancient textiles have provided information about the textile technology of Ancient Egypt, whilst the identification of insects and their life cycles in mummified remains has provided insights into both living conditions and the mummification process.

From the earliest days following the discovery of X-rays by Röntgen in 1895 there has been considerable interest in the value

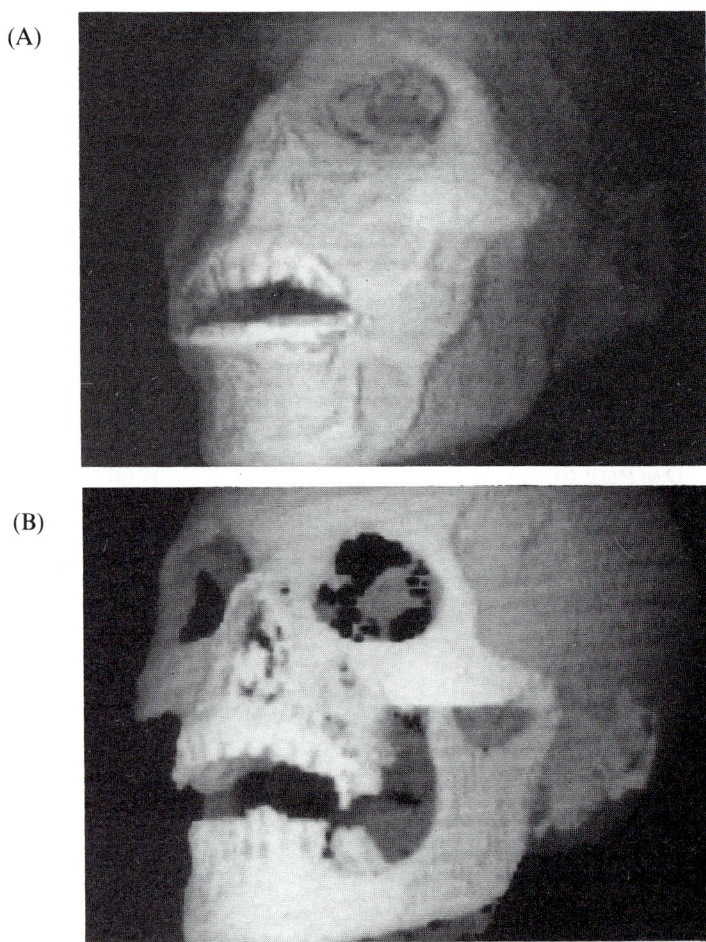

(A)

(B)

Figure 1. *THREE-DIMENSIONAL COMPUTED TOMOGRAPHY OF THE HEAD OF AN EGYPTIAN MUMMY FROM THE PTOLEMEIC PERIOD. (A) soft tissue detail. (B) bone detail (note the dental attrition).*

of Radiology in the investigation of mummified Egyptian remains. The first radiographs of mummified material were obtained in March 1896. A number of important radiological surveys have been carried out by several workers over the years, and detailed radiological studies have contributed significantly to the identification of historical Egyptian figures. Some of the techniques employed are now well established in forensic practice. Until recent years most recorded specimens were radiographed on site either in museums or at archaeological sites. Modern X-ray

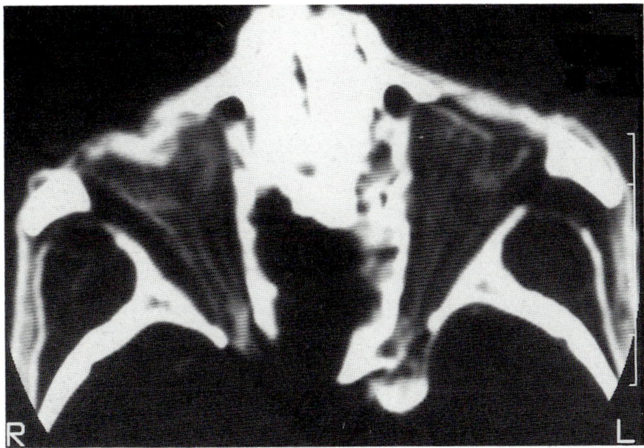

Figure 2. *COMPUTED TOMOGRAPHY OF A PTOLEMEIC EGYP-TIAN MUMMY DEMONSTRATING THE OPTIC NERVES AND THE OCULAR MUSCLES STILL IN SITU. Note the defect in the ethmoidal roof through which the brain was removed by the embalmer.*

techniques, including fluoroscopy, tomography and computed tomography, with reformatting and three-dimensional imaging, have provided new and rewarding opportunities in the study of ancient remains.

The NICER lecture will discuss the importance of the various scientific methods available and provide an account of a recent unwrapping of a human mummy from the Ptolemeic period.

References

1. David AR, ed. The Manchester Museum mummy project. Manchester Museum Publications 1974.
2. David AR, ed. Science in Egyptology. Manchester University Press 1986.

Author Index

Abbreviations

ADEM	see: Acute disseminated encephalomyelitis
AIDS	see: Acquired immune deficiency syndrome
ALD	see: Adrenoleukodystrophy
ARD	see: Anisotropic diffusion
AVM	see: Arteriovenous malformation
CMV	see: Cystomegalovirus
CSF	see: Cerebrospinal fluid
DNL	see: Disseminated necrotizing leukoencephalopathy
DVA	see: Developmental venous anomaly
MIP	see: Maximum Intensity Projection
MMC	see: Meningo-myelocele
MRA	see: Magnetic Resonance Angiography
MS	see: Multiple sclerosis
PKU	see: Phenylketonuria
PML	see: Progressive Multifocal Leukoencephalopathy
PNET	see: Primitive Neuroectodermal Tumor
PVL	see: Periventricular leukomalacia
SPECT	see: Single Photon Emission Computed Tomography
STIR	see: Short TI-IR Sequence

Keyword Index

O

P